# Epilepsies of Childhood

Dedicated to Barbara

# Epilepsies of Childhood

Third Edition

**Niall V. O'Donohoe** MD, FRCP(I), DCH
Formerly Professor of Paediatrics, Trinity College, Dublin

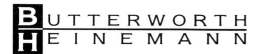

Butterworth-Heinemann Ltd
Linacre House, Jordan Hill, Oxford OX2 8DP

℞ A member of the Reed Elsevier plc group

OXFORD   LONDON   BOSTON
MUNICH   NEW DELHI   SINGAPORE   SYDNEY
TOKYO   TORONTO   WELLINGTON

First published 1979
Reprinted 1981
Second edition 1985
Third edition 1994
Reprinted 1994

© Butterworth-Heinemann Ltd 1994

**British Library Cataloguing in Publication Data**

O'Donohoe, Niall V.
    Epilepsies of Childhood.—3 Rev. ed
    I. Title
    618.92853

ISBN 0 7506 1598 2

Printed and bound in Great Britain by
The University Press, Cambridge

# Contents

# Foreword

The publication in 1979 of the first edition of Niall O'Donohoe's book was a landmark in paediatrics. As the late John Apley, General Editor of the series in which the book first appeared and an experienced general paediatrician of the kind rarely found today, pointed out, epilepsy looms large among the ailments of children, and yet until then the subject of childhood epilepsy had been sparsely treated in medical literature, usually being relegated to the status of a single chapter in books either on adult epilepsy or on paediatric neurology. The book remedied this neglect and gave the subject for the first time the coverage it deserves. The misconception still present in the mindset of many doctors, that children are little adults (I prefer the reverse concept that adults are obsolete children) is nowhere more dangerous than in the field of epilepsy. It is fascinating, when talking to 'general' neurologists or physicians on the topic of childhood epilepsy, to see their eyes opening on a whole new world.

On a personal note I must confess that when I was given a copy of the first edition to review I fell on it happily and had quickly marred its pages with those annotations, highlightings, asterisks, nota benes and underlinings, which indicate that the text is stimulating the reader to relate the writer's opinions to his own experience, to review his own cases and his practice and to delve more deeply into the literature. It was therefore with some embarrassment that I learned that, unusually, the reviewer was not entitled to keep the volume, but I had not a moment's hesitation in, or resentment at, buying my own personal copy, which served me well for seven years until replaced by the second edition in 1985.

The life of this classic work is now extended with the third edition. It has become a standard book which is depended on by many and should continue. The task of keeping up with the advances of the last fourteen years is no small one. These advances are documented in a legion of publications and in a few books. One thinks of Aicardi's (1986) volume and of the multi-author *Epileptic Syndromes* book first published in 1985 with a second edition in 1992; to both editions O'Donohoe contributed a scholarly chapter on febrile convulsions. In *Epilepsies of Childhood* we have the essence and a distillation of a vast corpus of knowledge, in manageable and user-friendly form and in elegant prose. We find, equally importantly, the *practical* approach of the expert who has experienced the common and the rarer problems of the child with epilepsy and of his family. The message gets across clearly to the reader because the medium is clear.

The author paid tribute in his first edition to his debt to the late Paul Sandifer at Great Ormond Street in the late 1950's. Those who were lucky enough to have this experience, as I did later, in the year before his tragically early death, will appreciate his contribution to this important field. Our mentor would be very proud of the continuing work and success of this book.

Edward Brett
Consultant Neurologist
The Hospital for Sick Children
Great Ormond Street
London

# Preface

The late Dr John Apley, who first suggested to me in 1975 that I should write this book for his Postgraduate Paediatrics Series, said that it should be of reasonable length, should emphasize basic concepts and should be written especially for those engaged in the care of children, particularly practising paediatricians. Seizures are among the most frequent symptoms presenting to the paediatrician and both the general paediatrician (and the general practitioner) have to learn to cope with their management. There will not be enough specialized paediatric neurologists to deal with this worldwide problem for the foreseeable future, if ever. I have been gratified by the way in which this book has been received in so many countries and by the responses from paediatric colleagues all over the world who have told me that they have found it useful and practical.

The book has been extensively revised and rewritten to take account of the remarkable advances in understanding, investigating and treating the childhood epilepsies. Two new chapters (Status Epilepticus and Intractable Epilepsy) have been added. At the same time, I have tried to keep it of reasonable length. I have emphasized basic concepts insofar as they are essential for the understanding of this, often difficult, subject. It seems to me so much more important to try to understand the condition and how it affects children than it is to become obsessional about the complexities of antiepileptic drug therapy – old and new. I have tried not to allow my own obsession with classification and categorization to gain the upper hand (I hope) although I am convinced that it is only by using the modern classification systems that we can communicate coherently with each other about the subject. As a good paediatrician should, I have tried to give a chronological account of the epilepsies from infancy through to adolescence. I hope that the book will be read as a continuous story, a biography of the child with epilepsy.

The book is as near 'state of the art' as I can make it. Inevitably, the subject will have moved on again by the date of publication, especially in the area of the rapidly proliferating new antiepileptic drugs. However, I hope that the latest journals and reviews will take care of that deficiency for the reader.

This Third Edition has been written in retirement. I look back gratefully on the many colleagues and friends (some sadly now deceased) who have helped me to learn about and understand this complex subject – Paul Sandifer, Christopher Ounsted, and David Taylor in Britain, Jean Aicardi and Henri Gastaut in France, Fritz Dreifuss in the United States, and many others. As in the Preface to the First

Edition, I acknowledge my special debt to the late Dr Ronald MacKeith, one of the greatest international paediatricians of his generation, who ensured that I joined the mainstream of British and European paediatric neurology.

I am most grateful to my old friend, Dr Edward Brett, for writing the Foreword. I would also like to acknowledge my special debt to Mr John French of Ciba-Geigy, Ireland, who has helped me so many times to travel from this small island to important meetings about childhood epilepsy in distant parts of the world.

Niall O'Donohoe

# Chapter 1

# Epilepsy: history and statistics

Epilepsy is not easily defined. The words 'epilepsy' and 'epileptic' are of Greek origin and have the same root as the verb meaning 'to seize' or 'to attack'. The word epilepsy means simply 'to be seized' in a passive sense. The idea of a disease seizing a man goes back to the old magic concept that all diseases were 'attacks' or seizures by gods or demons. Since epilepsy was the demoniac disease *par excellence*, the term gradually acquired a more particular meaning and came to signify an epileptic seizure. Epilepsy acquired its name because it attacked or seized both the senses and the mind. This concept of epilepsy is of ancient origin and was already in use, as were the terms 'epilepsy' and 'epileptic', in Hippocratic times (Temkin, 1971).

However, although 'epilepsy' and 'epileptic' were used in the earliest times as designations of both epileptic attacks and epileptic persons, the term epilepsy did not mean the underlying disease which the physicians preferred to refer to as 'the sacred disease' (morbus divinus). This name arose from the belief, common from antiquity to the relatively recent past, that diseases were phenomena more or less dependent on the supernatural and were considered to be a divine retribution for wickedness or a consequence of possession by spirits. Epilepsy, more than any other condition, was susceptible to explanation in these terms. Temkin (1971) wrote: 'In the struggle between the magic and the scientific conception, the latter has gradually emerged victorious in the western world. But the fight has been long and eventful, and in it epilepsy held one of the key positions.'

The battle was first joined around 400 BC when Hippocrates attacked the supernatural explanation of epilepsy in the book on 'The Sacred Disease' (Chadwick and Mann, 1950). The alleged divine character, the author or authors argued, was merely a shelter for ignorance and fraudulent malpractice. Epilepsy, it was claimed, was not more divine than any other disease, but, like all diseases, it was hereditary with its cause residing in the brain – a brain overflowing with a superfluity of phlegm, one of the four humours. Epilepsy, therefore, should be treated not by magic but by diet and drugs. Unfortunately the mythology surrounding epilepsy persisted, including a supposed link between epilepsy and lunacy and the idea that epilepsy could be caused by the influence of the cycle of the moon. The various ideas connecting epilepsy, madness, possession and similar states with the moon and other stars spawned a rich astrological literature through the centuries and even up to present day.

Having the sacred disease did not do the unfortunate sufferer much good. The epileptic was regarded as unclean; whoever touched him might become prey to the demon. It was thought that spitting would keep the demon away and throw back contagion, and thus one could escape infection. The magic concept, according to which epilepsy was a contagious disease, was one of the factors that made the epileptic's life a misery and gave him a social stigma. It was a disgraceful disease and the unfortunate person who felt an attack coming on rushed home or to a deserted place where he covered his head. To the ancients the epileptic was an object of horror and disgust, and throughout almost all of history those afflicted have been viewed with anxiety and fear. No other illness has set individuals apart so far, so often and so long, and these attitudes persist to the present day despite the quite frequent association of greatness and genius with the condition (Socrates, Julius Caesar, Napoleon, Dostoevski, Dante and Handel, to name a few).

From the time of Hippocrates physicians wrote about 'convulsions', particularly with reference to children, without clearly defining the meaning of the term and its relationship to epilepsy. There was an awareness in medical writing about children that convulsions in early childhood might have a different prognostic significance from epileptic seizures in older persons, but for a long time terminology remained confused. Attitudes to children with epilepsy were unenlightened and often cruel until well into the nineteenth century, and they frequently suffered the general fate of epileptics in being confined with insane persons.

The enlightenment of the eighteenth century and advances in neurology in the nineteenth century led to improved knowledge and understanding of epilepsy and to the final abandonment of the idea of demoniacal possession as a cause. The National Hospital for the Paralysed and Epileptic in London was opened in 1860 and during the early years of that decade the work of the great John Hughlings Jackson began in that hospital. In 1873 this produced a broad definition of epilepsy which is still perfectly valid: 'Epilepsy is the name for occasional, sudden, excessive, rapid and local discharges of grey matter.' According to his definition there was not just one form of the disease, but many epilepsies: one of these was a type of unilateral epilepsy with a characteristic march of clinical events which bears his name. Hughlings Jackson's former assistant W. R. Gowers published his important book *Epilepsy and Other Chronic Convulsive Diseases* in 1881, which incorporated many of Hughlings Jackson's ideas and attempted to differentiate epilepsy from conditions such as hysteria and migraine.

The epoch-making discovery of the human electroencephalogram (EEG) and the first publication of his observations on it by Hans Berger in 1929 (Gloor, 1974) provided the tool which facilitated the separation of epilepsy from other conditions and offered visual proof of Hughlings Jackson's theories. The subsequent explosion of knowledge about the EEG in epilepsy over the next two decades culminated in the publication of the classic *Atlas of Electroencephalography* by F. A. and E. L. Gibbs (1952). Other important milestones in the scientific understanding of epilepsy were Penfield and Jasper's (1954) *Epilepsy and the Functional Anatomy of the Human Brain*, which dealt in detail with the neuroanatomy and neurosurgery of epilepsy, and William Lennox's great book *Epilepsy and Related Disorders*, which was published in 1960 at the end of his long life devoted to the study of epilepsy and the care of its victims.

Lennox (1960) wrote that epilepsy was a disturbance of the normal rhythms of the brain. 'The rhythm of the body when orderly spells health. Dysrhythmia is a disease. Of all the systems of the body, the central nervous system is most nearly cyclic in function, and recurrent irregularity of its rhythm most profoundly disturbs the functions of both body and mind.' Lennox regarded epilepsy as an anarchy of cell function just as cancer is an anarchy of cell growth.

The manifestations of epilepsy are legion and no single symptom is essential. Lennox (1960) quoted Boerhaave (1724) as follows: 'For there is no one gesture, inflexion, or posture of the body known, which it has not shewn at some time, and it emulates all the motions of running, walking, turning, bending forwards, lying down, standing upright, or keeping the body in a very stiff and almost insuperable action.' The manifestations of epilepsy may appear as disturbances of consciousness or be evinced by sensory, visceral or motor signs, or present as perversions of ideation, emotion or mood. Some patients may experience all of these symptoms, others only one or two, and the symptomatology and intensity of the disturbances may vary from time to time. They may also experience what Lennox called the horror of epilepsy, quoting Margiad Evans (1953) as follows: 'Ever since a second convulsion I have been incredulous of all things firm and material. The light has held patches of invisible darkness. Time has become as rotten as worm-eaten wood, the earth under me is full of trap-doors and the sense of being, which is life and all that surrounds and creates it, a thing taken and given irresponsibly and without warning as children snatch at a toy.'

It is important to realize that all forms of epilepsy, as Hughlings Jackson wrote, arise from recurring excessive neuronal discharges occurring somewhere in the brain. Sometimes the site of origin can be easily identified while at other times no epileptic focus can be found. However, whatever their source the discharges frequently spread to other parts of the brain and even to the central nervous system as a whole. It must also be remembered that, as a rule, epilepsy is a chronic recurring disorder, and that many upsets in homoeostasis originating outside the central nervous system may provoke disturbances of the brain culminating in epileptic phenomena identical with those caused by epilepsy itself. Anyone may have a seizure given the right circumstances. These sporadic disturbances must be distinguished from epilepsy which is a recurring condition. Furthermore, the diagnosis must be made positively, based on careful history and clinical observations, and not just by exclusion. The label of epilepsy is, unfortunately, still too pejorative for mistakes to be made. In making a diagnosis, it is better to err on the side of 'not epilepsy' and subsequently to correct one's mistake than to apply a mistaken diagnosis of epilepsy which may be difficult to rectify later.

## Epidemiology: prevalence and incidence

The study of the epidemiology of epilepsy is beset with problems for many reasons. First of all, if epilepsy is associated with a social stigma, the presence of seizures may be denied and the disease remains hidden. The lack of a uniformly accepted definition and classification for epilepsy makes it difficult to compare the results of different epidemiological investigations. The study of epilepsy is further complicated by the fact that one is dealing with a symptom complex which may be a manifestation of a large number of diverse disease entities, each with a different cause of which some are known and some unknown. The definition of what constitutes epilepsy also varies. Some investigators include single, isolated seizures. Febrile convulsions may be included or excluded. The degree of case ascertainment also varies depending on the level of sophistication of medical and neurological services available. The ease of case ascertainment is also related to seizure type and frequency. Nocturnal seizures and absence seizures are more easily overlooked than are diurnal tonic–clonic seizures.

Epidemiology is the study of the natural history of disease, which includes its frequency, severity and course. Frequency of disease is best measured by population-based rates, which are ratios of the number of cases to the population at risk, expressed as cases per unit of population. Prevalence rate refers to the ratio of those people affected by a particular disorder at a given time per unit of population. Incidence refers to the number of new cases of a disorder arising within a given population in a given time period and may also be expressed as a percentage.

The survey of Pond, Bidwell and Stein (1960) gave an overall prevalence rate of 6.2/1000 population with an inception rate of new cases of 0.7/1000 per year. These authors included every type of epileptic seizure. Kurtzke *et al.* (1973) stated that the best evidence available at the time indicated a prevalence of convulsive disorders of about 4–6/1000 and emphasized that this must be considered a minimal estimate. Goodridge and Shorvan (1983), in a community based study of non-febrile seizures occurring among 6000 persons in a single general practice, found a lifetime prevalence of 20.3/1000 including single seizures and 17.0/1000 excluding single seizures. The prevalence of active epilepsy was 5.3/1000. Strict diagnostic criteria were employed and they considered that their unusually high prevalence rates were due to the inclusion of mild cases and those in prolonged remission. It is estimated that 1 in 20 of the population will have an epileptic seizure at some point in their lives and, at a conservative estimate, 1 in 200 will have epilepsy (Shorvon, 1990).

## Prevalence in childhood

Seizures are the commonest problem encountered in paediatric neurology. It has been estimated that 75% of cases of epilepsy have their onset before 20 years of age (Lennox, 1960). From data obtained through the National Child Development Study in Great Britain, Ross and Peckham (1983) found a prevalence of epilepsy of 4.1/1000 in children followed to the 11th birthday. In a study in Oklahoma, Cowan *et al.* (1989) established a prevalence rate of 4.71/1000 in children and adolescents followed to the 19th birthday. The incidence of epilepsy is greatest in the first year of life, remains high up to 4 years of age, falls during childhood and declines more slowly during adolescence and adult life and then rises sharply again after the age of 50 (Hauser, Annegers and Anderson, 1983). Early onset of epilepsy is considered by many authors to be associated with a poor neurological outcome (Chevrie and Aicardi, 1978), although the results of some large prospective studies do not support this (Ellenberg, Hirtz and Nelson, 1984).

Epilepsy in childhood and adolescence is, of course, much more than simply a matter of having seizures. Those affected are vulnerable medically and educationally and often face considerable social difficulties as a result of their seizures (Cooper, 1965). Epilepsy in childhood, just as in adults, is a family problem which will have an impact on and modify the lives of all the family members (Hoare, 1984). Looked at from the medical standpoint, the complexity of the problems facing the child with epilepsy and his parents is such as to make it impossible for any one discipline to deal adequately with all of them, and a team approach is essential (Hoare, 1988). The many facets of epilepsy make it difficult to define concisely. David Taylor (1969) wrote: 'Epilepsy is a phenomenon, it scarcely warrants being called a symptom and it is not a disease'. However, we need not take too much time trying to define epilepsy, but rather try to understand it. To do this, it is absolutely essential that we should first become familiar with and then use the continually evolving international classifications of the epilepsies and of seizures.

# References

BOERHAAVE, H. (1724) *Boerhaave's Aphorisms: Concerning the Knowledge and Cure of Diseases*, William and John Innys, London

CHEVRIE, J. J. and AICARDI, J. (1978) Convulsive disorders in the first year of life. Neurological and mental outcome and mortality. *Epilepsia*, **19**, 67–74

CHADWICK, J. and MANN, W. (1950) Translators. The sacred disease. In: *The Medical Works of Hippocrates*, Blackwell Scientific, Oxford

COOPER, J. E. (1965) Epilepsy in a longitudinal survey of 5000 children. *British Medical Journal*, **1**, 1020–1022

COWAN, L. D., BODENSTEINER, J. B., LEVITON, A. and DOHERTY, L. (1989) Prevalence of the epilepsies in children and adolescents. *Epilepsia*, **30**, 94–106

ELLENBERG, J. H., HIRTZ, D. G. and NELSON, K. B. (1984) Age of onset of seizures in young children. *Annals of Neurology*, **15**, 127–134

EVANS, M. (1953) *A Ray of Darkness*, Roy Publishers, New York, p. 191

GIBBS, F. A. and GIBBS, E. L. (1952) *Atlas of Electroencephalography*, Vol. 2: *Epilepsy*, Addison-Wesley, Cambridge, MA.

GLOOR, P. (1974) Hans Berger – Psychophysiology and the discovery of the human electroencephalogram. In: *Epilepsy. Proceedings of the Hans Berger Centenary Symposium* (eds P. Harris and C. Mawdsley), Churchill Livingstone, Edinburgh, London, New York, pp. 353–373

GOODRIDGE, M. G. and SHORVON, S. D. (1983) Epilepsy in a population of 6000. 1. Demography, diagnosis and classification. *British Medical Journal*, **287**, 641–644

GOWERS, W. R. (1881) *Epilepsy and Other Chronic Convulsive Diseases: Their Causes, Symptoms and Treatment*, Churchill, London

HAUSER, W. A., ANNEGERS, J. F. and ANDERSON, V. E. (1983) Epidemiology and the genetics of epilepsy. In: *Epilepsy* (eds A. A. Ward, J. R. Penry and D. Purpura), Raven Press, New York, pp. 267–294

HOARE, P. (1984) Psychiatric disturbances in the families of epileptic children. *Developmental Medicine and Child Neurology*, **26**, 14–19

HOARE, P. (ed.) (1988) *Epilepsy and the Family*. Symposium sponsored by Sanofi, UK and the Royal College of Physicians, London. Published by Sanofi, UK, Ltd, Withenshawe, Manchester M23 9NF

JACKSON, J. HUGHLINGS (1931–32) *Selected Writings of John Hughlings Jackson* (ed. J. Taylor), Hodder and Stoughton, London, p. 100

KURTZKE, J. F., KURLAND, L. T., GOLDBERG, I. D., CHOI, N. W. and REEDER, F. A. (1973) Convulsive disorders. In: *Epidemiology of Neurologic and Sense Organ Disorders*. APHA Monograph Series on Vital and Health Statistics (eds L. T. Kurland, J. F. Kurtzke and I. D. Goldberg), Harvard Press, Cambridge, Mass, pp. 15–40

LENNOX, W. G. (1960) *Epilepsy and Related Disorders*. 2 Vols. J. and A. Churchill, London

PENFIELD, W. and JASPER, H. (1954) *Epilepsy and the Functional Anatomy of the Human Brain*. Little, Brown, Boston, J. and A. Churchill, London

POND, D. A., BIDWELL, B. H. and STEIN, L. (1960) A survey of epilepsy in fourteen general practices. 1. Demographic and medical data. *Psychiatria, Neurologia, Neurochirurgia*, **63**, 217–236

ROSS, E. M. and PECKHAM, C. S. (1983) Seizure disorders in the National Child Development Study. In: *Research Progress in Epilepsy* (ed. F. C. Rose) Pitman, London, pp. 46–59

SHORVON, S. D. (1990) Epidemiology, classification, natural history and genetics of epilepsy. *Lancet*, **336**, 93–96

TAYLOR, D. C. (1969) Some psychiatric aspects of epilepsy. In: *Current Problems in Neuropsychiatry* (ed. R. N. Herrington), Headley Brothers, Ashford, Kent, pp. 106–109

TEMKIN, O. (1971) *The Falling Sickness*, 2nd Edition. Johns Hopkins, Baltimore and London

# Chapter 2

# Problems of classification and aetiology, including genetic aspects

Classification in general is a method of conveying information. The important components of any classification are accurate nomenclature, arrangement and grouping. The terminology and classification of epilepsy have evolved over many years, creating a profusion of interchangeable and confusing descriptive terms. Marsden and Reynolds (1982) have defined the problem of classification as a need to evolve a single code to cover three basically incompatible systems of classification; namely, that of clinical signs and symptoms of the seizure, that relating to the anatomical and electrophysiological evidence of the source of the seizure and that defining the aetiology of the seizure. Any classification employed must be useful and should reflect the needs of the user.

To the paediatrician and paediatric neurologist the chronological aspects of epilepsy through infancy, childhood and adolescence are particularly interesting, and a chronological approach will, to a large extent, be adopted in this book (*see Figures 3.1 and 4.1*). It is often difficult to convince doctors dealing exclusively or predominantly with adults that paediatrics is not just medicine (or neurology) in small people. The factors of age, growth and development exert their influences constantly and certainly not least in the problems of childhood epilepsy. Ounsted (1971) wrote that 'for all seizure disorders, maturation is the critical variable', and Lennox (1960) said that 'the type of epilepsy which occurs in a child represents a confluence of age, heredity, and structural brain abnormality'.

Hughlings Jackson's (1931) concept of a seizure as being due to 'an occasional, an excessive and a disorderly discharge of nerve tissue' has not been bettered as a description of the chronic recurrent paroxysmal disorder which constitutes epilepsy. A major problem in constructing classifications of the epilepsies and of seizures is, and has always been, the problem of aetiology. Why does nerve tissue behave abnormally in the way Jackson described? It is now widely accepted that the aetiology of an epilepsy is of equal or greater significance than the nature of the seizures it produces (Dreifuss, 1990). The seizure type is a product of the area of the nervous system involved, whereas the aetiology has implications in the areas of genetics, higher cortical function and intelligence. The natural history of the epilepsy, prognosis and response to medication are all closely linked to the nature of the epilepsy and its aetiology. Attempts to determine the exact aetiology of any particular epilepsy have been frustrated in the past by the complexity of the nervous system and the difficulties encountered in investigating it. The simple, time-honoured classification of epilepsy into idiopathic and symptomatic arose from this difficulty. Unfortunately, in the great majority of cases, an aetiology could not be determined. Hauser and Kurland (1975) were able to determine an aetiology in only 23.3% of the patients in the Rochester, Minnesota study. Since then, however, remarkable advances in genetics, neurophysiology and neuroimaging have made aetiological diagnosis increasingly possible. The simplistic, symptom-oriented approach to the epilepsies, with its concentration on seizures only, is no longer acceptable if we are to try to increase our understanding of them.

It has to be said, however, that it is easier to classify epileptic seizures than it is to classify the epilepsies on an aetiological basis. An international committee was convened by the International League Against Epilepsy in 1964 to formulate a comprehensive classification of epileptic seizures which would include the type of clinical seizure, the type of EEG seizure, the interictal EEG expression, the anatomical substrate and aetiology, and the age of the patient. This classification was published (Gastaut, 1970) and became known as the International Classification of Epileptic Seizures. Seizures were classified as:

1   Partial or those beginning locally.
2   Generalized or those which were bilaterally symmetrical and without local onset. These may be convulsive or non-convulsive in nature.
3   Unilateral seizures.
4   Unclassifiable seizures.

A revised version of the International Classification was published in 1981 (Commission on Classification, 1981) and is now in general use. It incorporated information derived from neurophysiological advances and from the use of simultaneous EEG and videotaping of patients during seizures. More accurate recognition of individual symptoms during seizures and their elaboration during the course of a seizure resulted from this intensive monitoring. The 1981 classification allows for the dynamic nature of some partial seizures by providing longitudinal descriptions of evolving seizure manifestations. This particularly relates to changes in awareness of and responsiveness to external stimuli. Subtle alterations of consciousness with impairment of awareness and responsiveness are much more easily discerned in videotape replay than by simply observing individual attacks. The Revised Classification of Epileptic Seizures (1981) will be used in this book and may be summarized as in Table 2.1. The main criticism of this revised classification has been that it has abandoned the use of some time-honoured terms, e.g. generalized tonic–clonic seizure instead of grand mal, absence instead of petit mal, complex partial seizure instead of temporal lobe or psychomotor seizure, myoclonic or atonic instead of minor motor seizure. However, these terms have been used in a loose or ambiguous manner in the past. The worst example of this has been the use by some of the term 'petit mal' to describe any seizure other than 'grand mal' and also the application of the term to all varieties of absence attacks. The terms psychomotor and temporal lobe are incorrect to describe all complex partial seizures, since these may arise elsewhere than in the temporal lobe, notably in the frontal lobe areas. However, many still prefer to use the descriptive anatomical terms temporal lobe seizures or frontal lobe seizures to describe these attacks (see Chapter 10). There are motor components in so many seizures, including non-convulsive attacks, that the term minor motor is meaningless and vague.

In 1989, the Commission on Classification proposed a new International Classification of Epilepsies, Epileptic Syndromes and Related Seizure Disorders (Commission

**Table 2.1 International classification of epileptic seizures**

---

I  Partial seizures (seizures beginning locally).
    A.  Simple partial seizures (consciousness not impaired).
        1.  With motor symptoms.
        2.  With somatosensory or special sensory symptoms.
        3.  With autonomic symptoms.
        4.  With psychic symptoms.

    B.  Complex partial seizures (with impairment of consciousness).
        1.  Beginning as simple partial seizure and progressing to impairment of consciousness.
        2.  With impairment of consciousness at onset.

    C.  Partial seizures becoming secondarily generalized.

II  Generalized seizures (bilaterally symmetrical and without local onset).
    A.  1.  Absence seizures.
        2.  Atypical absence seizures.
    B.  Myoclonic seizures.
    C.  Clonic seizures.
    D.  Tonic seizures.
    E.  Tonic-clonic seizures.
    F.  Atonic seizures.

III  Unclassified epileptic seizures.

---

(Adapted from Commission on Classification and Terminology, 1981)

on Classification, 1989). While some epilepsies are now known to have specific identifiable causes, many remain of unknown cause and have been categorized under the general rubric of 'idiopathic epilepsy'. This has encouraged a symptom-oriented approach which has inhibited understanding of epilepsy in the past. The symptoms of epilepsy, i.e. the seizures, are, however, to quote Dreifuss (1990), simply one of many pigments of which the whole picture of an epilepsy is painted, although they are the ones which usually draw attention to the existence of the condition. Individual seizure types are, in fact, rarely characteristic of any specific epilepsy or epileptic syndrome and some, such as the generalized tonic–clonic seizure, occur in many different types of epilepsy.

The term epileptic syndrome is used increasingly in paediatric epileptology to describe conditions in which a cluster of symptoms and signs, including seizures, are associated in a non-fortuitous manner (Roger *et al.*, 1992). These symptoms and signs include the presence or absence of a family history of epilepsy, the age of onset of the condition, the neurological and psychological findings, the features of the interictal and ictal EEG, the natural history of the disorder, the response to medication and any developmental complications. Some epileptic syndromes have also been shown to have specific pathological, chromosomal, or biochemical markers.

Two principal distinctions are used in the description of the epilepsies and epileptic syndromes. The first of these is the separation of epilepsies characterized by seizures that are generalized (generalized epilepsies) from those characterized by partial seizures which imply a focal cortical origin (partial or localization-related epilepsies). The second major subdivision is between epilepsies which are idiopathic or primary of 'non-lesional' from those which are symptomatic or secondary or 'lesional' (see Table 2.2).

**Table 2.2 Epilepsies and epileptic syndromes**

A. Generalized – with generalized seizures
B. Partial or localization-related – partial seizures.

A. Idiopathic, primary, non-lesional.
B. Symptomic, secondary, lesional.

The term cryptogenic is also used to refer to an epilepsy whose cause is hidden or occult, e.g. infantile spasms. In general cryptogenic epilepsy may be presumed to be symptomatic even though the aetiology is unknown. In the case of infantile spasms, for instance, the use of positron emission tomography is now revealing evidence of focal cortical dysgenesis in some cryptogenic cases (Chugani et al., 1990).

Primary epileptic syndromes occur in otherwise normal children, sometimes with a family history of a similar disorder, with no demonstrable underlying pathology and in whom the EEG shows a normal background interictal activity. In these children, the response to medication is usually good and remission is likely. In contrast, secondary or symptomatic syndromes are usually associated with underlying cerebral disease which may result in developmental abnormality. A positive family history is uncommon and there are abnormal neurological and investigative findings. In these children, the response to medication is unpredictable and spontaneous resolution is unlikely. It is important to recognize that similar seizures may occur in different syndromes and that some syndromes are characterized by multiple seizure types. Furthermore, the syndromes vary in specificity from those which represent broad concepts to those which are highly specific (Aicardi, 1988).

Although not all patients fit into the described syndromes, this approach to the epilepsies of childhood and adolescence has revolutionized the management of these disorders in recent years. It has led to more precise diagnostic, therapeutic and prognostic attitudes to the individual patient, it has improved communication and exchange of ideas about epilepsy and, inevitably, it is leading and will lead to more rational use of the newer and relatively specific antiepileptic drugs and thereby improve control of seizures (O'Donohoe, 1991, 1992).

An alternative neurobiological approach to the classification of the epilepsies has been advocated by the Montreal School which is complementary to the syndromic method (Berkovic et al., 1987). It is based on the evidence for the multifactorial origin of epilepsy, and on the recognition of a spectrum of clinical and EEG features in patients with both primary and secondary epilepsy. This method attempts to place the individual into a biological continuum which exists between the most genetically determined epilepsies on the one hand and the most clearly acquired forms on the other hand and to use clinical, EEG, radiological, and neuropsychological data to build a profile of the patient – an 'epileptic phenotype'.

## Age and epilepsy

As already mentioned, a chronological approach to the categorization of childhood epilepsies is particularly attractive to paediatricians. Age, growth, and development are not only of primary importance in determining whether or not epilepsy develops, but also influence the clinical and electrical manifestations of seizures and the types of epileptic syndromes which are encountered. Age is also an important factor in determining prognosis. Experimental evidence suggests that the immature brain is more susceptible to the development of seizures than is its mature counterpart (Moshé, 1987). This is best illustrated by the increased incidence of reactive seizures in response to high fever in the young. However, this susceptibility is coupled with a decreased potential for developing chronic epilepsy as the normal brain matures, best demonstrated by the fact that children who experience the common problem of febrile convulsions only relatively rarely develop epilepsy later. Recent research has demonstrated that the substantia nigra, which has strong inhibitory functions through its GABAergic output, functions inadequately in the immature organism but improves in this respect with the passage of time (Moshé et al., 1989).

Aicardi (1986) uses the chronological approach to the classification of epileptic syndromes and distinguishes four main periods or epochs in childhood and adolescent epilepsy. These are:

1   A neonatal period, which he extends to 3 months of age, during which seizures are related to structural pathology and the prognosis is poor.
2   A period from 3 months to 4 years in which the seizure threshold of the central nervous system is low and reactive seizures, especially with fever, are common. Serious epileptic syndromes such as infantile spasms (West's syndrome) and the Lennox–Gastaut syndrome occur in this epoch.
3   A period between 4 years and 9–10 years in which there is a predominance of primary or idiopathic generalized and partial epilepsies, for example, childhood absence epilepsy and benign partial epilepsy with centro-temporal spikes. Complex partial seizures secondary to structural brain abnormality also become better defined in this epoch.
4   From 9 to 10 years onwards, primary generalized epilepsies, such as the well-defined juvenile myoclonic epilepsy of Janz, occur while complex partial seizures are more frequently encountered.

This scheme is certainly useful to the paediatrician as a general diagnostic and prognostic framework.


## Pathophysiology and epileptogenesis

Epileptic seizures result from the sudden, excessive, electrical discharges of large aggregates of neurons, and the clinical components are determined by the site of origin of the discharge and by the pattern of spread. Neurons are rendered susceptible to abnormal electrical behaviour by inherited factors and/or disease. The varying convulsive threshold or inherent susceptibility to convulse at different ages depends on age and the state of maturation of the brain, on inherited genetic factors and on the degree of cerebral damage, if any, which is present. Triggering factors such as fever, illness, hypoxia, hypocalcaemia, hypoglycaemia, hyper- and hyponatraemia, overhydration, and alterations in acid–base balance may be involved in precipitating an individual seizure. Extraneous factors such as the administration of convulsant drugs, the too rapid withdrawal of anticonvulsant drugs, overdosage with various drugs producing drug toxicity and various toxins may also be responsible. Emotional disturbance, particularly when acute, and overfatigue due to lack of sleep may act as precipitants of seizures in those with a lowered convulsive threshold or with established epilepsy.

There is now evidence that epilepsy involves variations of the normal physiochemical mechanisms of nerve cells. *Epileptogenesis* is a term which refers to the dynamic processes underlying the development of epilepsy. It depends on the predisposition of neuronal aggregates to discharge when stimulated and on synchronization of firing within the neuronal substrate. The neocortex and hippocampus are uniquely likely to generate abnormal electrical activity of this nature because of their intrinsic organization and internal connections within the brain. Their excitability is modified both by interhemispheric events and by subcortical influences. The role of the substantia nigra has already been mentioned.

The neuronal membrane potential depends on its selective permeability to different ions. $Na^+$ and $Ca^{2+}$ influx is associated with excitatory depolarization and $K^+$ efflux and $Cl^-$ influx with inhibitory hyperpolarization. When depolarization occurs, an action potential is created which is a stimulus to neighbouring positions on the cell membrane from which it spreads along the axon, always away from the point of impulse generation. Nerve impulses arriving at the terminal bulb of the axon cause release of neurotransmitters which bind to receptors on the post-synaptic membrane and initiate a chain of events within the post-synaptic neuron. For most synapses the transmitter–receptor complex acts as a gate regulating the opening and closing of ion channels on the post-synaptic membrane, with resulting excitation and/or inhibition. Glutamate is the main excitatory neurotransmitter and every neuron has receptors for it. One pharmacologically identified glutamate receptor which binds with a glutamate analogue, N-methyl-D-aspartate, or NMDA, is of particular interest. When activated this receptor opens gated channels permeable to calcium ions. The NMDA receptor has a key role in the development of a process called long-term potentiation, a persistent change in the strength of synaptic connections which is thought to be involved in both the normal reorganization of neuronal connections which occurs with learning and experience and also in the process of epileptogenesis (Kalil, 1989). The action of the NMDA receptor–cation channel complex is a potential mechanism whereby recurrent epileptic events could induce widespread alterations in neuronal function. An exciting recent discovery has been the successful cloning of one of the glutamate receptors in the rat brain (Hollman *et al.*, 1989). It is expected that such research will lead to the identification of the structure of human glutamate receptors. It should then be possible to develop glutamate receptor blocking agents which might selectively control epileptic phenomena.

It is pertinent here to discuss the phenomenon of facilitation of seizures, a process called *kindling*. The term was introduced by Goddard (1967) and derives from the analogy of kindling a fire. Kindling may be defined as the facilitation of seizure pathways by repeated seizure discharges. In the experimental animal model, repeated brain exposures to localized repetitive low-intensity electrical stimuli induce an increasingly pathological response. Initially, the stimulus produces no effect, but, after a time, focal discharges develop and, eventually, behavioural automatisms and spontaneous seizures occur. This gradual alteration in brain function, once induced, is permanent. Since its discovery, kindling has been proposed as a possible mechanism whereby epileptogenesis in humans may be established. However, it is still not certain that the kindling process occurs in humans. If it does, then it could provide an explanation for the latent period that exists between the occurrence of a brain insult and the later onset of epilepsy. During this latent period, if one can extrapolate from the animal model, new neuronal connections may be formed which lead to increased local excitability, there is repetitive firing of neurons with progressive increments in the severity of the discharges, and eventually clinical seizures emerge. The kindling model is particularly attractive as an explanation for the chronic partial epilepsies, particularly those arising in the temporal lobe area. It might also provide an explanation for what is called secondary epileptogenesis. Chronic focal epileptogenic lesions can cause distant areas to become capable of generating abnormal electrical discharges and, in some cases, epileptic seizures. The best example of this is the formation of the so-called *mirror focus*, an independent epileptogenic area of cortex which is contralateral and homotopic to the primary epileptogenic lesion. This focus continues to function independently even after the ablation of the primary lesion, a fact which has important implications for the surgical treatment of epilepsy.

To summarize, there is still no certain evidence that the kindling mechanism is responsible for the establishment of epileptogenic foci in humans. Nevertheless, some progressive changes which occur in human epilepsy are reminiscent of the kindling process and it will continue to excite great interest among those interested in the pathophysiology of epilepsy (Reynolds, 1989). The review of the subject by Moshé and Ludvig (1988) is recommended to the reader.

The age-dependent appearance of spontaneous seizures in the primary epilepsies appears to depend on a critical period in cerebral maturation when the genetically determined defect is expressed clinically as a manifest change in behaviour. Since, by definition, the brain should be structurally normal in a primary epilepsy, it seems probable that, at a given maturational stage, alterations occur in the balance between excitatory and inhibitory brain systems and the convulsive threshold is lowered as a result of increased diffuse cortical excitability. The supposed normality of the brain in the primary generalized epilepsies has been challenged in recent years by those who claim that minor morphological changes may be found in brains of patients with these conditions (Meencke and Janz, 1984). These changes, called 'microdysgenesis' include an increase in cell density and abnormal arrangements of cortical neurons and an increase in white matter neurons. These changes have been reported more often in the cryptogenic epileptic syndromes such as West's syndrome of infantile spasms, in the Lennox–Gastaut syndrome and in severe myoclonic epilepsy of infancy (Renier and Renkawek, 1990). Whether these disorders of brain morphology are evidence of minor deviations in neuronal migration and glial cell production during the last trimester of intrauterine development, due to genetic or acquired intrauterine factors, is purely speculative at present. However, such changes could be associated with abnormal synaptic connections and resulting diffuse cortical hyperexcitability.

As far as the known pathological causes of epilepsy are concerned, it is recognized that a great variety of congenital and acquired structural lesions and also inflammatory, traumatic, vascular, neoplastic, degenerative, toxic and metabolic causes may be responsible for the eventual development of seizures (Hopkins, 1987; Meldrum, 1990). In a paediatric context and because of possible medicolegal implications, it is important to refer here to the work of Nelson and Ellenberg (1987) on the predisposing and causative factors in childhood epilepsy. Their results are based on the National Collaborative Perinatal Project in the US and are in agreement with the findings of the British National Child Development Study (Ross *et al.*, 1980). Both studies conclude that labour and delivery factors appear to contribute little to the subsequent development of childhood epilepsy. Maldevelopment, rather than damage at birth of an intact nervous system, appears to be a more common mechanism. The American authors commented that, among the hundreds of prenatal and perinatal factors which were explored as predictors of childhood epilepsy, the principal predictors identified were congenital malformations of the fetus (cerebral and non-cerebral), a family history of neurological disorders (epilepsy or mental retardation in the mother, epilepsy or motor deficits in a sibling), and neonatal seizures. The aetiology of most seizure disorders of early childhood which they examined by means of a large set of prenatal and perinatal variables remained unexplained.

## Genetics and epilepsy

One of the questions asked most frequently about epilepsy is 'Is it inherited?'. The fear of inheriting epilepsy has been present from earliest times and in all cultures. It is closely linked with the prejudice which many people have about individuals suffering from epilepsy. Much repressive legislation prohibiting marriage, prescribing sterilization, and limiting immigration has resulted. There is no doubt that, in some types of epilepsy, heredity plays a significant role and the doctor may be asked for genetic advice when a person with epilepsy is considering having a child, or when parents who have a child with epilepsy desire to have another child.

Genetic factors can act by causing the transmission of diseases of which seizures may be a symptom. There are over 100 single gene disorders which may have epilepsy as a symptom and most have other gross clinical characteristics also (McKusick, 1983). Together, however, they account for less than 2% of cases of epilepsy. Examples include autosomal dominant disorders such as tuberose sclerosis and neurofibromatosis, recessively inherited disorders such as the various degenerative lipid storage disorders of the central nervous system and disorders of amino acid and carbohydrate metabolism, and some X-linked conditions such as Menkes's syndrome. Seizures may also occur in clinical syndromes caused by chromosomal anomalies, for example Down's syndrome, and in syndromes due to sex chromosomal abnormalities.

In the great majority of patients with epilepsy, however, seizures are the only abnormal manifestation and in these, when inheritance plays a part, either a gene or possibly several genes must either increase the convulsive susceptibility of the individual or lower the convulsive threshold to epilepsy. In other instances, epilepsy may reflect the interaction of multiple genes, and the effects of environmental factors. Faced with this complex situation, there is intense research interest in attempts to discover a genetic linkage in certain well-defined and age-specific epileptic syndromes of childhood and adolescence. Two remarkable advances have been the demonstration of a genetic linkage for benign familial neonatal convulsions with chromosome 20 (Leppert et al., 1989) and for juvenile myoclonic epilepsy of Janz with chromosome 6 (Delgado-Escueta et al., 1989). A gene, once mapped in this way, will sooner or later be cloned and this will reveal the structure of the gene product (Editorial, 1987). The implications for the greater understanding of the pathophysiology of epilepsy and for therapeutic advances are clear.

A landmark in the study of genetic influences in the aetiology of epilepsy was the work of Metrakos and Metrakos (1961). They studied the relatives of patients with absence attacks and/or grand mal tonic-clonic seizures, not associated with any gross cerebral abnormality but manifesting a regular 3 Hz spike-wave abnormality of the EEG. They concluded that the spike-wave EEG trait, but not the epilepsy, was inherited as an autosomal dominant trait with age-dependent penetrance. This trait had the unusual characteristic of very low penetrance at birth, rising rapidly to nearly complete penetrance (expression in almost 50% of first degree relatives) around the age of 10 years, and declining rapidly to almost no penetrance after the age of 40. From this study, they concluded that the offspring and siblings of persons with this trait would have a 50% chance of carrying the gene, a 37% chance of having the typical EEG abnormality, a 12% chance of having one or more seizures, and an 8% chance of developing primary generalized epilepsy. An important aspect of their findings was the age dependency of both the seizures and the EEG abnormality, which were most frequently seen between the ages of 8 and 15 years, but diminished thereafter. It seems probable now that patients with the 3 Hz spike-wave EEG discharge do not represent a homogeneous population and that subgroups can be defined by clinical criteria. For example, other types of absence epilepsy occurring later than the classical childhood absence epilepsy may represent another phenotype (Delgado-Escueta, Treiman and Walsh, 1983). Two gene loci may need to interact to produce an appropriate phenotype, although analogy with gene identification in Duchenne and Becker muscular dystrophy (Rowland, 1988) and in the spinal muscular atrophies (Melki et al., 1990) make this unlikely. It seems probable that different types of the same disease are due to an allelic series of mutations at the same gene locus.

Another definable subgroup of primary generalized epilepsy is that of patients with photosensitivity. In these also, the EEG abnormalities are more frequent than the environmentally induced seizures, which are quite uncommon. The highest percentage of abnormalities occurs in early adolescence and females predominate. Febrile convulsions also provide strong evidence for the genetic influence on seizure susceptibility, and the incidence of a positive family history has ranged from 10 to 50%. In an important study Tsuboi (1977) showed that febrile convulsions occurred in 27.7% of siblings of probands with febrile convulsions. The incidence was only 6.2% among siblings of control children. The incidence among siblings of probands reached 45% when two family members had febrile seizures. The incidence among siblings was higher if one parent had a history of febrile convulsions (36.5%) and lowest if neither parent had such a history (18%). The genetic predisposition to convulse with fever may indirectly be responsible for the later development of secondary partial epilepsy if the child sustains temporal lobe damage during a prolonged febrile convulsion (Ounsted, Lindsay and Richards, 1987).

Andermann (1982) has suggested that, for each epileptic patient, one or more major genes or polygenes must interact with maturational, endocrine and environmental factors in order for a clinical epileptic syndrome to emerge. Even in the secondary of symptomatic epilepsies, where partial seizures are common and where one is less likely to obtain a family history of epilepsy, it has been demonstrated that the frequency of seizures and/or EEG abnormalities in other family members is higher than in control populations (Ottman et al., 1989), suggesting an interaction between genetic and acquired factors in these cases also. Gloor (1982) has written as follows:

> In spite of the multiplicity of exogenous factors which can cause epileptic seizures, most human epilepsies, whether generalized or partial, share a common genetic basis, which significantly contributes to epileptogenesis. By itself, the genetic predisposition is rarely, or perhaps never, sufficient to induce clinical epilepsy but may only be responsible for the expression of the EEG trait. For recurrent seizures to occur other aetiological factors must intervene. Some of these may also be genetic but the majority are exogenous and encompass the long list of pathological states long recognized as being capable of causing recurrent seizures. However, just as the genetic predisposition to seizures does not, by

itself, appear to be sufficient to cause clinically manifest epilepsy, these exogenous factors are also by themselves usually not capable of causing recurrent seizures. In order to do so, they must affect a brain which is genetically predisposed to hyperexcitability. In most cases of human epilepsy, therefore, the occurrence of seizures may reflect the interaction of a genetic predisposition to cortical hyperexcitability with the impact of an exogenous insult of some sort

The reviews by Hauser and Anderson (1986) and Bird (1987) are recommended to the reader. The role of genetic factors in the individual epileptic syndromes will be discussed further in the relevant chapters.

*Genetic counselling* may be sought by parents who have one child with epilepsy and who fear that other children they may have will be similarly affected. The risk depends on the nature of the proband's epilepsy, the risk being higher if it is primary or idiopathic in nature. The detailed long-term studies from Rochester, Minnesota (Annegers *et al.*, 1982) indicate that the risk of developing recurrent, non-febrile seizures in siblings is about 4%. When single seizures and febrile seizures are included, the total risk for epilepsy in siblings lies between 9 and 11%. Hauser, Annegers and Anderson (1983) showed that the risk of developing epilepsy in the siblings of probands having their onset of seizures in the first decade of life, was higher than if the probands developed seizures after the age of 10 years.

The prediction of risks for the offspring of individuals who have had epilepsy also depends on the nature of the parental epilepsy. For example, the incidence of seizures in the offspring of parents with absence epilepsy is much higher than in the offspring of parents with other seizure types. The risk also seems to increase when the proband has a generalized spike-wave EEG pattern or when such a pattern is found in another first-degree relative (Tsuboi and Endo, 1977). The risks to relatives and to offspring are usually much less when the proband has a partial epilepsy rather than a generalized epilepsy, since so many of these result from environmental causes. However, an exception must be made in the case of the common benign partial epilepsy with rolandic spikes where hereditary factors are of paramount importance in causation (15% of siblings have the same condition). Recent studies have suggested that the overall seizure risk in offspring of parents with partial epilepsy is not greatly different from the offspring of those with generalized epilepsy (Ottman et al., 1989) with the exception of a subgroup with absence seizures, where the incidence was three times as high as for partial cases.

The overall incidence of epilepsy in the offspring when one parent is affected is about 4%. When both parents are affected, it rises to 10% or more. If there are more than two affected family members, the risks are greater still. Unexplained is the fact that the children of epileptic mothers are more likely to develop epilepsy than are the children of epileptic fathers (Hauser and Anderson, 1986).

It will be appreciated that the role of the genetic counsellor in epilepsy is a difficult one, mainly because of the diversity of the epilepsies and the heterogeneous aetiological causes involved. When one or other parent has epilepsy secondary to acquired structural damage to the brain, the risk to future offspring will not usually be greater than in the general population with two normal parents.

# References

AICARDI, J. (1986) *Epilepsy in Childhood*, Raven Press, New York
AICARDI, J. (1988) Epileptic syndromes in childhood. *Epilepsia*, **29**, Supplement 3, S1–S5
ANDERMANN, E. (1982) Multifactorial inheritance of generalized and focal epilepsy. In: *Genetic Basis of*

*the Epilepsies* (eds V. E. Anderson, W. A. Hauser, J. K. Penry and C. F. Sing), Raven Press, New York, pp 355–374.

ANNEGERS, J. F., HAUSER, W. A., ANDERSON, V. E. and KURLAND, L. T. (1982) The risks of seizure disorders among relatives of patients with childhood onset epilepsy. *Neurology*, **32**, 174–179

BERKOVIC, S. F., ANDERMANN, F., ANDERMANN, E. and GLOOR, P. (1987) Concepts of absence epilepsies. Discrete syndromes or biological continuum? *Neurology*, **37**, 993–1000

BIRD, T. D. (1987) Genetic considerations in childhood epilepsy. *Epilepsia*, **28**, Supplement 1, S71–S81

CHUGANI, H. T., SHIELDS, W. D., SHEWMON, D. A. *et al.* (1990) Infantile spasms. I. PET identifies focal cortical dysgenesis in cryptogenic cases for surgical treatment. *Annals of Neurology*, **27**, 406–413

COMMISSION ON CLASSIFICATION AND TERMINOLOGY OF THE INTERNATIONAL LEAGUE AGAINST EPILEPSY (1981) Proposed revisions of clinical and electroencephalographical classification of epileptic seizures. *Epilepsia*, **22**, 480–501

COMMISSION ON CLASSIFICATION AND TERMINOLOGY OF THE INTERNATIONAL LEAGUE AGAINST EPILEPSY (1989) Proposal for revised classification of epilepsies and epileptic syndromes. *Epilepsia*, **30**, 389–399

DELGADO-ESCUETA, A. V., TREIMAN, D. M. and WALSH, G. O. (1983) The treatable epilepsies. I. *New England Journal of Medicine*, **308**, 1508–1514

DELGADO-ESCUETA, A. V., GREENBERG, D. A., TREIMAN, L. *et al.* (1989) Mapping the gene for juvenile myoclonic epilepsy. *Epilepsia*, **30**, Supplement 4, S8–S18

DREIFUSS, F.E. (1990) The epilepsies. Clinical implications of the International Classification. *Epilepsia*, **31**, Supplement 3, S3–S10

EDITORIAL (1987) Mapping the human genome. *Lancet*, **329**, 1121–1122

GASTAUT, H. (1970) Clinical and electroencephalographical classification of epileptic seizures. *Epilepsia*, **11**, 102–113

GLOOR, P. (1982) Towards a unifying concept of epileptogenesis. In: *Advances in Epileptology. The XIIIth Epilepsy International Symposium* (eds H. Akimoto, H. Kazamatsuri, M. Seino and A. A. Ward), Raven Press, New York, pp. 425–428

GODDARD, G. V. (1967) Development of epileptic seizures through brain stimulation at low intensity. *Nature*, **204**, 1020–1021

HAUSER, W. A. and KURLAND, C. T. (1975) The epidemiology of epilepsy in Rochester, Minnesota, 1935 through 1967. *Epilepsia*, **16**, 1–66

HAUSER, W. A. and ANDERSON, V. E. (1986) Genetics of epilepsy. In: *Recent Advances in Epilepsy*, No. 3 (eds T. A. Pedley and B. S. Meldrum), Churchill Livingstone, Edinburgh, London, pp. 21–36

HAUSER, W. A., ANNEGERS, J. F. and ANDERSON, V. E. (1983) Epidemiology and the genetics of epilepsy. In: *Epilepsy* (eds A. A. Ward, J. K. Penry and D. Purpura), Raven Press, New York, pp. 267–294

HOLLMAN, M., O'SHEA-GREENFIELD, A., ROGERS, S. W. and HEINEMANN, S. (1989) Cloning by functional expression of a member of the glutamate receptor family. *Nature*, **342**, 643–648

HOPKINS, A. (1987) The causes and precipitation of seizures. In: *Epilepsy* (ed. A. Hopkins), Chapman and Hall, London, pp. 115–136

JACKSON, J. HUGHLINGS (1931) *Selected Writings of John Hughlings Jackson* (eds J. Taylor, G. Holmes and F. M. R. Walshe), **Vol. I**, P. 8. Hodder and Stoughton, London

KALIL, R. E. (1989) Synapse formation in the developing brain. *Scientific American*, **261**, 38–45

LENNOX, W. G. (1960) *Epilepsy and Related Disorders*. J. and A. Churchill, London

LEPPERT, M., ANDERSON, V. E., QUATTLEBAUM, T. *et al.* (1989) Benign familial neonatal convulsions linked to genetic markers on chromosome 20. *Nature*, **337**, 647–648

MCKUSICK, V. A. (1983) Mendelian inheritance in man. *Catalogs of Autosomal Dominant, Autosomal Recessive and X-Linked Phenotypes*, 6th Edition, Johns Hopkins University Press, Baltimore

MARSDEN, C. D. and REYNOLDS, E. H. (1982) Neurology. In: *A Textbook of Epilepsy*, 2nd Edition (ed. J. Laidlaw and A. Richens), Churchill Livingtone, Edinburgh, London, pp. 97–131

MEENCKE, H. J. and JANZ, D. (1984) Neuropathological findings in primary generalized epilepsy: a study of eight cases. *Epilepsia*, **25**, 8–21

MELDRUM, B. S. (1990) Anatomy, physiology and pathology of epilepsy. *Lancet*, **336**, 231–234

MELKI, J., SHETH, P., ABDELHAK, S. et al. and FRENCH SPINAL MUSCULAR INVESTIGATORS (1990). Mapping the acute (Type 1) spinal muscular atrophy to chromosome. 5q12–q14. *Lancet*, **336**, 271–273

METRAKOS, J. D. and METRAKOS, K. (1961) Genetics of convulsive disorders. II. Genetic and electroencephalographic studies in centrencephalic epilepsy. *Neurology*, **11**, 474–483

MOSHÉ, S. L. (1987) Epileptogenesis and the immature brain. *Epilepsia*, **28**, Supplement I, S3–S15

MOSHÉ, S. L. and LUDVIG, N. (1988) Kindling. In: *Recent Advances in Epilepsy*, No. 4 (eds T. A. Pedley and B. S. Meldrum) Churchill Livingstone, Edinburgh, London, pp. 21–44

MOSHÉ, S. L., SPERBER, E. F., BROWN, L. L. *et al.* (1989) Experimental epilepsy: developmental aspects. *Cleveland Clinic Journal of Medicine*, **56**, Supplement Part 1, S92–S99

NELSON, K. B. and ELLENBERG, J. H. (1987) Predisposing and causative factors in childhood epilepsy. *Epilepsia*, **28**, Supplement 1, S16–S24

O'DONOHOE, N. V. (1991) The epilepsies. In: *Paediatric Specialty Practice for the 1990s* (eds J. Eyre and R. Boyd), Royal College of Physicians of London, London, pp. 51–61

O'DONOHOE, N. V. (1992) Delineation of epileptic syndromes. *Current Paediatrics*, **2**, 68–72

OTTMAN, R., ANNEGERS, J. F., HAUSER, W. A. and KURLAND, L. T. (1989) Seizure risk in offspring of parents with generalized versus partial epilepsy. *Epilepsia*, **30**, 157–161

OUNSTED, C. (1971) Some aspects of seizure disorders. In: *Recent Advances in Paediatrics* (eds D. Gairdner and D. Hull), J. and A. Churchill, London, p. 365

OUNSTED, C., LINDSAY, J. and RICHARDS, P. (1987) *Temporal Lobe Epilepsy 1948–1986: A Biographical Study*. Clinics in Developmental Medicine, No. 103. Cambridge University Press, Cambridge

RENIER, W. O. and RENKAWEK, U. (1990) Clinical and neuropathological findings in a case of severe myoclonic epilepsy of infancy. *Epilepsia*, **31**, 287–291

REYNOLDS, E. H. (1989) The process of epilepsy: is kindling relevant? In: *The Clinical Relevance of Kindling* (eds T. G. Bolwig and M. R. Trimble), John Wiley and Sons, Chicester, New York, pp. 149–160

ROGER, J., BUREAU, M., DRAVET, C. *et al.* (1992) *Epileptic Syndromes in Infancy, Childhood and Adolescence*, 2nd Edition, John Libbey, London, Paris

ROSS, E. M., PECKHAM, C. S., WEST, P. B. and BUTLER, N. R. (1980) Epilepsy in childhood: findings from the National Child Development Study. *British Medical Journal*, **1**, 207–210

ROWLAND, L. P. (1988) Clinical concepts of Duchene muscular dystrophy. The impact of molecular genetics. *Brain*, **111**, 479–495

TSUBOI, T. (1977) Genetic aspects of febrile convulsions. *Human Genetics*, **38**, 169–173

TSUBOI, T. and ENDO, S. (1977) Incidence of seizures and EEG abnormalities among offspring of epileptic patients. *Human Genetics*, **36**, 173–189

Chapter 3

# Neonatal seizures

Seizures occur in just over 1% of neonates. Statistics vary with the population studied; 3% of babies admitted to neonatal intensive care facilities have seizures and, if only high-risk admissions are considered, the frequency is much higher. Like so much else in the newborn, they present special problems in recognition, in determining their cause and in treatment. It is often extremely difficult to distinguish between normal and abnormal behaviour in newborns, and this particularly applies to disorders of movement.

Neonatal seizures are usually partial and always symptomatic. Although there are very many possible causes of convulsions at this age, in practice over 90% are due to birth complications, to hypocalcaemia, to hypomagnesaemia or hypoglycaemia or to meningitis. Of the birth complications, brain anoxia and ischaemia are the most important factors and usually cause seizures in the first 24–72 hours of life (*see Figure 3.1*). Hypoxic–ischaemic brain injury is the single most important neurological problem occurring in the neonatal period, and produces damage by depriving the central nervous system of oxygen. Hypoxaemia diminishes the amount of oxygen available for the brain and ischaemia diminishes the amount of cerebral blood perfusion. The combination of both can lead to death or to the production of one of the serious chronic brain syndromes, namely mental handicap, cerebral palsy and epilepsy. Hypoxaemia leads to profound biochemical changes in the brain and ischaemia may lead to infarction of the brain (Levy *et al.*, 1985). Brain swelling can occur with both, and this may further reduce cerebral perfusion. Cerebral necrosis may be another consequence of hypoxaemia and ischaemia.

The causes of hypoxia in the newborn are many and may operate before delivery in about half the cases, during delivery in the majority of the remainder and postpartum in about 10% of the infants. Seizures may begin within 6–12 hours of birth in asphyxiated babies.

## Seizure patterns in neonates

Seizure patterns in the neonate are different from those in older infants and children. Generalized tonic–clonic convulsions, so often seen later, are rarely encountered. Usually, the seizure patterns are fragmentary, resembling parts of a generalized seizure. There may be shifting clonic convulsive movements migrating

18

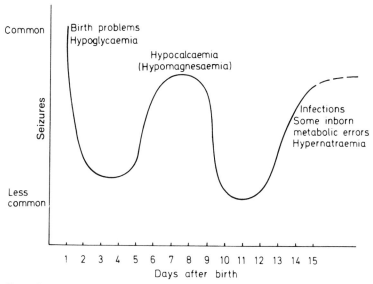

*Figure 3.1* Neonatal convulsions. Timing in relation to cause. (From N. V. O'Donohoe. *Growing Points in Childhood Epilepsy*, 1: *The First Six Months*, by courtesy of Geigy Pharmaceuticals, Horsham, West Sussex)

rapidly and in a non-Jacksonian disorderly fashion from one part of the body to other ipsilateral or contralateral areas. Focal clonic convulsions may occur and remain localized to one area or spread to involve one half of the body. Alternating hemiconvulsive seizures, involving first one and then the other half of the body, can occur. Generalized tonic seizures, sometimes resembling episodes of decerebrate rigidity, are not uncommon and may be the presenting clinical feature of intracranial haemorrhage, especially when they occur in premature infants.

Finally, there is a group of motor automatisms also called 'subtle' seizures because the clinical correlates are so slight (Volpe, 1977). These motor automatisms include one or more of the following: tonic horizontal deviation of eyes with or without jerking of the eyes; repetitive blinking or fluttering of the eyelids; drooling, sucking, or other oral-buccal-lingual movements; 'rowing' or 'swimming' movements of the upper limbs or, less commonly, 'pedalling' movements of the lower limbs; less frequently, vertical deviation of the eyes (usually down) with or without jerking; hyperpnoea and vasomotor phenomena or tonic posturing of a limb or portion of a limb may occur. It is important to realize that, although slight, these clinical changes may signify serious underlying brain injury. There may also be momentary changes in the respiratory rate or even periods of apnoea. Nevertheless, it should be emphasized that apnoeic spells, particularly in the premature infant, are more likely to be related to mechanisms other than seizures. When apnoea is a manifestation of a seizure, the spell is almost always accompanied or preceded by one or more of the other subtle manifestations of a seizure (Watanabe *et al.*, 1982).

During the past decade, intensive study of abnormal neonatal behaviour by means of portable time-synchronized EEG/polygraphic/video monitoring systems in the newborn nursery has led to a reappraisal of what are and what are not genuine epileptic events at this age (Mizrahi and Kellaway, 1987; Mizrahi, 1989). It has been demonstrated that generalized tonic seizures and motor automatisms can occur without associated EEG seizure activity or even when no electrical activity of cerebral origin can be demonstrated in the EEG. This implies that these phenomena are generated and elaborated at a brainstem level by non-epileptic mechanisms. Tonic posturing and motor automatisms may be evoked by tactile stimulation and suppressed by restraint or repositioning of the body or affected limbs, manoeuvres which do not usually affect epileptic motor activity. Such characteristics are, in fact, more typical of reflex behaviour than of epileptic seizures. Primitive reflex mechanisms are normally mediated by spinal mechanisms and facilitated by centres within the brainstem. These centres are inhibited by the forebrain and may be stimulated by proprioceptive stimuli. When the forebrain is depressed, brainstem centres are disinhibited and primitive reflexes may occur spontaneously or be evoked by stimulation. It has been proposed that tonic posturing and motor automatisms, as a group, should now be designated 'brainstem release phenomena' rather than epileptic seizures (Mizrahi and Kellaway, 1987). Neonates with these motor phenomena usually have clinical and EEG evidence of forebrain depression. They are obtunded or comatose and their background EEG activity is depressed and undifferentiated. This subdivision of neonatal seizures into epileptic and non-epileptic events has a practical importance, since it may mean that antiepileptic drug therapy is not appropriate for all types of seizures and, in the case of non-epileptic seizures, the drugs may add insult to injury by further depressing higher brain centres.

### Jitteriness

It is important to distinguish the movement disorder usually called jitteriness from convulsive movements. The dominant movement in jitteriness is tremor, i.e. the alternating movements are rhythmic and of equal rate and amplitude. The dominant movement in seizures is clonic jerking, i.e. the movements have a fast and slow component. Jitteriness is not accompanied by abnormalities of gaze or by extraocular movements and it is frequently provoked by external stimuli. Gently flexing the affected limb will abolish the fast jittery movement whereas clonic jerking will continue to be transmitted through the examiner's hand.

Jitteriness is the most common involuntary movement of the newborn and is often observed during the examination of full-term healthy neonates. It is common in infants over 12 hours old and diminishes markedly in the second week of life. Jittery infants are more likely to be difficult to console when crying and to be less visually alert. Jitteriness in an otherwise healthy full-term infant is of uncertain clinical significance. It has been associated with a variety of pathological conditions including hypoglycaemia, hypocalcaemia, prenatal exposure to narcotics, hypoxic encephalopathy and intracranial haemorrhage. It is also commoner in infants who are smaller and shorter than average. However, such problems are infrequent in association with jitteriness and the cause is usually not apparent (Parker et al., 1990).

## Developmental explanation

The reasons for the difference in seizure types in the neonate compared with later infancy and childhood must relate to the developmental state of the nervous system.

For a generalized seizure to be possible there must be a certain degree of cortical organization existing to propagate and sustain the electrical discharge, and this is not present in the newborn. Neonatal EEG studies have shown that convulsions are usually of focal cerebral origin, that discharges are frequently limited to one region of the hemisphere and diffuse slowly in the ipsilateral hemisphere or to the contralateral hemisphere, and that bilateral synchrony is rare. The reasons for these characteristics are related to the immaturity of the forebrain. The intercellular connections of cortical ganglion cells are incomplete and myelination is deficient in the hemispheres and in the corpus callosum, reducing the chances of contralateral spread. Surrounding any epileptic focus there is a population of neurons which develops inhibitory potentials during paroxysmal discharges produced by a mass of cells in the focus. This 'inhibitory surround' limits the local cortical spread of epileptic activity. It has been demonstrated, using intracellular recordings, that these inhibitory postsynaptic potentials are common in immature neocortical neurons, and this physiological situation has an influence in creating the high convulsive threshold which exists in the neonate and in early infancy (Purpura, Shofer and Scarff, 1967). In addition, neurotransmitter function at the synaptic level is different in the neonatal brain. It has been demonstrated that inhibitory neurotransmitters have a predominant effect over excitatory transmitters (Johnson and Singer, 1982).

Hill and Volpe (1981) point out that the relatively advanced degree of development of the limbic system and its connections to the diencephalon and brain-stem may account for the frequent occurrence of clinical manifestations originating in those structures; for example, oral-buccal-lingual movements, ocutomotor phenomena and apnoea.

## Timing and causes of neonatal seizures

Seizures may occur early in the neonatal period, i.e. in the first 24–72 hours, or later at the end of the first week of life. The timing of seizures is closely related to their cause. Volpe (1973, 1976) has consistently emphasized that the *hypoxic–ischaemic brain insult* is the single most common cause of neonatal convulsions in both premature and full-term infants; in his series, it accounted for just over 60% of the cases. Characteristically, the attacks begin in the first 24 hours and indeed, in the majority of cases, in the first 12 hours of life. The attacks are usually frequent and severe and may be continuous. Overt seizures are also nearly always associated with subtle attacks. In the premature infant generalized tonic seizures may occur and in the full-term baby multifocal clonic attacks take place. The vast majority of these infants will have shown clinical evidence indicating the occurrence of fetal distress due to intrauterine asphyxia. The common manifestations of this situation are slowing of the fetal heart and/or meconium-stained liquor and a very low Apgar score at birth. Failure to breathe spontaneously at birth adds a postnatal hypoxic-ischaemic insult to the intrauterine insult.

As already emphasized, seizures due to hypoxic–ischaemic insult develop early and are usually severe. Seizures resulting from *cerebral contusion*, which are usually secondary to a traumatic labour (precipitate or prolonged labour, transverse arrest, high forceps extraction, difficult breech delivery, etc.) commonly occur on the second postnatal day and are often truly partial or focal in type. Primary subarachnoid haemorrhage in the term infant probably originates from tearing of the superficial veins by shearing forces during a prolonged delivery with the head engaged. The newborn is usually well until an unexpected seizure occurs on the first or second day. Lumbar puncture reveals the presence of blood-stained cerebrospinal fluid. Most affected newborns will be neurologically normal later (Fenichel, Webster and Wong, 1984). In the preterm infant with primary subarachnoid haemorrhage, seizures usually present on the second day and, between attacks, the baby may seem well, giving rise to the description of the 'well baby with seizures'. *Periventricular intracerebral haemorrhage* with intraventricular spread, arising from the subependymal veins in the germinal matrix, is almost exclusively a lesion of the very small premature infant. It may occur from 1 to 3 days after severe hypoxia and present with generalized tonic seizures, coma, rapid deterioration; respiratory arrest follows within a few hours. A milder, so-called saltatory, course is also described. *Subdural haemorrhage*, due to a tear of falx tentorium or superficial cortical veins, is a traumatic lesion of large babies and is now uncommon. Seizures are secondary to associated cerebral contusion and are usually partial or focal in type. They occur in about half the cases and present usually in the first 48 hours of life.

The other important cause of seizures arising in the early neonatal period is *hypoglycaemia*. This is usually considered to be present when the blood glucose level falls below 1 mmol/l (20 mg/100 ml) in the premature baby and below 1.5 mmol/l (30 mg/100 ml) in the full term infant. However, it should be realized that the actual level of glucose which is required to prevent neurological damage in the neonate is unknown and may be higher than these levels (Koh, Eyre and Aynsley-Green, 1988). Hypoglycaemia is most common in small babies (especially those small for gestational age), in the smaller of twins where there is a marked discrepancy in birth weights and in the infants of diabetic or prediabetic mothers. Late feeding of small infants was a contributory cause of hypoglycaemia in the past. The most important factor in the occurrence of neurological damage due to hypoglycaemia is the duration of the hypoglycaemia; therefore early diagnosis and treatment are vital. The neurological symptoms of hypoglycaemia consist of irritability, drowsiness, hypotonia and, occasionally, apnoea, and these symptoms commonly develop in the second postnatal day. Approximately half the small babies who become hypoglycaemic develop neurological symptoms and about one-quarter of these go on to develop actual seizures. In the larger babies of diabetic mothers neurological symptoms, including seizures, are much less common, possibly because the duration of hypoglycaemia may be only one aetiological factor in causing convulsions in a small infant; hypoxic damage, hypocalcaemia and even infection may all be associated causes in the same infant. Symptomatic hypoglycaemia should be preventable by monitoring glucose levels, by the early feeding of small infants (particularly prematures) or by the administration of intravenous dextrose where early feeding is impossible. As already emphasized, early and vigorous treatment of symptomatic hypoglycaemia, if and when it occurs, is essential to prevent the occurrence of brain damage, although this is one instance where prevention is certainly better than cure because symptomatic hypoglycaemia is followed by neurological sequelae, even despite vigorous therapy at the time, in perhaps half of those affected.

*Hypocalcaemia*, i.e. serum calcium below 1.7 $\mu$mol/l (7 mg/100 ml), may occur in the first 2–3 days of life either in low birth weight infants (premature or dysmature), or in association with the complications of birth asphyxia. It may then contribute to the production of seizures but is rarely the primary cause. On the other hand, hypocalcaemia occurring later, i.e. at the age of 6–8 days, is usually the primary cause of the clinical features of neonatal tetany which include jitteriness, jaw, knee and ankle clonus, and partial or focal seizures. There may be associated

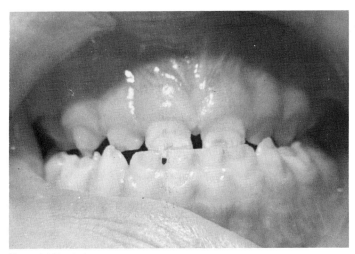

*Figure 3.2* Teeth from a child with enamel hypoplasia. Note the typical 'shelf' on the lower incisors and canines (*Courtesy of Dr R. J. Purvis*)

*hypomagnesaemia* or even hypomagnesaemia without hypocalcaemia causing tetany. The incidence of *neonatal tetany* due to hypocalcaemia and/or hypomagnesaemia has shown wide variations in different countries, reaching 55% in one Scottish survey (Cockburn *et al.*, 1973). In Volpe's (1977) series, there was only a 13% incidence of hypocalcaemia which was always complicated by other factors and no single case of typical neonatal tetany of later onset was found. He ascribed these differences to the fact that his unit was receiving selected referrals and to the recent widespread changes in cow's milk preparations with emphasis on their formulas being comparable with human milk. There has been a similar steep fall in the incidence of neonatal hypocalcaemia in Britain in the last 15 years. Classic neonatal tetany tended to develop in large full-term infants who fed avidly on a cow's milk mixture in which the ratios of phosphorus to calcium and phosphorus to magnesium were four times higher than in human milk. Hypocalcaemia is rare in breast-fed infants and in infants fed with the modern 'humanized' milks. Infants who have had neonatal tetany may later show enamel hypoplasia of the teeth, the timing of which suggests an antenatal insult during the last trimester (*Figure 3.2*) (Purvis *et al.*, 1973). Maternal vitamin D deficiency may also be the cause of the seasonal variations in the incidence of tetany, which is more common in babies born in spring after the relatively sunless months of winter, and may also explain geographical variations in incidence.

Alterations in sodium levels may also lead to neonatal seizures. *Hypernatraemia* may be associated with dehydrating illnesses, may follow the accidental administration of salt for sugar in a milk feed, or may result from the accidental administration of an unsuitable saline intravenous solution to the newborn. Dehydration in the salt-losing syndrome of congenital adrenal hyperplasia is associated with *hyponatraemia* and this imbalance may also lead to seizures. Hyponatraemia may also occur in association with overhydration in infants with meningitis who develop water retention as a result of increased secretion of antidiuretic hormone, and a similar situation may complicate neonatal asphyxia. Water intoxication may occur in the treatment of hypoglycaemia with intravenous glucose infusions, resulting in hyponatraemia and a low serum osmolality. Oedema, both peripheral and cerebral, may follow, with jitteriness, extensor tonic seizures, and even a decerebrate state can be seen. If a correct diagnosis is not made, further glucose and water solutions may mistakenly be given, with disastrous results. Even excessive oral administration of water to the neonate is capable of producing a dilutional hyponatraemia and seizures as a consequence (Vanapruks and Prapaitrakul, 1989) and Keating, Schears and Dodge (1991) have reported what they describe as an epidemic of oral water intoxication in very small infants living in poor and deprived circumstances where supplies of milk formula may be inadequate.

The possibility of infections causing seizures in the newborn should always be considered, even in the presence of another potential cause. Intrauterine or postnatal central nervous system infections may be responsible and septicaemic infants, even without meningitis, may develop seizures. Apart from the commoner varieties of neonatal meningitis, neonatal encephalitis may be caused by the herpes simplex virus (HSV2). The most frequent reason is contamination by the virus during the second stage of labour as a result of contact with maternal genital herpes. The EEG is always abnormal and demonstrates a periodic pattern with mutifocal discharges (Mizrahi and Tharp, 1982).

*Structural abnormalities of the brain* may be associated with neonatal seizures but account for less than 5% of cases. Disorders of neuronal migration are particularly likely to be associated with abnormal neurological behaviour and seizures and the attacks may be difficult to control. Such disorders include lissencephaly (Aicardi, 1989), pachygyria and polymicrogyria. Porencephaly, hydranencephaly and holoprosencephaly are other causes. Incontinentia pigmenti is a rare inherited neurocutaneous syndrome involving the skin and central nervous system. The female-to-male ratio is 20:1. Neurological disturbances, especially neonatal seizures on the second or third day of life, occur in under half the cases. The erythematous and vesicular rash on the flexor surface of the limbs and lateral aspect of the trunk should alert the clinician to the diagnosis (O'Doherty and Norman, 1968).

*Pyridoxine (vitamin B_6) deficiency*, transmitted as an autosomal recessive trait, is a rare disorder caused by defective binding of pyridoxine to its apoenzyme, glutamate decarboxylase. The result is a failure of conversion of glutamic acid to gamma-aminobutyric acid (GABA), the main inhibitory neurotransmitter in the central nervous system. The typical clinical presentation is the occurrence of almost continuous seizures beginning within hours of birth and unresponsive to antiepileptic drugs. There may be a history of intrauterine convulsive movements by the fetus. The EEG shows severe continuous abnormalities. In a typical case, the intravenous administration of pyridoxine in a dosage of up to 100 mg will abolish the seizures after a variable interval of up to 10 minutes and, coincidentally, the EEG should return to its normal pattern. In many cases, the diagnosis is made because a sibling has been similarly affected and has died. A lifelong dietary supplement of the vitamin, in doses ranging from 2 to 30 mg/kg per day is necessary, and withdrawal of pyridoxine leads to rapid relapse. Mental development may be normal but is frequently impaired despite vitamin supplementation. Bankier, Turner and Hopkins (1983) have drawn attention to the considerable variation in the clinical presentation of this disorder and stress that the diagnosis needs to be considered in any infant with intractable seizures, even after the neonatal period. Goutières and Aicardi

(1985) advise that the diagnosis of pyridoxine dependency should be carefully considered in every infant with convulsions in the first 18 months of life and list the following suggestive clinical features: (1) cryptogenic seizures in a previously normal infant, especially if they are severe and prolonged; (2) the history of a severe convulsive disorder, often leading to death during status epilepticus, in a previous sibling; (3) long-lasting focal or unilateral seizures often with partial preservation of consciousness; (4) irritability, restlessness, crying and vomiting preceding the actual seizures. They note that even infantile spasms have been reported in association with pyridoxine dependency.

*Disorders of amino acid metabolism* may occasionally present with neonatal seizures, and maple syrup urine disease is the one most likely to do so. In a case not already detected by metabolic screening at birth and treated appropriately, seizures may begin after several days in which feeding difficulty and increasing lethargy have been observed. The *ketotic hyperglycinaemias* constitute a heterogeneous group of disorders, also recessively inherited, in which there are defects in the degradation of branch-chained amino acids. Seizures are a feature of the clinical presentation and, biochemically, they demonstrate metabolic acidosis, ketosis, hyperammonanaemia and hyperglycinaemia. *Primary enzyme defects in urea synthesis* may also present very soon after birth with vomiting and increasing drowsiness, followed by the later onset of seizures. Biochemically, they show hyperammonaemia without organic acidaemia. The diagnosis and management of these and other inborn errors of metabolism in the newborn period are reviewed by Wraith (1988), Collins (1990) and Menkes (1990). The rare *inherited peroxisomal disorders affecting the nervous system*, including Zellweger's syndrome and neonatal adrenoleukodystrophy, have dysmorphic features and seizures among their clinical manifestations, and biochemically, show defects in the oxidation of very-long-chain fatty acids. The reader is referred to the review by Stephenson (1988).

Seizures in the newborn may be caused by the *withdrawal of drugs*, usually hypnotics or analgesics and including alcohol, taken by the mother during late pregnancy. However, they are unusual after withdrawal of long-acting barbiturates such as phenobarbitone. Maternal heroin addiction results in a neonatal syndrome of jitteriness but seizures are uncommon. The newborn may inadvertently receive significant amounts of *local anaesthetic agents* given to the mother during labour and delivery. The infants on delivery are meconium-stained, flaccid and apnoeic and may be thought to have suffered the effects of intrapartum anoxia. Seizures, commencing between 1 and 3 hours after birth, are a common feature of this type of intoxication. Treatment consists of diuresis and acidification of the urine while conventional antiepileptic drugs are of limited benefit (Hillman, Hillman and Dodson, 1979). Clonic convulsions are a feature of *kernicterus due to hyperbilirubinaemia* in a small proportion of cases. This condition is now most likely to be seen in small premature infants with a low serum albumin and a poor bilirubin-binding capacity who develop septicaemia and acidosis or who suffer from the respiratory distress syndrome.

It is important to realize that, despite the great increase in knowledge of the newborn in recent times, there remains a small group of infants whose seizures have no attributable cause. This amounted to 8% in the series of Levene and Trounce (1986). Furthermore, seizures are not disease specific in the neonate and may be due to a variety of disturbances in an individual infant. For example, although asphyxia is an important primary cause of neonatal seizures, hypoglycaemia, hypocalcaemia, haemorrhage or infarction may occur as associated secondary causes. Since the great majority of seizures occurring in the intermediate neonatal period are the result of anoxic–ischaemic insult, it has been proposed that the incidence of early seizures in the neonate may be used as an index of the quality of perinatal care (Derham, Matthews and Clarke, 1985).

Two neonatal epileptic syndromes remain to be mentioned. The first of these is termed *benign idiopathic neonatal convulsions*, also known as 'fifth-day fits'. This condition presents between the third and seventh day of life in otherwise normal newborns, without known aetiology or concomitant metabolic disturbance. The seizures are frequent, clonic in type, multifocal in distribution and characterized especially by jerking of limbs and face, often unilateral with alternation from side to side, and sometimes associated with apnoea or cyanosis. Interictal EEGs may show focal sharp waves unilaterally or bilaterally. The seizures usually recur for less than 48 hours and are apparently benign (Pryor, Don and McCourt, 1981). Seizures do not recur later and subsequent psychomotor development is normal.

The other important though rare syndrome is entitled *benign familial neonatal convulsions* (Carton, 1978). This is inherited as an autosomal dominant disorder and presents with clonic or apnoeic seizures but with no specific EEG criteria. The seizures may begin as early as the second or third day of life or as late as 3 months old. The attacks are brief, recur frequently up to the seventh day and then infrequently for weeks or months. Those affected appear otherwise normal. Although the outcome of this syndrome is favourable as regards psychomotor development, about 14% of reported cases have developed epilepsy later (Dreifuss, 1989) although no case of severe epilepsy has been reported. This syndrome has now been shown to have a genetic linkage with chromosome 20 (Leppert *et al.*, 1989).

The development of intractable seizures during the neonatal period is a feature of early infantile epileptic encephalopathy or Ohtahara's syndrome, discussed in Chapter 4.

## Diagnostic evaluation

The diagnostic evaluation of a newborn with seizures should include a complete prenatal and natal history and a comprehensive physical examination, with emphasis on a neurological examination appropriate to a neonate. The presence of skin lesions may be a clue to both infection and neurocutaneous syndromes. Fundoscopy is difficult in the neonate but can be of diagnostic importance if it reveals haemorrhages indicative of trauma or choroidoretinitis resulting from intrauterine infection. The first laboratory tests should be directed against the two diseases that are especially dangerous but treatable, i.e. hypoglycaemia and bacterial meningitis. Serum electrolytes, urea, calcium, phosphorus and magnesium should also be measured and a blood culture should be started. The place of the EEG examination will be discussed later. When attempting to make an aetiological diagnosis it should be remembered that several factors may be operating in the same patient, for example hypoxia–ischaemia, hypocalcaemia and infection, so therefore investigation must be detailed. The rarer causes of neonatal seizures may require more elaborate tests for their elucidation. The reader is referred to the handbook by Stephenson and King (1989) for information about these investigations.

# Therapy

The treatment of neonatal seizures depends on establishing the cause as quickly as possible and acting appropriately. The question of prevention is of great importance, especially in the case of anoxic–ischaemic brain injury. Careful monitoring of the fetus and prompt and skilled intervention at the first signs of fetal distress are critical.

Symptomatic hypoglycaemia should also be completely preventable today. Continuous or frequent seizures of themselves can result in brain injury because they are often accompanied by serious hypoventilation and/or apnoea which results in hypoxaemia and hypercapnia and because neuronal necrosis may result from the increased neuronal energy requirement during prolonged seizure activity. Hypoxaemia may result in cardiovascular collapse and ischaemic injury to the brain. A diminution in cerebral blood flow can also occur with increased intracranial pressure which can be aggravated by hypercapnia. Consequently, vigorous support of ventilation and blood pressure is important in the sick convulsing neonate.

# Drugs and other treatment

Many of the established antiepileptic drugs have been used in the treatment of frequent severe and continuous seizures in the newborn. Phenobarbitone is the one most frequently chosen as the initial therapeutic agent. Apart from its anticonvulsant properties, there is the possibility that it may have a protective effect on neurons by decreasing their rate of metabolism. In order to obtain therapeutic but non-toxic levels rapidly, the drug should be administered intravenously as a loading dose. Therapeutic levels will usually be achieved by a mean loading dose of 15 mg/kg given intravenously (or intramuscularly) followed by a maintenance dose of 5–6 mg/kg per day (Ouvrier and Goldsmith, 1982). However, loading doses of up to 30 mg/kg have been used by some. Since the plasma half-life of phenobarbitone in the first weeks of life may be twice that of adults (Holden and Freeman, 1975), it is important to watch for signs of respiratory depression because ventilatory support may be necessary. Monitoring of serum levels is essential when these high doses are being used. Relative bradycardia may be a consequence of high phenobarbitone dosage in neonates and result in significant decreases in cardiac output and diminished cerebral blood flow (Painter, 1989).

Phenytoin is the second most frequently used antiepileptic drug in the treatment of neonatal seizures, either alone or as an adjunct to phenobarbitone. Loading doses of 10–15 mg/kg have been used and produce therapeutic non-toxic serum levels. However, the subsequent metabolism of phenytoin in the neonate is unpredictable and frequent monitoring of serum levels is required in order to titrate the maintenance dose and to avoid toxicity. The major acute toxic effect of intravenous phenytoin is a cardiac arrhythmia, but there is also the possibility that toxic levels of the drug may damage the developing cerebellum.

Intravenous diazepam has been used in a regimen of 0.1 mg every 2 minutes up to a maximum of 1 mg repeating this dose at 1 to 3h intervals. Continuous infusion rates of 0.5–2.75 mg/h have also been employed. However, this drug does not seem to be particularly effective in controlling neonatal seizures, is short acting in its effect, may carry an increased risk of respiratory depression when used with phenobarbitone and has been criticized for use intravenously in the neonate because its vehicle (sodium benzoate) is an effective uncoupler of the bilirubin–albumin complex and may increase the risk of kernicterus. Paraldehyde has been used intravenously in a 3–10% solution injected slowly, but it has the disadvantage that it is excreted through the lungs and may produce a pneumonitis. Gamstorp (1985) advocated the use of lignocaine (xylocaine) in an intravenous infusion, and recommended 3–4 mg/kg per hour for 12–24 h initially, continuing in gradually diminished doses over the next few days provided the infant was seizure free Dodson (1983) has published a comprehensive review of antiepileptic drug use in newborns and infants and more recent information may be found in the reviews of Painter (1989) and in the *Lancet* (1989) Unfortunately, despite the number of drugs available for treating neonatal seizures, it has to be said that they may be of limited benefit only and all have side-effects (Connell *et al.*, 1989b).

Volpe (1976) stressed the importance of maintaining an adequate supply of glucose to the brain in asphyxiated infants. He pointed out that work with newborn animals had shown that glucose reduced mortality and brain cell loss and prevented the fall in brain glucose which occurred during continuous seizures. However, as already mentioned, this manoeuvre has to be balanced against the risks of fluid overload increasing oedema.

Dexamethasone 0.5 mg/kg intravenously, followed by the same dose given in four divided doses every 24 h for approximately 3 days, has been used to reduce cerebral oedema, but its use is still controversial. Similarly, there is some dispute over the use of hypertonic solution, such as mannitol, in the treatment of cerebral oedema because of the fear that these hyperosmolar preparations may increase the risk of intracranial haemorrhage, especially in premature infants. It is important to emphasize that infrequent or mild seizures may not need to be treated. Holden and Freeman (1975) stressed that, in general, more harm may be done by the side effects of the anticonvulsants used for treatment of the infrequent 'twitches' than by the seizures themselves. If necessary, they can be treated with oral phenobarbitone in a dosage of 5–7 mg/kg per day or with chloral hydrate 50 mg/kg per day in divided doses.

Hypoglycaemia is likely to cause convulsions only if it is severe, which usually means a blood glucose concentration of less than 1 mmol/l (20 mg/100 ml). In an emergency situation glucose may be given as a bolus injection of 2 ml/kg of a 50% solution. However, a bolus injection of this kind is not helpful in the long term because it causes a sudden peaking of blood glucose which leads to insulin release followed by a rapid fall in blood glucose. A suitable regimen is a continuous infusion of 10% dextrose, 65 ml/kg in the initial 24 h with increasing amounts subsequently as the infant's fluid needs increase, bearing in mind the danger of water intoxication. Occasionally, stronger concentrations of dextrose (up to 15%) are used by infusion but they carry a risk of producing venous thrombosis. Resistant hypoglycaemia may require treatment with glucagon, steroids or ACTH, or even diazoxide.

The treatment of hypocalcaemia is less urgent, since neonatal tetany is a more benign condition. Calcium gluconate may be given as a 10% solution before each feed, even though the effect on the serum calcium may be slow. Alternatively, 0.2 ml/kg of 10% calcium gluconate may be given slowly intravenously, but intravenous calcium can be dangerous and its effect is brief. Perhaps the most important therapeutic measure is to reduce the phosphate load by using a low phosphate milk such as breast milk or a humanized dried milk formula or a dilute cow's milk formula (e.g. evaporated milk 1 part and water 4 parts). Associated hypomagnesaemia may be treated by giving 0.2 mg/kg of 50% magnesium sulphate intramuscularly and repeating this dose if necessary while monitoring the serum magnesium at the same time.

When hyponatraemia is the cause of neonatal seizures, for whatever reason, it may be treated by the slow infusion of normal saline accompanied by careful monitoring of serum sodium levels.

## Prognosis

The prognosis of neonatal convulsions depends on various factors, including birth weight and aetiology of the seizures. Seizures occurring in the first few days of life in general carry a poor prognosis. Brown, Cockburn and Forfar (1972) had 11 deaths among 60 babies with seizures commencing 1–4 days after birth. Of these babies, 15 subsequently developed severe or moderate handicap, both physical and mental, and 34 babies had a mild handicap or were normal. The number of days of seizure activity is also an important predictor of neurological impairment. In contrast, of 60 babies developing seizures from 5–7 days after birth, virtually all were normal subsequently and none died. Many of the earlier surveys of neonatal seizures grouped together early and late-onset seizures and consequently found a better overall prognosis. Knauss and Marshall (1977) reviewed the prognosis for babies in a neonatal intensive therapy unit who developed seizures, and more than half the convulsions occurred in the first 72 h of life. The type of seizure was predominantly multifocal clonic (50%) but 16% had tonic seizures and half of the babies with this latter type died. Perinatal events were the most prevalent aetiological factors in infants with seizures in the first 72 h of life, irrespective of birth weight. Hypoglycaemia was an infrequent primary cause but was associated with other aetiologies in approximately a third of the cases. Infections were an important cause of convulsions in babies weighing less than 2500 g at birth. In infants weighing less than 1500 g at birth who developed seizures the mortality was 61% and the morbidity was 43% in the survivors. In those weighing between 1501 and 2500 g at birth the mortality rate was 44% and the morbidity was 46% in the survivors. In infants whose birth weights were greater than 2500 g the mortality rate was 35% and the morbidity was 40% in the survivors. In other words, low birth weight infants with a short period of gestation had a higher mortality rate, but the rates of morbidity among all the survivors did not vary significantly with birth weight. In general a poor prognosis (i.e. death or survival with moderate to severe sequelae, such as cerebral palsy, mental retardation, epilepsy) is likely when there is a serious underlying aetiology and when the infant displays marked clinical neurological impairments. These impairments include coma, accompanied by a markedly abnormal EEG background with numerous seizures. Conversely, a favourable outcome may be anticipated with milder underlying pathology, normal mental status and activity, and when the number of clinical and electrographical seizures are few and the interictal EEG background activity is preserved (Legido, Clancy and Berman, 1988). The importance of the EEG in assessing prognosis is discussed in the next section.

There is controversy about the need to keep infants who have had significant neonatal seizures on maintenance antiepileptic drug therapy and also concerning the duration of such therapy. The duration of such therapy will depend on the aetiology of the seizures and the possible risk of recurrence. Newborn infants with cerebral malformations have a risk of recurrence of up to 80% and others at high risk are the survivors from neonatal meningitis and hypoxic cerebral insults (about 30%). Early neurological development, the persistence of neurological deficits, and the evolution of the EEG also determine decisions about duration of treatment. Volpe (1989) recommends stopping all drugs, except phenobarbitone, as soon as the acute illness is over – in practice, when the intravenous lines are discontinued. Phenobarbitone is also stopped if the neurological examination is normal. If it is abnormal, the EEG is assessed and the drug is continued if seizure discharges are present. The infant is reassessed at 1 month and, if the neurological examination is still abnormal, an EEG is obtained. If this does not show electrographic seizure discharges, phenobarbitone is discontinued, even in the presence of an abnormal neurological examination. In practice, only a few infants need phenobarbitone beyond the first 1–2 months of life. There is concern by many about the possible deleterious effects of long-term phenobarbitone and other drugs on the infant's rapidly developing brain.

## Electroencephalography

The value of the interictal EEG in prognosis has been stressed by many authors, especially Rose and Lombroso (1970). In their series infants with seizures and a normal interictal EEG had an 86% chance for normal development at the age of 4 years, whereas an EEG with multifocal abnormalities was associated with only a 12% chance for normal development. In 10% of the patients in their series they demonstrated a periodic burst/suppression pattern consisting of alternating periods of flatness in the tracing interrupted by bursts of high-voltage sharp waves and spikes and also slow waves. This pattern was correlated with severe cerebral disease and a poor prognosis in the full-term baby, but a similar pattern can occur normally in young premature infants with a gestational age of less than 34 weeks. It must always be remembered that the interpretation of the EEG in the newborn is difficult, and most experienced electroencephalographers are aware that in about a quarter to a third of full-term neonates with seizures doubtful or borderline abnormalities occur which are difficult to relate to either short-term or long-term prognosis. Scher and Painter (1989) have written an excellent review of the use of the EEG in the investigation of neonatal seizures.

It is essential for diagnostic and prognostic purposes that the initial EEG should be recorded within 10 days of birth because many EEG abnormalities will have resolved after that time. The intermittent use of standard EEGs presents problems in neonatal intensive care units. The recorders are bulky, the application of multiple electrodes is required, other electronic equipment causes electrical interference, and nursing and medical procedures may be obstructed. Continuous EEG monitoring allows earlier recognition of seizures and is superior to clinical observation in this respect. Continuous EEG recording is possible using the 'Medilog' (Oxford Medical Systems) which allocates two channels to EEG, one to ECG and one to monitoring respiration or as an event marker. Cerebral function monitoring (CFM) is used for a similar purpose in neonatal intensive care. Its signal is derived from a single pair of parietal electrodes and a processed EEG signal is produced continuously. Information from either method is usually sufficient to fulfil the prognostic role already proven for standard EEG recordings, and has been shown to be prognostically significant in the great majority of infants who either die or have serious neurological impairment. Continuous monitoring has also shown a high frequency of electrographic seizures without clinical manifestations in high-risk infants and those ventilated and therapeutically paralysed (Connell *et al.*, 1989a, b). Synchronized video-EEG monitoring is also being used increasingly to study the clinical patterns of abnormal motor behaviour in the newborn and to establish an epileptic aetiology where that is relevant.

Non-invasive imaging of the brain is used increasingly to investigate neonates with seizures, particularly when cerebral haemorrhage is suspected. Cranial ultrasound imaging of the brain through the anterior fontanelle has gained wide acceptance and is not known to be associated with biological hazards. The equipment is easily portable and causes minimal disturbances to the infant, who is often being nursed in an intensive care area. Real-time imaging with ultrasound allows continuous viewing of intracranial structures in a manner comparable to X-ray fluoroscopy. Other non-invasive techniques using the physiological 'window to the neonatal brain' provided by the anterior fontanelle (Volpe, 1982) include the measurement of intracranial pressure by sensors applied to the skin over the fontanelle and measurement of cerebral blood flow velocity in the anterior cerebral arteries using the Doppler technique (Perlman, McMenamin and Volpe, 1983). All these methods can be employed repeatedly without risk or disturbance to the sick newborn. Computerized tomographic (CT) scanning is also used for visualizing the neonatal brain for evidence of haemorrhage or developing hydrocephalus, but the long-term effects of repeated radiation on the immature brain are unknown and CT should therefore be employed with discretion in the neonate.

## References

AICARDI, J. (1989) The lissencephaly syndromes. *International Pediatrics* (Miami), **4**, 127–132

BANKIER, A., TURNER, M. and HOPKINS, I. J. (1983) Pyridoxine-dependent seizures – a wider clinical spectrum. *Archives of Disease in Childhood*, **58**, 415–418

BROWN, J. K., COCKBURN, F. and FORFAR, J. O. (1972) Clinical and chemical correlations in convulsions of the newborn. *Lancet*, **1**, 135–139

CARTON, D. (1978) Benign familial neonatal convulsions. *Neuropädiatrie*, **9**, 167–171

COCKBURN, F., BROWN, J. K., BELTON, N. R. and FORFAR, J. O. (1973) Neonatal convulsions associated with primary disturbance of calcium, phosphorus and magnesium metabolism. *Archives of Disease in Childhood*, **49**, 99–108

COLLINS, J. (1990) A practical approach to the diagnosis of metabolic disease in the neonate. *Developmental Medicine and Child Neurology*, **32**, 79–83

CONNELL, J., OOZEER, R., DE VRIES, L., DUBOWITZ, L. M. S. and DUBOWITZ, V. (1989a) Continuous EEG monitoring for neonatal seizures: diagnostic and prognostic considerations. *Archives of Disease in Childhood*, **64**, 452–458

CONNELL, J., OOZEER, R., DE VRIES, L., DUBOWITZ, L. M. S. and DUBOWITZ, V. (1989b) Clinical and EEG response to anticonvulsants in neonatal seizures. *Archives of Disease in Childhood*, **64**, 459–464

DERHAM, R. J., MATTHEWS, T. G. and CLARKE, T. A. (1985) Early seizures indicate quality of perinatal care. *Archives of Disease in Childhood*, **60**, 809–813

DREIFUSS, F. E. (1989) Classification of epileptic seizures and the epilepsies. *Pediatric Clinics of North America*, **36**, No. 2, 265–279

FENICHEL, G. M., WEBSTER, D. T. and WONG, W. K. T. (1984) Intracranial haemorrhage in the term newborn. *Archives of Neurology*, **41**, 30–34

GAMSTORP, I. (1985) *Paediatric Neurology*, 2nd Edition, Butterworths, London, Boston, p. 108

GOUTIÈRES, F. and AICARDI, J. (1985) Atypical presentations of pyridoxine-dependent seizures. A treatable cause of intractable epilepsy in infants. *Annals of Neurology*, **17**, 117–120

HILL, A. and VOLPE, J. J. (1981) Seizures, hypoxic-ischaemic brain injury, and intraventricular haemorrhage in the newborn. *Annals of Neurology*, **10**, 109–121

HILLMAN, L., HILLMAN, R. and DODSON, W. E. (1979) Diagnosis, treatment and follow-up of neonatal mepivacaine intoxication secondary to paracervical and pudendal blocks during labour. *Journal of Paediatrics*, **95**, 472–477

HOLDEN, K. R. and FREEMAN, J. M. (1975) Neonatal seizures and their treatment. *Clinics in Perinatology*, **2**, 3–13

JOHNSON, M. V. and SINGER, H. S. (1982) Brain neurotransmitters and neuromodulators in pediatrics. *Pediatrics*, **70**, 57–68

KEATING, J. P., SCHEARS, G. J. and DODGE, P. R. (1991) Oral water intoxication in infants. An American epidemic. *American Journal of Diseases of Children*, **145**, 987–990

KNAUSS, T. A. and MARSHALL, R. E. (1977) Seizures in a neonatal intensive care unit. *Developmental Medicine and Child Neurology*, **19**, 719–728

KOH, T. H. H. G., EYRE, J. A. and AYNSLEY-GREEN, A. (1988) Neonatal hypoglycaemia – the controversy regarding definition. *Archives of Disease in Childhood*, **63**, 1386–1388

LEADING ARTICLE (1989) Neonatal seizures. *Lancet*, **334**, 135–137

LEGIDO, A., CLANCY, R. R. and BERMAN, P. H. (1988) Recent advances in the diagnosis, treatment and prognosis of neonatal seizures. *Pediatric Neurology*, **4**, 79–86

LEPPERT, M., ANDERSON, V. E., QUATTLEBAUM, T., STAUFFER, D., O'CONNELL, P., NAKAMURA, Y., LABOUEL, J. and WHITE, P. (1989) Benign familial neonatal convulsions linked to genetic markers on chromosome 20. *Nature*, **337**, 647–648

LEVENE, M. I. and TROUNCE, J. Q. (1986) Cause of neonatal convulsions. Towards more precise diagnosis. *Archives of Disease in Childhood*, **61**, 78–79

LEVY, S. R., ABROMS, I. F., MARSHALL, P. C., and ROSQUETA, E. E. (1985) Seizures and cerebral infarction in the full-term newborn. *Annals of Neurology*, **17**, 366–370

MENKES, J. H. (1990) Metabolic disorders of the nervous system. In: *Textbook of Child Neurology*, 4th Edition, Lea and Febiger, Philadelphia, London; pp. 28–138

MIZRAHI, E. M. (1989) Clinical and neurophysiological correlates of neonatal seizures. *Cleveland Clinic Journal of Medicine*, **56**, Supplement Part I, S100–S111

MIZRAHI, E. M. and KELLAWAY, P. (1987) Characterization and classification of neonatal seizures. *Neurology*, **37**, 1837–1844

MIZRAHI, E. M. and THARP, B. R. (1982) Characteristic EEG pattern in neonatal herpes simplex encephalitis. *Neurology*, **32**, 1215–1220

O'DOHERTY, N. J. and NORMAN, R. M. (1968) Incontinentia pigmenti (Bloch–Sulzberger syndrome) with cerebral malformations. *Developmental Medicine and Child Neurology*, **10**, 168–174

OUVRIER, R. A. and GOLDSMITH, R. (1982) Phenobarbitone dosage in neonatal convulsions. *Archives of Disease in Childhood*, **57**, 653–657

PAINTER, M. J. (1989) Therapy of neonatal seizures. *Cleveland Clinic Journal of Medicine*, **56**, Supplement Part I, S.124–S.131

PARKER, S., ZUCKERMAN, B., BAUCHNER, H., FRANK, D., VINCI, R. and CABRAL, H. (1990) Jitteriness in full-term neonates: prevalence and correlates. *Pediatrics*, **85**, 17–23

PERLMAN, J. M., MCMENAMIN, J. B. and VOLPE, J. J. (1983) Fluctuating cerebral blood-flow velocity in respiratory distress syndrome. *New England Journal of Medicine*, **309**, 204–209

PRYOR, D. S., DON, N. and MACOURT, D. C. (1981) Fifth-day fits: a syndrome of neonatal convulsions. *Archives of Disease in Childhood*, **56**, 753–758

PURPURA, D. F., SHOFER, R. J. and SCARFF, T. (1967) Intracellular study of spike potentials and synaptic activity of neurons in immature neocortex. In: *Regional Development of the Brain in Early Life* (ed. A. Minkowski), F. A. Davis, Philadelphia, pp. 297–325

PURVIS, R. J., MACKAY, G. S., COCKBURN, F., BARRIE, W. J. MCK, WILKINSON, E. M. and BELTON, N. R. (1973) Enamel hypoplasia of the teeth associated with neonatal tetany: a manifestation of maternal vitamin D deficiency. *Lancet*, **2**, 811–814

ROSE, A. L. and LOMBROSO, C. T. (1970) Neonatal seizure states. *Pediatrics*, **45**, 404–425

SCHER, M. S. and PAINTER, M. J. (1989) Controversies concerning neonatal seizures. *Pediatric Clinics of North America*, **36**, 281–310

STEPHENSON, J. B. P. (1988) Inherited peroxisomal disorders involving the nervous system. *Archives of Disease in Childhood*, **63**, 767–770

STEPHENSON, J. B. P. and KING, M. D. (1989) *Handbook of Neurological Investigations in Children*. John Wright, London, Boston

VANAPRUKS, V. and PRAPAITRAKUL, K. (1989) Water intoxication and hyponatraemic convulsions in neonates. *Archives of Disease in Childhood*, **64**, 734–735

VOLPE, J. J. (1973) Neonatal seizures. *New England Journal of Medicine*, **289**, 413–416

VOLPE, J. J. (1976) Perinatal hypoxic-ischaemic brain injury. *Pediatric Clinics of North America*, **23**, 383–397

VOLPE, J. J. (1977) Neonatal seizures. *Clinics in Perinatology*, **4**, 43–46

VOLPE, J. J. (1982) Anterior fontanel: window to the neonatal brain. *Journal of Pediatrics*, **100**, 395–398
VOLPE, J. J. (1989) Neonatal seizures: current concepts and revised classification. *Pediatrics*, **84**, 422–428
WATANABE, K., HARA, K., MIYAZAKI, S., HAKAMADA, S. and KUROYANAGI, M. (1982) Apnoeic seizures in the newborn. *American Journal of Diseases of Children*, **136**, 980–984
WRAITH, J. E. (1988) Diagnosis and management of inborn errors of metabolism. *Archives of Disease in Childhood*, **64**, 1410–1415.

# Chapter 4

# Convulsions in early infancy and infantile spasms

After the neonatal period and up to the age of 5 or 6 months convulsions are a relatively uncommon symptom, and this time of life could be called the silent period for epilepsy, particularly when it is remembered that convulsions are commoner during the first 5 years of life than at any other time. Furthermore, convulsions in the early months are difficult to recognize and are often partial, fragmented and disorganized. There may be only localized jerking movements at irregular intervals. The reasons for these characteristics have already been discussed in Chapter 3 and are connected with the slow transmission of discharges in the brain at this age. There is a high 'convulsive threshold' in early infancy and this is why even clinically trivial epilepsy at this age may, in fact, be symptomatic of a serious underlying brain disorder or abnormality.

In an unpublished personal series (O'Donohoe, unpublished) of 20 infants presenting with partial seizures between 1 and 3 months of age and followed prospectively for 8 years, only 4 patients were later found to be of normal intelligence and 14 patients were mentally handicapped, usually to a moderate or a severe degree. While five patients had probably suffered perinatal brain damage, nine had an apparently normal birth history and it was assumed that the seizures were probably symptomatic of some generalized abnormality of the brain.

Ohtahara (1978) described a severe epileptic syndrome with onset before 3 months characterized by frequent tonic spasms, marked psychomotor retardation, a burst-suppression pattern in the EEG and a very poor prognosis. The condition, which can be familial, may be associated with major brain malformations or with metabolic errors including non-ketotic hyperglycinaemia (Dalla Bernardina *et al.*, 1979). It has been entitled Ohtahara's syndrome or early infantile epileptic encephalopathy (EIEE syndrome). Ohtahara (1984), reviewing his ten personal cases of the condition, observed that the onset of the brief generalized tonic spasms occurred within 20 days of birth in eight cases. In some cases, focal clonic spasms preceded the tonic spasms and series of spasms were also seen. The most characteristic feature in each case was the presence of a burst-suppression pattern in the EEG in both the waking and sleeping states. This pattern disappeared after 3 months of age and was replaced by a hypsarrhythmic EEG pattern. The prognosis in his cases was uniformly poor with all showing severe mental defect and with early death occurring in four. CT scanning showed severe developmental abnormalities in some cases. Ohtahara (1984) proposed that the term 'age-dependent epileptic

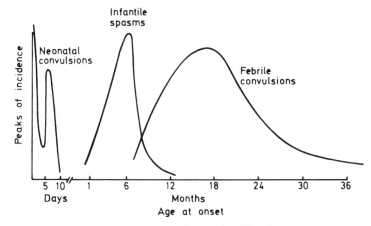

*Figure 4.1* Chronology of epilepsy in infancy and childhood

encephalopathy' be given to the three disorders of EIEE, West's syndrome and the the Lennox–Gastaut syndrome because they share the characteristics of age dependency, frequent and intractable minor seizures, severe and almost continuous epileptic EEG abnormality, aetiological heterogeneity, and the association of mental defect, refractoriness to treatment and a grave prognosis.

## Infantile spasms (West's syndrome)

Inhibitory influences in the brain gradually decline and the conduction of discharges improves so that by 5–6 months of age generalized epilepsy becomes possible, and the very serious disorder known as *infantile spasms* has its peak time of onset during this period (*Figure 4.1*). The first description of this remarkable condition appeared in the *Lancet* in 1841 when Dr. W. J. West wrote a letter to the editor under the heading 'On a peculiar form of infantile convulsions'. He described both the onset of the attacks in his own son at the age of 4 months and the subsequent intellectual regression in the child who had been developing normally up to the onset of the epilepsy. Over 100 years later Gibbs and Gibbs (1952) described the chaotic EEG pattern in the condition and gave it the title of hypsarrhythmia. The triad of spasms, retardation and hypsarrhythmia is frequently called West's syndrome and appears to be an age-specific convulsive disorder of infancy. In 1958 Sorel and Dusaucy-Bauloye described the results of treatment with ACTH. The International Classification of Epileptic Seizures (Gastaut, 1969) recognized infantile spasms as one of the types of generalized seizures, i.e. bilaterally symmetrical seizures without focal onset. The Commission on Classification and Terminology of the Epilepsies and Epileptic Syndromes (1989) preferred the term West syndrome (infantile spasms) for the condition and categorized it with the generalized epilepsies and syndromes. A subdivision was made into cryptogenic and symptomatic types. Lennox–Gastaut syndrome and some of the myoclonic epilepsies were similarly categorized. Cryptogenic epilepsy refers to a disorder whose cause is hidden or occult. The term does not necessarily mean that a lesion is not present but rather that the fundamental aetiology is as yet undetermined by diagnostic methods currently available.

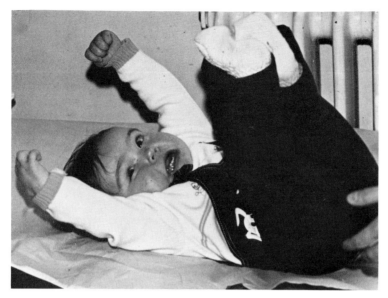

*Figure 4.2* A flexor spasm

## Clinical aspects

Clinically, infantile spasms involve sudden bilateral symmetrical contraction of muscles. In the commonest type, flexor spasm, simultaneous flexion of neck and trunk occurs. Flexion, abduction or adduction of the upper limbs and flexion and adduction of the lower limbs occur simultaneously. The flexor spasm (*Figure 4.2*) may be confused with sudden colic or even with a Moro reflex. In the rarer extensor spasm, the neck and trunk extend and again there may be a resemblance to a Moro reflex. Sometimes, the neck and trunk may flex and the lower limbs extend.

There is no relationship between the type of spasm and the seriousness or otherwise of the condition. Perhaps the most characteristic feature of these attacks is their tendency to occur in a repetitive series in which each attack is brief, lasting only seconds or less, and there are probably brief interruptions of consciousness, although this is not certain. A cry or scream is common just after a spasm and the child may be very irritable between series of attacks. At the onset of the illness the attacks may be relatively infrequent, becoming very frequent at the height of the illness. Attacks tend to be more frequent during periods of drowsiness, either when dropping off to sleep or on awakening, and may also be provoked by handling the baby. Other types of seizure, including generalized tonic-clonic attacks, may sometimes occur concurrently in patients with infantile spasms.

It is generally agreed that infants who develop spasms demonstrate a cessation of normal psychosocial development and frequently show a marked developmental deterioration as the spasms continue to occur. Motor performance may be affected to a lesser degree than adaptive behaviour. It is, of course important to realize that a large proportion of infants will already have shown evidence of developmental delay prior to the onset of their illness, but the association between infantile spasms and intellectual deterioration is irrefutable.

Males predominate among patients with infantile spasms. In the author's personal series of 100 cases studied from 1960 through to 1975 57 males presented with this condition (O'Donohoe, 1976). Others have described a male to female ratio of 2:1. A familial occurrence of infantile spasms is rare, and the familial incidence of epilepsy is low in patients with infantile spasms.

## Cryptogenic and symptomatic infantile spasms

Consideration of any large number of cases of infantile spasms reveals that there are three groups of patients, namely, cryptogenic, symptomatic and doubtful. This subdivision was used in the classic monograph on the subject by Jeavons and Bower (1964). They defined the cryptogenic group as having 'normal birth and development until the onset of spasms, usually around five months, and no known aetiology'. One third of their series of 112 cases fell into this category. A further 60% of patients in whom a definite predisposing aetiological factor could be identified were described as symptomatic. A small remaining group was labelled as doubtful. This has constituted less than 10% of most series.

The impact of modern diagnostic neuroimaging has been to make categorization of these patients more precise. At present, patients are classified on the basis of medical history, developmental history, neurological examination and computed tomographic (CT) scan findings. A patient is classified as cryptogenic if there is no known aetiological factor, if development has been normal prior to onset of the spasms, if the neurological examination is normal, and if the CT scan is normal prior to therapy. Using these strict criteria, about 15% or fewer of all patients will qualify as truly cryptogenic and the rest are classified as symptomatic (Hrachovy and Frost, 1989). Doubts about the nature of any particular case are usually resolved by further clinical observation and by investigation.

### Aetiology

The cryptogenic group is particularly important because it is now fully realized that early diagnosis and vigorous treatment of these children may reverse whatever process is causing the illness, and may even bring about subsequent normal intellectual development. On the other hand, treatment of symptomatic cases, even after early diagnosis, is very disappointing. It is now recognized that infantile spasms represent a non-specific reaction on the part of the brain to a wide variety of insults. *It seems likely that the condition is more age specific than disease specific.* The insult may be prenatal and follow a complication of pregnancy, a congenital cerebral defect or an intrauterine infection, or it may occur in an infant who has been small for dates. Perinatal birth injury, particularly anoxic injury, is a frequent forerunner of the disorder. After birth a neonatal meningitis may injure the brain and be followed by infantile spasms. Metabolic disorders, such as untreated phenylketonuria, are not infrequently complicated by infantile spasms, and damage produced by neonatal hypoglycaemia can also be causative. The hypoglycaemia resulting from unrecognized leucine sensitivity may cause brain damage in much the same way (Lacy and Penry, 1976).

Two conditions merit special attention, namely the association with *tuberose sclerosis* and the cases associated with *triple immunization*. Infantile spasms are a common early manifestation of the tuberose sclerosis syndrome, which may be the

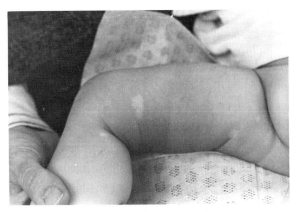

*Figure 4.3* 'White patches' in tuberose sclerosis

cause where the infantile spasms are of doubtful aetiology. In a review of individuals with tuberose sclerosis who had epilepsy, infantile spasms were the presenting symptom in 68% of cases (Hunt, 1983). Clues to the diagnosis may be the presence of poorly pigmented areas on the trunk and limbs, the so-called 'white or ash-leaf patches' (*Figure 4.3*), and the later development of the rash of adenoma sebaceum on the face (*Figure 4.4*) (Pampiglione and Moynahan, 1976). The diagnosis of tuberose sclerosis in any individual requires a careful clinical examination, particularly a thorough examination of the skin, including the use of ultraviolet light in a darkroom to highlight any white patches which may be present. Unfortunately, 2–3 per 1000 of apparently normal newborn infants also show these patches (Alper and Homes, 1983). Intracranial calcification in infancy is rarely visible on plain radiography but may be revealed by CT scanning (*Figures 4.5 and 4.6*). Apart from CT scanning, careful ophthalmoscopy and, less frequently, renal ultrasound and echocardiography may be required in the diagnostic evaluation. It is now known that the gene for tuberose sclerosis is located on chromosome 9 and this discovery will doubtless produce further diagnostic requirements. Excellent reviews of diagnostic problems by Osborne (1988) and of the special problems of children with infantile spasms and tuberose sclerosis by Riikonen and Simell (1990) are recommended to the reader.

In previous editions of this book, consideration was given to a possible causal relationship between the use of diphtheria-tetanus-pertussis vaccine and the onset of infantile spasms. The pertussis component has been identified by some as responsible for various acute neurological events. Febrile convulsions are the most frequent of these (Hirtz, Nelson and Ellenberg, 1984). Such seizures have the usual clinical characteristics of febrile convulsions from whatever cause and there is no evidence that they produce central nervous system injury, herald the onset of epilepsy, or worsen pre-existing neurological disease. Although there is an increased risk of postimmunization seizures in a child with a personal or family history of febrile convulsions, there is no evidence that other neurological problems will develop after immunization in this group (Golden, 1990). Because of the age at which triple immunization is given is also the peak age for the onset of infantile spasms, a cause-and-effect association has been suspected. The author is satisfied, however, both from his own experience and from reading the voluminous literature on this topic,

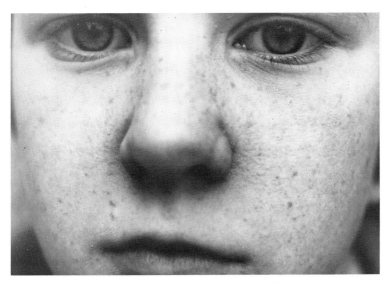

*Figure 4.4* The rash of adenoma sebaceum in tuberose sclerosis

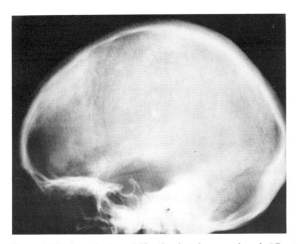

*Figure 4.5* Periventricular calcification in tuberose sclerosis (*Courtesy of Dr J. Toland*)

that the relationship between the two events is a purely temporal and coincidental one. Furthermore, his experience agrees with that of Shields *et al.* (1988) and Cherry (1990) in regarding the so-called post-pertussis-vaccine-encephalopathy as a myth. Consistent neuropathological findings have never been produced to support such a specific pathophysiological process, nor has any acceptable animal model been found (Golden, 1990).

The syndrome of infantile spasms, agenesis of the corpus callosum and atrophic areas in the choroid described by Aicardi in 1969 and now bearing his name, should also be mentioned. It seems to be confined to females and is usually fatal (Aicardi, Chevrie and Rouselle, 1969; Chevrie and Aicardi, 1986). Other gross abnormalities

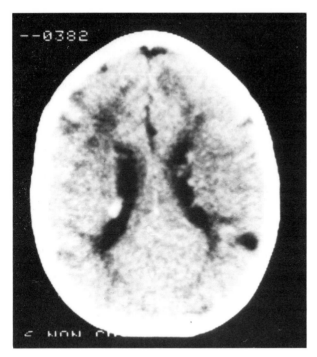

*Figure 4.6* CT scan. Nodules of tuberose sclerosis projecting into lateral ventricles

of the brain may also be associated with the development of infantile spasms. These include hydranencephaly, porencephaly and agenesis of the corpus callosum. More subtle abnormalities indicating disturbances during the period of neuronal migration are also found. Migration starts when immature neurons from the germinal neuroepithelium after final mitosis leave the periventricular area to move outwards into their future positions in the developing cortical plate. They are supported by radiating glial fibres extending from the ventricular zone to the pial surface. In the cerebral cortex, the deepest layers are formed first and later arriving neurons migrate past them to form more superficial layers whereby synaptic contacts can be formed. Disturbances during the migratory process will cause neuronal heterotopias and mild varieties of cortical dyslamination. More comprehensive malformations include lissencephaly, pachygyria and polymicrogyria. Early development may appear normal up to the onset of spasms in the presence of milder heterotopias (Palm, Blennow and Brun, 1986). It is unlikely that heterotopic neurons per se have a pathophysiological role, but they may lead to defects in the synaptic networks by their presence. Such defective networks could be involved in the genesis of infantile spasms.

## Diagnosis and investigation

The diagnosis of infantile spasms is based on clinical suspicion aided by EEG examination (*Figures 4.7 and 4.8*). The EEG nearly always shows a total disorganiza-

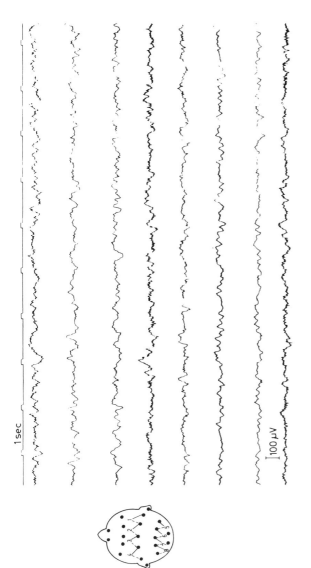

*Figure 4.7* Normal EEG in a 5-month-old male infant who is awake with eyes open

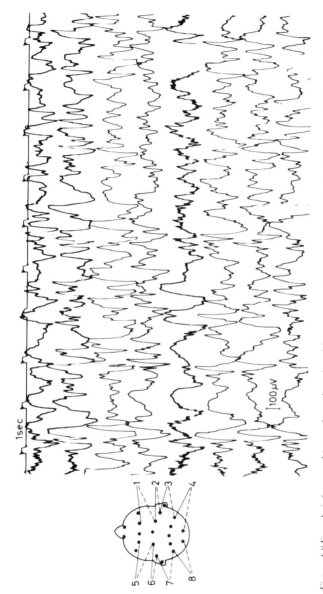

*Figure 4.8* Female infant aged 6 months and awake with eyes open. EEG shows hypsarrhythmia. Note the high-voltage irregular activity and frequent spike discharges.

tion of the record with almost continuous spikes and polyspike discharges present bilaterally forming the general abnormality called hypsarrhythmia. Like infantile spasms, hypsarrhythmia is an age-specific abnormality and may be found in severely abnormal children in the same age group who do not have the clinical syndrome of infantile spasms. The abnormality is usually present during sleeping and waking but may be more marked during sleep in certain cases. Hypsarrhythmia persists for a time and then disappears with advancing age of the child and maturation of the nervous system and is replaced by a less disorganized pattern. An upper age limit for hypsarrhythmia has not been established but it is uncommon beyond the age of 3 years. The presence of hypsarrhythmia in an infant during the first year of life is a physical sign of grave prognostic significance, even if unassociated with infantile spasms, and implies that the later incidence of mental subnormality will be at least 80% (Friedman and Pampiglione, 1971). Some patients with infantile spasms have periods of relatively organized brain activity separating the periods of hypsarrhythmia in their EEGs. This periodic pattern is entitled 'modified hypsarrhythmia'. In some patients, hypsarrhythmia is seen only in the sleep EEG and in others, hypsarrhythmia may be unilateral or show consistent foci of abnormal discharge in the temporal regions (Hrachovy, Frost and Kellaway, 1984). Very rarely patients with infantile spasms may have normal EEGs, particularly early in the course of the illness. Lombroso and Fejerman (1977) described 16 infants, aged 3–8½ months, with seizures which resembled infantile spasms, but the infants were without arrest or regression in psychomotor development and with normal EEGs throughout. The prognosis was excellent with or without therapy and the abnormal movements ceased in all cases by the age of 18 months. They called the condition 'benign myoclonus of early infancy'.

## Mental retardation

The most important feature of infantile spasms is the association with intellectual retardation. The majority of patients in the symptomatic group will usually have shown evidence of developmental delay prior to the onset of the spasms. Further intellectual deterioration may occur when the spasms commence, but this may not be particularly marked. Patients in the cryptogenic group, however, will usually have been developmentally normal prior to the onset of spasms and will then, as a rule, show striking developmental regression. It appears that the same process which leads to the occurrence of spasms also halts normal development and then leads to regression. As the spasms are treated or gradually disappear with the passage of time developmental progress picks up again to a greater or lesser degree.

## Therapy

Therapy for infantile spasms was extremely disappointing prior to the apparently successful use of ACTH in 1958. Since then there has been controversy about the efficacy or otherwise of this method of treatment. In the reported series there has been considerable variability in the therapeutic agents employed (ACTH or steroids), the dosages used and the duration of therapy. Most workers have favoured ACTH rather than steroids for initial therapy because it was claimed that a more rapid response was obtained, but Hrachovy et al. (1983), in a controlled study, were unable to find any major differences in the effectiveness of the two agents. The dosage of ACTH has varied from fairly moderate daily dosages (20–40 units) up to very high dosages (80–120 units per day). The initial administration of 40 units per day for 1–2 weeks, followed by 20 units per day or 40 units on alternate days for a further 2–3 weeks, followed by oral steroid therapy for up to 3 months, has been a widely recommended regimen. Others have recommended continuing ACTH for 3–6 months or even longer after the initial month of treatment, using 20–80 units on alternate days (Singer, Rabe and Haller, 1980). Riikonen (1982), in a retrospective analysis of high-dosage (120–160 units/day) versus low dosage (20–40 units/day) ACTH, was unable to show any differences in the results obtained by the two regimes. Prednisolone in an initial dose of 2 mg/kg per day or dexamethasone in a dose of 0.3 mg/kg per day have been used with gradual reductions in dosage to a maintenance level for a variable duration of therapy (Lacy and Penry, 1976).

Controversy has centred around the question of whether this form of treatment really benefits the patient. There is fairly general agreement that patients who have normal development up to the onset of spasms and who have normal CT scans, i.e. the cryptogenic group, are most likely to respond to treatment and are least likely to relapse subsequently (Singer et al., 1982). Another point about which there is some agreement concerns the time-lag between onset of spasms and commencement of treatment. The shorter this is, and particularly if it is less than 1 month, the better the response and the outlook. But again, this mainly applies to the cryptogenic cases and, in the National Child Encephalopathy Study, cases treated within 1 month of onset fared no better in the long term than cases treated within 1 month with a non-steroid drug (Bellman, 1983). A rapid clinical response to ACTH or steroid therapy is also accepted as another good prognostic indicator. However, in various series nearly 70% of cases responded well initially but over half of these subsequently relapsed, and a sustained improvement was reported in just under a third of the total number of patients treated. Furthermore, Jeavons and Bower (1964), in their classic report on a large series, stressed that patients with relapsing infantile spasms are unlikely to respond to additional courses of treatment, although repeated courses are usually given. Riikonen (1984) reported that, when relapse occurs after a primarily good response, a new course of ACTH was again effective in 74% of cases in her series. Usually EEG improvement parallels clinical improvement, and this usually becomes apparent in the second week of therapy. However, it is important to stress that clinical improvement can occur without EEG improvement and vice versa. Relapses are usually accompanied by a return of the severe EEG abnormality, and the frequency of these relapses has led many to question whether ACTH or steroid therapy has anything other than a transient beneficial effect, and to ask whether they confer any long-term benefit. Despite these doubts, most physicians confronted with a patient with infantile spasms, especially if these are of recent onset and occurring in a previously normal child, would hesitate to withhold ACTH or steroid therapy.

Even if it is accepted that treatment stops the spasms and improves the EEG, there still remains the most important question of intellectual improvement. Again, many would contend that the cryptogenic group, especially if diagnosed and treated early, probably does benefit intellectually in the short term and in the long term from ACTH or steroid therapy. Some would argue that those cases which improve would do so anyway without treatment or with antiepileptic drug therapy. There is no agreement about the effect on intellectual development in those infants with symptomatic spasms, and probably the majority would contend that ACTH or steroids do no more than improve the epilepsy and the EEG temporarily (Hrachovy and Frost, 1989). There is a feeling that this group should not be given this type of therapy but should have conventional antiepileptic drugs only. It should be emphasized that ACTH and steroids used in large doses at this age lead to obesity, electrolyte disturbances, fluid retention and increased susceptibility to infection, particularly pneumonia and septicaemia. Death during treatment is not uncommon (Riikonen and Donner, 1980). One particular hazard, in the author's experience, is profound depletion of body potassium, and this can be fatal if unrecognized.

The hazards of hormone therapy have led to a search for alternative methods of treatment. The benzodiazepine drugs, particularly nitrazepam and clonazepam, and also sodium valproate, have been used with some success in controlling the spasms but with no significant beneficial effect on intellectual retardation. Most clinicians would prefer to use ACTH or steroids as primary therapy, particularly in cryptogenic spasms, while reserving the benzodiazepines for the occasional child with cryptogenic spasms, but without evidence of psychomotor regression, a clinical situation which is difficult to establish with certainty. These drugs are also used in those children with symptomatic spasms where hormone therapy is considered to be futile, and also as maintenance therapy after treatment with hormones. The reader will notice that this short account of the benzodiazepines seems to imply that ACTH and steroids confer some extra, perhaps physiological, benefit on the patient which cannot be achieved by a chemical medication. Such a suggestion is, however, purely speculative and has never been proven.

## Prognosis

There have been relatively few studies of the long-term prognosis of infantile spasms. Probably the most informative is the study of Jeavons, Bower and Dimitrakoudi (1973), which was concerned with 150 children seen between 1954 and 1970. Just over two-thirds of the cases received hormone therapy. There were 44 cryptogenic cases, 96 symptomatic cases of which 21 were then considered to be related to immunization, and 10 doubtful cases. The criterion of normality was considered to be attendance at a normal school. The length of follow-up was 2–12 years.

The study of Jeavons, Bower and Dimitrakoudi (1973) confirmed that the most important factor associated with complete mental recovery was normal development prior to the onset of spasms. This group of patients had a 37% chance of complete recovery in this series. However, in the total series only 16% achieved complete recovery, and of the rest 34% were severely subnormal, 47% had neurological abnormalities (usually a spastic hemiplegia, diplegia or tetraplegia) and 22% died. The greatest mortality occurred before the age of 4 years and reference has already been made to the causes of this high death rate.

In the author's series (O'Donohoe, 1976), 100 consecutive cases seen between 1960 and 1970 were analysed and only 21 were found to be normal physically and intellectually on follow-up. Nearly half of the children were severely mentally retarded and many of these had severe neurological handicaps also. In this series 19 children died and a third of the deaths occurred during ACTH therapy. Over 90 patients had received this form of treatment, so a comparison between treated and untreated cases was not possible. However, Jeavons, Bower and Dimitrakoudi (1973) were able to make such a comparison and were not convinced that treatment had influenced the long-term prognosis. It should certainly not be assumed that, because ACTH may stop the seizures in an individual case, long-term improvement in mental development will follow (Gordon, 1981). Matsumoto *et al.* (1981) reported complete recovery in only 19 of 200 cases (9.5%), again predominantly in cryptogenic cases, and Glaze *et al.* (1988) reported only 5% as normal. In general, the longer the period of follow-up of cases of this condition, the fewer are the totally normal survivors.

In the light of such gloomy long-term results and despite the evidence that ACTH and corticosteroids have no influence on the ultimate developmental status and only transient effects on the seizures and EEG abnormalities, it must again be asked why these agents continue to be used. The answer at present appears to be that since ACTH and steroid therapy undoubtedly has a beneficial, although often temporary, effect on the spasms and the EEG and since the prognosis is generally so bad, it seems reasonable to continue to use this form of therapy, particularly in those cases where there may be hope of a successful outcome.

The essential pathological change in this remarkable age-related condition remains a mystery. It has not been possible to find a suitable animal model for study. Investigations using special staining methods and microscopic techniques have suggested that there may be a decreased number of synaptic sites in the brains of these children, particularly at certain cortical levels (Huttenlocher, 1974). A disturbance of synaptogenesis or in development of neurotransmitter mechanisms at a critical stage of cortical maturation has also been suggested and ACTH and corticosteroids, which accelerate certain normal developmental events in immature animals, could act by altering the functional activity of neurotransmitter systems at the synapses. It is hoped that future neuropathological and neurochemical research along these lines will shed more light on this tragic and, as yet, little understood type of generalized epilepsy in early infancy. In this regard, the remarkable work reported by Chugani *et al.* (1990) must be mentioned. Using positron emission tomographic scanning (PET) in a small group of children with infantile spasms, they identified focal cortical abnormalities in some which were not visible by magnetic resonance imaging (MRI). These areas were resected surgically with encouraging immediate results. Histologically, the tissue removed showed microscopic cortical dysplasia. The authors were hopeful that PET might be capable of delineating a subgroup of children with infantile spasms who might obtain long-term benefit from surgery.

Computerized tomographic (CT) scanning should, if possible, be done on all cases. Gastaut *et al.* (1978) reported cerebral abnormalities in 81% of those scanned, including cortical atrophy, agenesis of the corpus callosum and calcifications in the lesions of tuberose sclerosis. Singer *et al.* (1982) found cerebral abnormalities in 73% of their patients and emphasized that, in children who were developmentally normal before spasms began and in whom the CT scan was normal, a good prognosis for normal mental development later could be expected provided treatment was begun early in the course of the disease. It is important to note that, if possible, CT scanning should be done before commencing ACTH therapy since this treatment may cause a reversible ventricular dilatation which may be mistaken for irreversible cortical atrophy with an implied poor prognosis (Deonna and Voumard, 1979; Ito *et al.*, 1983).

## References

AICARDI, J., CHEVRIE, J. J. and ROUSELLE, F. (1969) Le Syndrome spasmes en flexion, agénesie calleuse, anomalies chorio-rétiniennes. *Archives Francaises de Pediatrie*, **26**, 1103–1120

ALPER, J. C. and HOMES, L. B. (1983) The incidence and significance of birthmarks in a cohort of 4141 newborns. *Paediatric Dermatology*, **1**, 58–68

BELLMAN, M. (1983) Infantile spasms. In: *Recent Advances in Epilepsy, No. 1.* (eds T. A. Pedley and B. S. Meldrum), Churchill Livingstone, Edinburgh, London, pp. 113–138

CHERRY, J. D. (1990) 'Pertussis encephalopathy': It is time to recognize it as the myth that it is. *Journal of the American Medical Association*, **263**, 1679–1680

CHEVRIE, J. J. and AICARDI, J. (1986) The Aicardi Syndrome. In: *Recent Advances in Epilepsy, No. 3* (eds T. A. Pedley and B. S. Meldrum), Churchill Livingstone, Edinburgh, London, pp. 189–210

CHUGANI, H. T., SHIELDS, W. D., SHERMON, D. A. *et al.* (1990) Infantile spasms. I. PET identifies focal cortical dysgenesis in cryptogenic cases for surgical treatment. *Annals of Neurology*, **27**, 406–413

COMMISSION ON CLASSIFICATION AND TERMINOLOGY OF THE INTERNATIONAL LEAGUE AGAINST EPILEPSY (1989) Proposal for revised classification of epilepsies and epileptic syndromes. *Epilepsia*, **30**, 388–389

DALLA BERNARDINA, B., AICARDI, J., GOUTIÈRES, F. and PLOUIN, P. (1979) Glycine encephalopathy. *Neuropädiatrie*, **10**, 209–225

DEONNA, T. and VOUMARD, C. (1979) Reversible cortical atrophy and corticotrophin (Letter). *Lancet*, **2** 207

FRIEDMAN, E. and PAMPIGLIONE, G. (1971) Prognostic implications of electroencephalographic findings of hypsarrhythmia in first year of life. *British Medical Journal*, **4**, 323–325

GASTAUT, H. (1969) Clinical and electroencephalographical classification of epileptic seizures. *Epilepsia*, **10**, Supplement, 2–21

GASTAUT, H., GASTAUT, J. L., REGIS, H. *et al.* (1978) Computerized tomography in the study of West's syndrome. *Development Medicine and Child Neurology*, **20**, 21–27

GIBBS, F. A. and GIBBS, E. L. (1952) *Atlas of Electroencephalography.* Vol. 2, Addison-Wesley, Cambridge, Mass

GLAZE, D. G., HRACHOVY, R. A., FROST, J. D. *et al.* (1988) Prospective study of outcome of infants with infantile spasms treated during controlled studies of ACTH and prednisone. *Journal of Pediatrics*, **112**, 389–396

GOLDEN, G. S. (1990) Pertussis vaccine and injury to the brain. *Journal of Pediatrics*, **116**, 854–861

GORDON, N. (1981) Long-term prognosis after infantile spasms. *Developmental Medicine and Child Neurology*, **23**, 260

HIRTZ, D. G., NELSON, K. B. and ELLENBERG, J. H. (1983) Seizures following childhood immunizations. *Journal of Pediatrics*, **102**, 14–18

HRACHOVY, R. A. and FROST, J. D. (1989) Infantile spasms. *Cleveland Clinical Journal of Medicine*, Supplement, Part I. S. 10–S. 16

HRACHOVY, R. A., FROST, J. D. KELLAWAY, P. and ZION, T. (1983) Double-blind study of ACTH vs. prednisone therapy in infantile spasms. *Journal of Pediatrics*, **103**, 641–645

HRACHOVY, R. A., FROST, J. D. and KELLAWAY, P. (1984) Hypsarrhythmia: variations on a theme. *Epilepsia*, **25**, 317–325

HUNT, A. (1983) Tuberous sclerosis: a survey of 97 cases. I. Seizures, pertussis immunization and handicap. *Developmental Medicine and Child Neurology*, **25**, 346–349

HUTTENLOCHER, P. R. (1974) Dendritic development in neocortex of children with mental deficit and infantile spasms. *Neurology*, **24**, 203–210

ITO, M., TAKAO, T., OKUNA, T. and MIKAWA, H. (1983) Sequential CT studies of 24 children with infantile spasms on ACTH therapy. *Developmental Medicine and Child Neurology*, **25**, 475–480

JEAVONS, P. M. and BOWER, B. D. (1964) Infantile Spasms: a review of the literature and a study of 112 cases. *Clinics in Developmental Medicine*, **No. 15**, Spastics Society/Heinemann Medical, London; pp. 50–63

JEAVONS, P. M., BOWER, B. D. and DIMITRAKOUDI, M. (1973) Long-term prognosis of 150 cases of 'West' syndrome. *Epilepsia*, **14**, 153–164

LACY, J. R. and PENRY, J. K. (1976) *Infantile spasms.* Raven Press, New York

LOMBROSO, C. T. and FEJERMAN, N. (1977) Bening myoclonus of early infancy. *Annals of Neurology*, **1**, 138–143

MATSUMOTO, A., WATANABLE, K., NEGORO, T., *et al.* (1981) Long-term prognosis after infantile spasms: a statistical study of prognostic factors in 200 cases. *Developmental Medicine and Child Neurology*, **23**, 57–65

O'DONOHOE, N. V. (1976) A 15-year follow-up of 100 children with infantile spasms. *Irish Journal of Medical Science*, **145**, 138

OHTAHARA, S. (1978) Clinico-electrical delineation of epileptic encephalopathies of childhood. *Asian Medical Journal*, **21**, 7–17

OHTAHARA, S. (1984) Seizure disorders in infancy and childhood. *Brain and Development*, **6**, 509–519

OSBORNE, J. P. (1988) Diagnosis of tuberous sclerosis. *Archives of Disease in Childhood*, **63**, 1423–1425

PALM, L., BLENNOW, G., and BRUN, A. (1986) Infantile spasms and neuronal heterotopies. *Acta Paediatrica Scandinavica*, **75**, 855–859

PAMPIGLIONE, G. and MOYNAHAN, E. J. (1976) Tuberous sclerosis syndrome: clinical and EEG studies in 100 children. *Journal of Neurology, Neurosurgery and Psychiatry*, **39**, 666–673

RIIKONEN, R. (1982) A long-term follow-up study of 214 children with the syndrome of infantile spasms. *Neuropediatrics*, **13**, 14–23

RIIKONEN, R. (1984) Infantile spasms: modern practical aspects. *Acta Paediatrica Scandinavica*, **73**, 1–12

RIIKONEN, R. and DONNER, M. (1980) ACTH therapy in infantile spasms: side effects. *Archives of Disease in Childhood*, **55**, 664–672

RIIKONEN, R. and SIMELL, O. (1990) Tuberous sclerosis and infantile spasms. *Archives of Disease in Childhood*, **32**, 203–209

SHIELDS., W. D., NIELSEN, C., BUCH, D. *et al.* (1988) Relationship of pertussis immunization to the onset of neurologic disease. A retrospective epidemiological study. *Journal of Pediatrics*, **113**, 801–805

SINGER, W. D., RABE, E. F. and HALLER, J. S. (1980) The effect of ACTH upon infantile spasms. *Journal of Pediatrics*, **96**, 485–489

SINGER, W. D., HALLER, J. S., SULLIVAN, L. R., *et al.* (1982) The value of neuroradiology in infantile spasms. *Journal of Pediatrics*, **100**, 47–50

SOREL, L. and DUSAUCY-BAULOYE, A. (1958) A propos de 21 cas d'hypsarhythmie de Gibbs: son traitment spectaculaire par l'ACTH. *Acta Neurologica et Psychiatrica Belgica*, **58**, 130–140

WEST, W. J. (1841) On a peculiar form of infantile convulsions. *Lancet*, **1**, 724–725.

# Chapter 5

# Myoclonic epilepsies of early childhood

It has been seen in the preceding chapter how infantile spasms represent a nonspecific reaction on the part of the brain to a variety of insults occurring at a particular developmental stage which lead to a severe and often intractable type of generalized epilepsy. Lennox (1960) originally pointed out that the type of epilepsy which occurs in a child represents a confluence of age, heredity and structural brain abnormality. The syndrome of infantile spasms illustrates this concept, even though heredity does not seem to play a significant role. The heterogeneous group of disorders, now usually called the myoclonic epilepsies of childhood, represents another set of age and developmental dependent conditions and is one in which various brain insults and heredity may be involved. The term myoclonus is used in neurology to describe a variety of phenomena, most of which are not epileptic in nature. The myoclonic phenomena which occur in epilepsy are believed to be caused by cortical epileptic mechanisms.

The history of the myoclonic epilepsies is a confused one. Lennox (1945) recognized that they were distinct from true petit mal and he described their earlier time of onset as being in the age group of 1–6 years. He noted the male predominance, the common association with structural brain abnormality, the high incidence of mental handicap, the variety of seizures which could occur, the fact that hyperventilation did not provoke attacks and the lack of response to the then specific therapy for petit mal with the dione drugs. He also described their frequent association with an EEG pattern of slow spike-wave discharges occurring at a rate of 1.5–2.5 complexes per second. The term 'petit mal variant' was coined but this has since been abandoned because it tended to compound the confusion about terminology. Gastaut *et al.* (1966) reviewed the problem in a classic article and proposed the title 'childhood epileptic encephalopathy with diffuse slow spike waves'. He also proposed an alternative title of the 'Lennox syndrome' which was subsequently altered by others to the 'Lennox–Gastaut syndrome'. These eponymous titles are in wide use and have been applied rather loosely to a heterogeneous group of disorders of diverse aetiology, occurring at different ages in early childhood. The general title 'myoclonic epilepsies of early childhood' is, in the author's opinion, to be preferred to describe this group of epilepsies. The Lennox-Gastaut syndrome is increasingly regarded as a distinct epileptic syndrome among these epilepsies and an attempt will be made to define it more precisely later in this chapter.

The resemblances between the clinical characteristics as defined by Lennox (1945) and the clinical features of the infantile spasms syndrome will be apparent to the reader. Indeed, infantile spasms are sometimes referred to as infantile myoclonic epilepsy. Furthermore, between one-fifth and one-third of the patients with infantile spasms go on to develop clinical myoclonic epilepsy, with or without a seizure-free interval, and they may show the typical slow spike-wave patterns in their EEGS.

## Primary and secondary groups

Myoclonic epilepsies in early childhood are generalized epilepsies and can conveniently be regarded as falling into two groups in much the same way as infantile spasms, namely a primary group (cryptogenic or idiopathic) and a secondary group (symptomatic). As with infantile spasms the secondary group is always the larger group, forming at least two-thirds of most series, and, on closer inspection, many apparently primary cases will be found to have had suspect neurodevelopmental history prior to the onset of epilepsy. However, there are certainly primary cases which have a completely normal history up to the time of onset of the epilepsy, and with those one is in the same state of puzzlement with regard to aetiology as with cryptogenic infantile spasms, i.e. are they due to a metabolic cause, to an autoimmune reaction to infection, to a neurotransmitter failure of some kind, or to hereditary factors influencing neurological development in some way? For example, Doose (1992) described a group of children, predominantly boys, with myoclonic and drop attacks, absences and absence status, and sometimes tonic–clonic seizures, who have a strong family history of epilepsy in close relatives and usually no evidence of an organic brain lesion. The onset of epilepsy is between the ages of 2 and 5 years and the neurodevelopmental background is normal prior to onset. He has called this syndrome *myoclonic–astatic epilepsy of early childhood* and has concluded that a genetically determined susceptibility to epilepsy is of prime aetiological significance. The outcome is variable but remission of seizures and normal psychomotor development later are not uncommon. This close relationship between idiopathic or primary myoclonic epilepsy and an improved long-term prognosis can be observed in most of the myoclonic epileptic syndromes but there are exceptions (see severe myoclonic epilepsy in infants later).

## Varieties of myoclonic seizures

A variety of seizures occurs in the myoclonic epilepsies, the commonest being the following:

1  Atonic-akinetic attacks in which violent falls occur suddenly with immediate recovery and resumption of activity, the duration being less than 1 second (*Figure 5.1*); multiple injuries may occur, particularly to the forehead, lips, teeth and chin.
2  Tonic attacks, occurring during the waking and sleeping states, which may consist of sudden flexion of the head and trunk, elevation and abduction of the upper limbs or sudden falls. They may show asymmetrical or unilateral features. Clusters of attacks are common and automatic behaviour may follow one or several attacks.

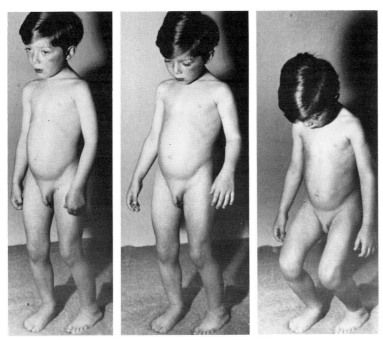

*Figure 5.1* An atonic-akinetic seizure (*Courtesy of Prof. H. Doose*)

3  Head-dropping or head-nodding attacks, which are a partial form of the generalized atonic–akinetic or tonic seizures. The patient may drop the head or fall
either because he or she becomes floppy (atonic) or rigid (tonic).
4  Atypical absences, consisting of a brief interruption of consciousness which is
often incomplete and which has a gradual onset and cessation, perhaps accompanied by automatisms; consciousness is usually clouded rather than
completely lost.
5  Myoclonic phenomena, consisting of symmetrical and synchronous flexion movements; asymmetrical shock-like myoclonic jerks also occur infrequently. A
massive myoclonic flexion of the trunk may even cast the patient to the ground.
6  Major tonic–clonic generalized seizures may occur, particularly in sleep.
7  Episodes of minor epileptic status (Brett, 1966) in which recurring atypical
absences, atonic–akinetic attacks and myoclonic jerks are repeated over hours or
days may also be seen.

The term 'minor motor seizures' is no longer recommended for use in describing
these various attacks.

Sometimes the onset of a myoclonic epilepsy may appear in an innocent way with
the occurrence of a grand mal seizure, perhaps precipitated by fever. Weeks may
then go by before the more serious manifestations of myoclonic epilepsy appear,
including the characteristic atonic–kinetic attacks. Patients frequently manifest a
variety of different types of seizure.

With regard to the *aetiology of the secondary or symptomatic group*, the conditions
producing the cerebral insult are as diverse as they are in symptomatic infantile

spasms, and in a small proportion of cases the aetiology may not be obvious. It seems likely that multifocal or diffuse brain damage is at play in all the secondary cases. Perinatal difficulties, intrauterine infections and acquired brain damage from whatever cause may all precede the condition. Tuberose sclerosis may also be a cause. As with those severely affected by infantile spasms, neurological abnormalities such as spasticity are common in the severely affected cases of myoclonic epilepsy.

## Mental retardation

Although mental handicap is very frequently associated with the myoclonic epilepsies, the degree of handicap is variable. There is a definite correlation between the age of onset of the epilepsy and later intelligence. The earlier the onset the more mentally retarded the patient. Those beginning under 3 years of age do far worse than those at 3 years or over. The younger age group contains a larger number of definite secondary cases and also those who have previously had infantile spasms, whereas in the older group there are more primary cases. Aicardi (1973) estimated that the proportion of severely mentally retarded patients may be three times higher in the secondary group when compared with the primary group.

## Prognosis

The reasons for the differences in prognosis between the primary and secondary groups are not clear. However, in the secondary group an earlier age of onset probably reflects the greater severity of the cerebral insult, whereas in the primary group hereditary factors are probably more important than the underlying brain abnormality. Therefore, one may say with a certain amount of confidence that the later the onset and the more blameless the history antedating the disorder, the better the response to therapy and the better the prognosis for mental development. Whatever the type of case, the long-term outlook for these epilepsies is always uncertain and a seizure-free recovery from the more severe Lennox–Gastaut syndrome is rare. In those who continue to have epilepsy a fluctuating course is characteristic and the pattern of the seizures usually changes with the years. In the Lennox–Gastaut syndrome, diurnal and particularly nocturnal tonic–clonic attacks predominate later on, and brief tonic attacks occurring in slow-wave sleep but not in rapid-eye-movement (REM) sleep continue to be a characteristic feature (Gastaut *et al.*, 1966).

## Subgroups of the myoclonic epilepsies

Many authorities now prefer to divide the large general group of myoclonic epilepsies in early childhood into two groups (Aicardi and Gomes, 1989) as follows:

(a)  A group featuring mainly tonic and atonic seizures, associated usually with interictal slow spike-wave complexes in the EEG. This group corresponds to what most people call the Lennox–Gastaut syndrome.

(b)  A group characterized by true myoclonic seizures, i.e. the occurrence of brief shock-like muscle contractions, and associated usually with ictal or interictal fast spike-wave complexes in the EEG.

## The Lennox–Gastaut syndrome

The myoclonic epilepsies represent a heterogeneous group of disorders and not a single entity (Aicardi, 1973). Gastaut (1985) referred to 'the minestrone of myoclonic syndromes'! Most confusion and controversy surrounds the precise definition of the Lennox–Gastaut syndrome. Lennox and Davis (1949) described the slow spike-wave complexes in these epilepsies and emphasized the lack of temporal relationship between the EEG paroxysms and the clinical seizures. They also noted the mental retardation and described three types of seizures, viz, myoclonic jerks, atypical absences, and head nods and drop attacks which they called akinetic or astatic seizures. In fact, genuine brief myoclonic jerks are relatively uncommon in this syndrome (Gastaut, 1985). Gastaut et al. (1966) emphasized the importance of tonic seizures as a characteristic feature. These occur in the majority of patients, both during the day and especially during sleep when they may pass unnoticed. They are associated with loss of impairment of consciousness but not with clonic activity. Head flexion or extension, opisthotonos, tonic extension of the limbs may be observed in these attacks. They are characterized in the EEG by the occurrence of either flattening of the tracing or by the presence of rhythmic fast spike discharges. Atypical absences are a feature in the great majority of cases and may be difficult to detect clinically because both onset and termination occur in a progressive fashion and incomplete loss of consciousness may allow the patient to continue normal activities to some extent. Slight myoclonic movements of the eyelids and around the mouth, drooling, and a glazed look may alert the observer to their occurrence. More prolonged episodes of this kind, perhaps lasting hours or even days, constitute minor epileptic status (Brett, 1966), another characteristic feature of the condition. When atypical absences or minor status or other seizures are frequent in this syndrome, transient cerebellar syndromes with ataxia may occur and ataxia may even be an initial presenting symptom of this epilepsy (Aicardi and Chevrie, 1971). The EEG is a vital diagnostic tool in such a situation and shows continuous slow spike-wave complexes or polyspikes and slow waves or sometimes a pattern resembling hypsarrhythmia. The ataxia is usually reversible if and when the epilepsy responds to treatment.

Gastaut (1985) lists three diagnostic criteria for the Lennox–Gastaut syndrome. These are:

(a)  Mental retardation, not necessarily present at the onset.
(b)  Diffuse slow spike-wave complexes in the EEG, present in 95% of cases (*Figure 5.2*), and also fast discharges during sleep which may be associated with tonic seizures.
(c)  A variety of seizures including especially drop attacks and tonic seizures.

The natural history of the Lennox–Gastaut syndrome is very variable (Roger, Dravet and Bureau, 1989). In about 30% of cases, children without any relevant previous history, without previous epilepsy, without any clinical or radiological evidence of brain abnormality and with normal psychomotor development up to the time of onset, develop the syndrome. These are entitled cryptogenic cases. The remainder are deemed to have symptomatic Lennox–Gastaut syndrome and may have evidence of pre-, peri-, or postnatal brain abnormality or of an inherited

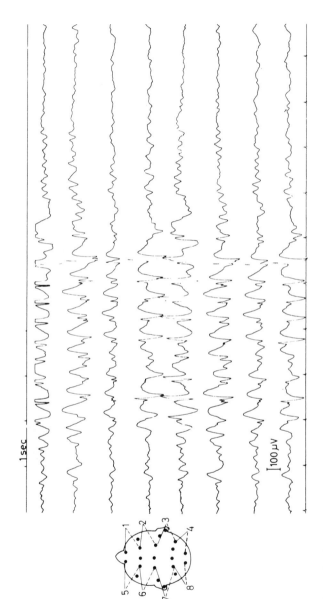

*Figure* 5.2 Girl aged 10 years and awake with eyes open. EEG shows a short burst of slow spike–wave complexes

disorder such as tuberose sclerosis. Psychomotor retardation and a history of previous epilepsy (including infantile spasms in up to a third of cases) are present. CT scans are frequently abnormal, cerebral atrophy being the commonest finding. In very many cases, both cryptogenic and symptomatic, no cause can be identified. A positive family history of epilepsy is present more frequently in cryptogenic cases. In some cryptogenic cases, the onset of the syndrome may coincide with the onset of an apparently unrelated disorder, as in a remarkable case of the author's where the epilepsy started in close temporal relationship with the development of a sympathetic ophthalmia following eye injury. Recently reported findings in Lennox–Gastaut syndrome using positron emission tomography (PET) are described in the section on treatment.

The age of onset is between 1 and 6 years, rarely later, and perhaps most often between 18 months and 3 years. As mentioned earlier, it may begin in an apparently innocent fashion with a tonic–clonic seizure, perhaps precipitated by fever, and the characteristic drop attacks may not appear for several weeks. The appearance of the characteristic EEG pattern may also be delayed. It may, however, begin explosively with an episode of status epilepticus or with very frequent seizures and the rapid development of psychomotor retardation. In such circumstances, Ohtahara's term 'age-dependent epileptic encephalopathy' is particularly applicable (Ohtahara, 1984). Once the typical clinical syndrome has developed, its evolution is usually rapid and severe. Seizures are frequent, remissions short, episodes of status epilepticus occur and psychological deterioration develops. Patients may demonstrate the type of 'autistic' withdrawn behaviour with bizarre mannerisms which is also seen in children with infantile spasms. Severe behavioural disturbances are common.

There is a progressive deterioration in learning ability and psychological difficulties tend to worsen unless some effective treatment can be found.

The prognosis for children with the Lennox–Gastaut syndrome is poor. In a Japanese follow-up of 116 cases (Ohtahara, Yamatogi and Ohtsuka, 1977), 98 cases (84.5%) were shown to have some degree of mental defect and 71 patients (61.2%) continued to have seizures. Both cryptogenic and secondary cases were included. The resemblance to the usual figures quoted for mental defect and epilepsy after infantile spasms should be noted; this similarity is borne out by the results of a large comparative Japanese study (Kurokawa et al., 1980), in which those with infantile spasms fared slightly better. Truly, these two epilepsies are the most terrible which afflict babies and young children. Roger, Dravet and Bureau (1989) have enumerated the main factors for a bad prognosis as follows:

(a)  Symptomatic cases of Lennox–Gastaut syndrome, particularly when the condition evolves from infantile spasms (about 20% of cases).
(b)  Early onset of the syndrome before the age of 3 years is associated with a poor prognosis in the symptomatic type but also in the cryptogenic type.
(c)  High frequency of seizures and repeated episodes of status, associated with infrequent periods of remission.
(d)  Constantly slow background activity in the EEG, without periods of improvement; the presence of focal changes in the EEG.

This epileptic syndrome was the subject of an international symposium in 1987 and the interested reader is referred to the excellent summary of current opinion about the condition by Oller-Daurella and Oller (1988) in the published proceedings.

## Other myoclonic epilepsies of early childhood

As already noted, it is permissible to regard the myoclonic epilepsies of early childhood as composed of two groups consisting first of the Lennox–Gastaut syndrome and, secondly, of a group characterized by brief shock-like myoclonic jerks and associated with rather different EEG features to the Lennox–Gastaut syndrome. Unfortunately, the distinctions between these two groups are not sharply defined, since different kinds of attack may occur in the same patient and EEG patterns may show both slow and fast spike-wave activity. It is the presence of this grey area around the Lennox–Gastaut syndrome which causes so much confusion, controversy and debate.

Epilepsies in which myoclonic jerks are the most dramatic and characteristic clinical feature may present in children from the age of 6 months up to 5 or 6 years of age. These children do not have evidence of previous brain abnormality and have developed normally prior to the illness. Some, however, will have a history of previous seizures, especially febrile convulsions. Other seizure types, including tonic–clonic convulsions, occur as the disease progresses. This epileptic syndrome has been called 'cryptogenic myoclonic epilepsy of childhood' and 'true myoclonic epilepsy' by Aicardi and Chevrie 1971 or simply 'myoclonic epilepsy of childhood' (Jeavons, 1977). Dravet, Bureau and Roger (1992) have used the title '*benign myoclonic epilepsy in infants*' when the condition begins in infancy. At whatever age it begins, its clinical course is difficult to predict, although it is certainly better than that of the Lennox–Gastaut syndrome. It is probably fair to say that, the more purely myoclonic the syndrome and the more it corresponds to a truly primary generalized epilepsy, the better the prognosis. A ready response to antiepileptic medication is also a good augury. However, the occurrence of other types of seizures (except for brief febrile convulsions) before the onset of the myoclonic attacks, the association of other types of seizures with the myoclonic attacks, and a suspect mental development before the onset of the illness suggest an unfavourable outcome (Aicardi, 1980). Nevertheless, even when myoclonic jerks, drop attacks, and generalized tonic–clonic seizures are associated, the response to treatment and the eventual outcome can be better than expected, especially when the child's development has been normal previously and when there is a strong family prevalence of epilepsy (Doose *et al.*, 1970). Later onset may also be a good omen in such a situation, in the author's experience.

Dravet (1978) and others have drawn attention in recent years to another sinister epileptic syndrome with some myoclonic features. This has been entitled *severe myoclonic epilepsy in infants*. It presents as a primary or cryptogenic epilepsy with severe seizures beginning during the first year of life, often around 5–6 months of age. There is frequently a family history of epilepsy, but no previous personal history of disease and development prior to onset is normal. The epilepsy begins with generalized or unilateral tonic-clonic or clonic seizures, usually precipitated by minor febrile illnesses. These attacks are often prolonged and may include episodes of status. Myoclonic seizures and partial seizures resembling complex partial seizures appear later, usually after the first birthday. The EEG is usually normal initially but, during the second year, paroxysmal abnormalities consisting of rapid, generalized spike-waves or polyspike waves appear, and perhaps also focal abnormalities. Paroxysmal abnormalities in the EEG in response to photic stimulation appear early, regarded by some as an ominous finding (Aicardi and Gomes, 1989). Psychomotor development is retarded from the second year onward and all those affected are mentally handicapped later. In a personal case, the affected girl was found dead in her cot during the second year after surviving several attacks of status epilepticus. This epilepsy is very resistant to all forms of therapy. No definite aetiology has been identified although unfavourable genetic factors seem likely in view of the strong family history of epilepsy in many cases (Dravet *et al.*, 1992). An autopsy report of a 19-month-old boy with the disorder revealed several developmental brain abnormalities, including microdysgenesis of cerebellum and cerebral cortex (Renier and Renkawek, 1990).

The quintessential primary myoclonic epilepsy, namely, juvenile myoclonic epilepsy of Janz, is discussed in Chapter 13.

## Diagnosis and differential diagnosis

The diagnosis of a myoclonic epilepsy is usually not difficult if the characteristic drop attacks occur. However, in the event of the condition beginning with a major generalized seizure in a setting of fever, the clinician may be misled. In the early stages of a myoclonic epilepsy, even in the severe Lennox–Gastaut syndrome, the EEG may be normal or show only mild diffuse slowing and dysrhythmia. There is a further diagnostic difficulty when absence attacks are a prominent feature, especially in cases of later onset. It is most important to distinguish such absences from those of childhood absence epilepsy (petit mal), since treatment and prognosis for the two conditions are so different. One should always be wary of a child with apparent petit mal presenting under 5 years of age, who has a history suggesting a structural lesion of the brain, where there is a possibility of associated mental handicap even of mild degree and where the EEG patterns are atypical and irregular. Simultaneous video and EEG monitoring is of considerable value in differential diagnosis here and also in distinguishing epileptic from non-epileptic head drops in young children (Brunquell, McKeever and Russmann, 1990).

Transient cerebellar syndromes with ataxia may occur in the myoclonic epilepsies when attacks are frequent and ataxia may even be the initial presenting symptom (Aicardi and Chevrie, 1971). There is frequently a close temporal relationship between the episodes of ataxia and temporary worsening of the epileptic disorder and patients in minor epileptic status may present with ataxia. Once again, the EEG is the vital diagnostic tool in such a situation with video-EEG monitoring an added refinement. The ataxia usually improves if and when the epilepsy responds to treatment.

The occurrence of a clinical feature such as ataxia may also suggest the possible existence of a progressive neurodegenerative disorder. Myoclonic phenomena are a feature of two such conditions, namely, subacute sclerosing panencephalitis (SSPE) and neuronal ceroid lipofuscinosis or Batten–Vogt disease. The EEG is of diagnostic assistance in both these diseases, showing repetitive polyspike complexes in SSPE and abnormal responses to photic stimulation at slow flash frequencies in Batten–Vogt disease (Pampiglione and Harden, 1977). Non-epileptic myoclonus characterized by sudden limb and eye movements occurs in the 'dancing-eye syndrome' (Kinsbourne, 1962) and in this condition the EEG is normal.

Aicardi and Chevrie (1982) drew attention to a group of children who may be misdiagnosed as having severe myoclonic epilepsy. The onset in their cases was always after 2 years of age. Partial motor seizures occurred on falling asleep or on awakening, reminiscent of those seen in benign partial epilepsy of childhood with centro-temporal spike discharges (see Chapter 9). Some generalized tonic–clonic seizures also occurred in sleep. Brief absences, similar to petit mal, and tonic or myoclonic seizures causing repeated falls were also observed. EEGs showed intense slow spike-wave activity in sleep and much less marked abnormality, often focal discharges, when awake. Neither neurological deficit nor intellectual deterioration were observed and, even though resistance to drug treatment was usual initially, eventual remission of the seizures and return of the EEG to normal were the rule. The authors entitled this epileptic syndrome 'atypical benign partial epilepsy of childhood'.

## Therapy

In line with their heterogeneity, one might expect that the treatment of myoclonic seizures would be difficult and indeed it is notoriously so. There is hardly another group of epilepsies in childhood which so often proves as unyielding to medication as do the myoclonic seizures. Drugs used in major generalized epilepsy in older children and adults, for example phenobarbitone, primidone, phenytoin and carbamazepine, are usually ineffective and, indeed, both phenobarbitone and primidone often tend to exacerbate the overactivity and aggressiveness which are common accompaniments of these epilepsies. However, in the author's experience, primidone may be worth a cautious trial in some cases. Occasionally, even ethosuximide may prove surprisingly successful, especially in so-called 'true myoclonic epilepsy'. ACTH has been used in some severe cases of the Lennox–Gastaut syndrome and sometimes brings about a measure of control in much the same rather inexplicable way in which it benefits children with infantile spasms (Snead, Benton and Myers, 1983). When this regimen is beneficial it usually has to be continued for many months, and the author has used empirical doses of 40 units on alternate days, gradually lengthening the intervals between doses to twice weekly.

The most important advances, however, have been the use of the benzodiazepines and sodium valproate in treatment. It is now customary to use one or other of these initially. The *benzodiazepine drugs* which have been used are nitrazepam, clonazepam and clobazam. Diazepam has also been used orally in large doses (between 5 and 30 mg per day) but side effects such as drowsiness, ataxia, diplopia and extrapyramidal movements have largely precluded its widespread use. Nitrazepam has been used more successfully than diazepam and, if it is introduced in a small dose (2.5–5 mg at night, depending on the age of the child) and if increments are made very slowly until attacks cease or until side-effects occur, then it may be quite well tolerated. However, clonazepam is probably the benzodiazepine most widely used in the myoclonic epilepsies. Hanson and Menkes (1972) treated 59 patients with 'minor motor seizures', selected because they did not respond to the usual medications. The series included some patients who had had infantile spasms. Of the 59 patients in the series, 45 derived significant benefit from clonazepam after a 3-month trial and 39 continued to receive benefit for periods of 3–18 months. Hanson and Menkes concluded that clonazepam appeared to be the most useful anticonvulsant available in the management of the myoclonic epilepsies. Roussounis and Rudolf (1977), on the basis of their results, also regarded the response to clonazepam as encouraging. In their myoclonic–akinetic group control was achieved in 14 out of 22 patients. O'Donohoe and Paes (1977) also reported good results with the drug (i.e. better than 50% control of attacks) in 8 out of 10 patients with myoclonic akinetic attacks, and good control in 3 out of 7 patients with more severe and intractable myoclonic epilepsy (Lennox–Gastaut syndrome). Many of their patients had previously been taking a variety of other drugs without success. The arbitrary maximum dosage for infants under 1 year was 0.3 mg/kg per day, and for those over 1 year the dose was 0.25 mg/kg per day. The drug was introduced extremely slowly, beginning with 0.25 mg at bedtime and increasing by small increments every fifth day until the epilepsy responded or serious side effects were encountered. These included drowsiness, hypersecretion and drooling, ataxia and, in older children, hyperactivity. Most people using the benzodiazepines as anticonvulsants have noted the development of tolerance to the drugs which develops in up to 25% of those treated (Brown and Penry, 1973), usually 1–6 months after the commencement of treatment. This is due to a reduction in benzodiazepine receptor binding. It has been suggested that this is less of a problem with clonazepam than with the other benzodiazepines. Gastaut (1982) considers the benzodiazepines, including clobazam, more effective than all other anticonvulsants in the treatment of seizures in the secondary generalized myoclonic epilepsies, especially in the Lennox–Gastaut syndrome. Despite their disadvantages, he recommends them as drugs of first choice in these epilepsies, although in other epilepsies they should be used only after failure of more appropriate drugs.

The use of intermittent antiepileptic therapy with benzodiazepines is now an accepted treatment strategy in preventing the development of tolerance to the drugs. Clobazam has been used in this way for 10 days each month to treat catamenial epilepsy and alternate-day clonazepam has been used for intractable seizures (Sher, 1985). Clobazam may be added on to existing therapy for short periods to control clusters of seizures, or prescribed intermittently on a regular basis.

*Sodium valproate* is also used for treating these epilepsies and is discussed in greater detail in a later chapter on drug therapy (*see* p.271). It may act by increasing the level of GABA in the brain by inhibiting enzymes responsible for its synthesis and breakdown. GABA is a known inhibitor at certain synapses. Jeavons, Clarke and Maheshwari (1977) have reported on its use in the myoclonic epilepsies. They reported good results (control or marked improvement) in 16 of their 32 patients with atonic–akinetic seizures. Similar responses were obtained in 10 of their 11 patients with true myoclonic epilepsy. They concluded that, in their opinion, sodium valproate was superior to all other drugs in the treatment of the myoclonic epilepsies. Jeavons again reported favourably on his considerable experience with the drug in 1982. In the author's experience it has been particularly successful in primary or cryptogenic myoclonic epilepsy, beginning in the child of 3 years or older, in those with atypical absences, and in true myoclonic epilepsy. However, like most other drugs it is unpredictable in its effects on the secondary myoclonic epilepsies, including the severe Lennox–Gastaut syndrome, and makes some patients worse. It does not appear to be superior to the benzodiazepines in these patients. However, combined treatment with one of the benzodiazepines may sometimes be effective.

It is important to avoid the use of carbamazepine in treating these epilepsies, especially the multiple seizure types and atypical absences of the Lennox–Gastaut syndrome, since this drug may exacerbate the condition (Snead and Hosey, 1985). On the other hand, the new antiepileptic drug vigabatrin should certainly be considered as adjunctive or add-on therapy for cases of the Lennox–Gastaut syndrome with refractory seizures. The response is usually unpredictable, but good

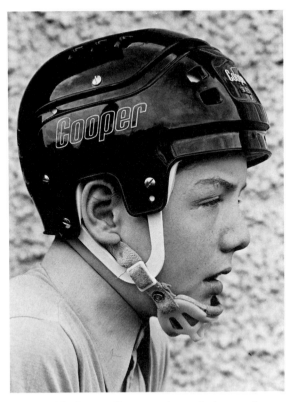

*Figure 5.3* The Lennox-Gastaut syndrome. Patient wearing protective headgear and having an absence attack

to excellent results have been reported in some patients (Livingston *et al.* 1989). The recommended dosage is 40–80 mg per kg daily. A novel method of treatment, for which some success has been claimed, is the use of high-dosage intravenous gammaglobulin therapy (Sandstedt, Kostulas and Larsson, 1984). This is extremely expensive and quite unpredictable in its effects.

The effects of a *ketogenic diet* on intractable epilepsy have been known since the early 1920s, and the diet appears to act by increasing the concentrations of acetoacetate and $\beta$-hydroxybutyrate levels in the plasma. It is suggested that the availability and use of ketones by the brain result in certain biochemical changes which reduce the tendency for neurons to discharge and also inhibit the spread of discharges in the brain. The diet has been regarded as expensive, difficult to manage, unpalatable and even nauseating. Huttenlocher, Wilbourn and Signore (1971) brought about a significant practical advance in the use of this dietetic regimen when they used medium-chain triglycerides (MCT) to induce ketosis. This made the diet easier to manage and more palatable, and also meant that carbohydrates need not be so rigidly restricted. This modification of the ketogenic diet has been found to be most effective in younger children, but is probably worth considering at any age. The author has had both dramatic successes and dismal failures with the diet, and the outcome cannot be predicted in any case

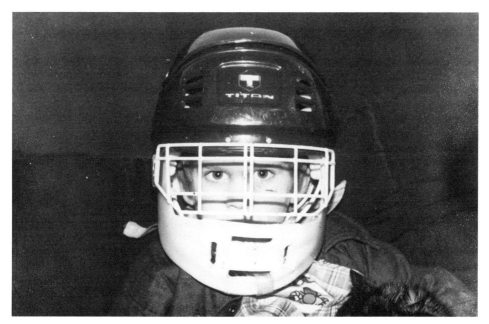

*Figure 5.4* This child is wearing a junior ice-hockey helmet. The parents found that this was the only device which provided complete protection to the face, teeth and chin

without a trial. The success of the method depends on both the understanding and cooperation of the mother and on the acceptance of the diet by the child. Strict adherence to the diet and the maintenance of persistent ketosis are essential. Full details of the diet are given in Appendix 1 (*see also* Gordon, 1977; Schwartz *et al.*, 1989).

The operation of section of the corpus callosum (callosotomy) is being advised for some cases of the Lennox–Gastaut syndrome with intractable seizures, particularly when there is a focal abnormality in the EEG (Wyllie, 1988). Taylor (1990) has expressed his reservations about such procedures. The author has referred only two such cases for this procedure. Both were in early adult life. Both have benefited in seizure control and in other respects and neither has shown significant new deficits postoperatively. Whether the finding of focal regions of depressed cerebral glucose metabolism by positron emission tomography (PET) in some patients with the Lennox–Gastaut syndrome (Ferrendelli, 1987) will lead to treatment by local ablative surgery is still a matter for speculation.

Finally, the *general care* of the child with these chronic and disabling epilepsies is of the utmost importance. They present an enormous challenge to the paediatrician or paediatric neurologist dealing with them. The parents need regular advice and support. Parent support groups have been formed in some countries (e.g. Australia). Protective headgear is frequently necessary (*Figures 5.3 and 5.4*), particularly when the atonic–akinetic drop seizures are frequent. This particular type of epilepsy, as Lennox (1960) remarked in his classic work on the subject, is surely the charter member of the ancient order of 'Falling Sickness'. Further discussion of the educational and other problems which beset these patients will be found in Chapter 21.

## References

AICARDI, J. (1973) The problem of the Lennox syndrome. *Developmental Medicine and Child Neurology*, **15**, 77–81

AICARDI, J. (1980) Course and prognosis of certain childhood epilepsies with predominently myoclonic seizures. In *Advance in Epileptology*, The Xth International Epilepsy Symposium (eds J. A. Wada and J. K. Penry), Raven Press, New York, pp. 159–163

AICARDI, J. and CHEVRIE, J. J. (1971) Myoclonic epilepsies of childhood. *Neuropädiatrie*, **3**, 177–190

AICARDI, J. and CHEVRIE, J. J. (1982) Atypical benign partial epilepsy of childhood. *Development Medicine and Child Neurology*, **24**, 281–292

AICARDI, J. and GOMES, A. L. (1989) The myoclonic epilepsies of childhood. *Cleveland Clinic Journal of Medicine*, **56**, Supplement Part 1, S34–S39

BRETT, E. M. (1966) Minor epileptic status. *Journal of the Neurological Sciences*, **3**, 52–75

BROWN, T. R. and PENRY, J. K. (1973) Benzodiazepines in the treatment of epilepsy: a review. *Epilepsia*, **14**, 277–310

BRUNQUELL, P., MCKEEVER, M. and RUSSMAN, B. S. (1990) Differentiation of epileptic from non-epileptic head nods in children. *Epilepsia*, **31**, 401–405

DOOSE, H. (1992) Myoclonic astatic epilepsy of early childhood. In *Epileptic Syndromes in Infancy, Childhood and Adolescence*, 2nd Edition (eds J. Roger, M. Bureau, C. Dravet *et al*.), John Libbey, London, Paris, pp. 103–114

DOOSE, H., GERKEN, H., LEONHARDT, R., *et al.* (1970) Centrecephalic myoclonic-astatic petit mal. Clinical and genetic considerations. *Neuropädiatrie*, **2**, 59–78

DRAVET, C. (1978) Les épilepsies graves de l'enfant. *Vie Médicale*, **8**, 543–548

DRAVET, C., BUREAU, M. and ROGER, J. (1992) Benign myoclonic epilepsy in infants. In *Epileptic Syndromes in Infancy, Childhood and Adolescence*, 2nd Edition (eds J. Roger, M. Bureau, C. Dravet, *et al*.), John Libbey, London, Paris, pp. 67–74

DRAVET, C., BUREAU, M., GUERRINI, R. *et al.* (1992) Severe myoclonic epilepsy in infants. In *Epileptic Syndromes in Infancy, Childhood and Adolescence*, 2nd Edition (eds J. Roger, M. Bureau, C. Dravet, *et al*.), John Libbey, London, Paris, pp. 75–88

FERRENDELLI, J. A. (1987) Lennox–Gastaut syndrome and positron emission tomography. *Annals of Neurology*, **21**, 3

GASTAUT, H. (1982) The effects of benzodiazepines on chronic epilepsies in man (with particular reference to clobazam). In *Clobazam*. Royal Society of Medicine International Congress and Symposium Series. No. 43, Academic Press/ Royal Society of Medicine, London, pp. 141–150

GASTAUT, H. (1985) Discussion of myoclonic epilepsies and Lennox–Gastaut syndrome. In *Epileptic Syndromes in Infancy, Childhood and Adolescence*, 1st edition (eds J. Roger, C. Dravet, M. Bureau, *et al*.), John Libbey Eurotext, London, Paris, pp. 100–104

GASTAUT, H., ROGER, J., SOULAYROL, R. *et al.* (1966) Childhood epileptic encephalopathy with diffuse slow spike-waves (otherwise known as 'petit mal variant' or Lennox syndrome). *Epilepsia*, **7**, 139–179

GORDON, N. S. (1977) Medium-chain triglycerides in a ketogenic diet. *Developmental Medicine and Child Neurology*, **19**, 535–538

HANSON, R. A. and MENKES, J. H. (1972) A new anticonvulsant in the management of minor motor seizures. *Developmental Medicine and Child Neurology*, **14**, 3–14

HUTTENLOCHER, P. R., WILBOURNE, A. J. and SIGNORE, J. M. (1971) Medium-chain triglycerides as therapy for intractable childhood epilepsy. *Neurology*, **21**, 1097–1103

JEAVONS, P. M. (1977) Nosological problems of myoclonic epilepsies in childhood and adolescence. *Developmental Medicine and Child Neurology*, **19**, 3–8

JEAVONS, P. M. (1982) Myoclonic epilepsies: therapy and prognosis. In: *Advances in Epileptology*. The XIIIth Epilepsy International Symposium (eds H. Akimoto, H. Kazamatsuri, M. Seino and A. A. Ward), Raven Press, New York, pp. 141–144

JEAVONS, P. M. CLARK, J. E. AND MAHESHWARI, M. C. (1977) Treatment of generalized epilepsies of childhood and adolescence with sodium valproate (Epilim). *Developmental Medicine and Child Neurology*, **19**, 9–25

KINSBOURNE, M. (1962) Myoclonic encephalopathy of infancy. *Journal of Neurology, Neurosurgery and Psychiatry*, **25**, 271–276

KUROKAWA, T., GOYA, N., FUKAYAMA, Y., SUZUKI, M., SEKI, T. AND OHTAHARA, S. (1980) West syndrome and Lennox–Gastaut syndrome: a survey of natural history. *Pediatrics*, **65**, 81–88

LENNOX, W. G. (1945) The petit mal epilepsies: their treatment with Tridione. *Journal of the American Medical Association*, **129**, 1069–1074

LENNOX, W. G. (1960) *Epilepsy and Related Disorders*, Vol. 1 J. and A. Churchill, London, Little Brown, Boston

LENNOX, W. G. AND DAVIS, J. P. (1949) Clinical correlates of the fast and slow spikewave electroencephalogram. *Transactions of the American Neurological Association*, **74**, 194–197

LIVINGSTON, J. H., BEAUMONT, D., ARZIMANOGLOU, A. AND AICARDI, J. (1989) Vigabatrin in the treatment in epilepsy in children. *British Journal of Pharmacology*, **27**, Supplement 1: S. 109–S. 112

O'DONOHOE, N. V. AND PAES, B. A. (1977) A trial of clonazepam in the treatment of severe epilepsy in infancy and childhood. In *Epilepsy, proceedings of the Eighth International Symposium* (ed J. K. Penry) Raven Press, New York, pp. 159–162.

OHTAHARA, S. (1984) Seizure disorders in infancy and childhood. *Brain and Development*, **6**, 509–519.

OHTAHARA, S., YAMATOGI, Y. AND OHTSUKA, Y. (1977) Prognosis of the Lennox syndrome. A clinical and electroencephalographic study. *Epilepsia*, **18**, 130–131

OLLER-DAURELLA, L. AND OLLER, F-V. L. (1988) The Lennox-Gastaut syndrome: synopsis. In *The Lennox-Gastaut syndrome* (eds. E. Niedermeyer and R. Degen) Alan R. Liss, Inc., New York

PAMPLIGLIONE, G. AND HARDEN, A. (1977) So-called neuronal ceroid lipofuscinosis. Neurophysiological studies in 60 children. *Journal of Neurology, Neurosurgery and Psychiatry*, **40**, 323–330

RENIER, W. O. and RENKAWEK, K. (1990) Clinical and neuropathological findings in a case of severe myoclonic epilepsy of infancy. *Epilepsia*, **31**, 287–291

ROGER, J., DRAVET, C. and BUREAU, M. (1989) The Lennox–Gastaut syndrome. *Cleveland Clinic Journal of Medicine*, **56**, Supplement, Part 2. S.172–S.180

ROUSSOUNIS, S. and RUDOLF, N. de M. (1977) Clonazepam in the treatment of children with intractable seizures. *Developmental Medicine and Child Neurology*, **19**, 326–334

SANDSTEDT, P., KOSTULAS, V. and LARSSON, L. E. (1984) Intravenous gammaglobulin for post-encephalitic epilepsy. *Lancet*, **324**, 1154–1155

SCHWARTZ, R. H., EATON, J., BOWER, B. D. and Aynsley-Green, A. (1989) Ketogenic diets in the treatment of epilepsy. Short-term clinical effects. *Developmental Medicine and Child Neurology*, **31**, 145–151

SHER, P. K. (1985) Alternate-day clonazepam treatment of intractable seizures. *Archives of Neurology*, **42**, 787–788

SNEAD, O. C. and HOSEY, L. C. (1985) Exacerbation of seizures in children by carbamazepine. *New England Journal of Medicine*, **313**, 916–921

SNEAD, O. C., BENTON, J. W. and MYERS, G. J. (1983) ACTH and prednisone in childhood seizure disorder. *Neurology*, **33**, 966–970

TAYLOR, D. C. (1990) Callosal section for epilepsy and the avoidance of doing everything possible. *Developmental Medicine and Child Neurology*, **32**, 267–270

WYLLIE, E. (1977) Corpus callosotomy for intractable generalized epilepsy. *Journal of Pediatrics*, **113**, 255–261

# Chapter 6

# Febrile convulsions

## Aetiology of febrile convulsions

These occur in young children who have an individual susceptibility to convulse in a setting of acute fever. The incidence of these seizures is about 3% in the population at risk; they are rare below 6 months and above 5 years of age and the peak incidence occurs from 9 to 20 months. The term 'febrile convulsions' should be confined to those occurring solely with fever and should not be applied to seizures which occur in young children with an infection of the nervous system such as meningitis.

The typical febrile convulsion is brief, generalized, tonic–clonic in sequence and the body temperature is high. It occurs more frequently when the child is asleep, and the illness which causes the fever is commonly an acute upper respiratory tract infection (Millichap, 1968). The convulsion is usually the first indication that the child is ill, since 90% of febrile convulsions occur in the first 24 hours of fever (Anderson *et al.*, 1989). The parents almost invariably find the seizure very frightening if they witness it and are apprehensive that the child may be dying. The convulsion is usually single, but repeated ones can occur in the same illness. The attack is followed by sleep as a rule and parents, when asked about the duration of the episode, may give a false impression about its length by including the postictal sleep. This may be important when the clinician is attempting to judge the seriousness of an attack retrospectively.

## Raised temperature and the infective agent

The convulsion is more likely to occur when the temperature is rising rapidly, and this situation is associated with the onset of the illness in about half the cases. However, further convulsions are uncommon even though the temperature remains elevated, and this fact casts doubt on the proposition that the fever is primarily or solely responsible for triggering the seizure. The actual rate of the rise in temperature may be the important factor, but the temperature achieved is not thought to be of primary importance. It is possible that fever causes some other change in the young individual which may then be the triggering factor; for example, the increased oxygen demand consequent on fever may overtax the cerebral oxidative mechanisms.

Viral illnesses causing upper respiratory tract infection are perhaps the commonest cause of fever leading to febrile seizures. Wallace and Zealley (1970), in a careful study of children with proven viral illnesses and febrile convulsions, concluded that seizures associated with viral infections were more likely to be long, repeated or focal than were those associated with non-viral illnesses. Lewis *et al.* (1979) identified a virus infection in over 80% of their cases. Urinary tract infections and other bacterial infections may also be responsible at times. Immunizations which result in fever, especially with the pertussis and measles vaccines, may trigger a febrile convulsion, most frequently in a child with a personal history of febrile convulsions or with such a history in first-degree relatives (Hirtz *et al.*, 1983).

## Age dependency

As with so many types of childhood epilepsy, febrile convulsions are highly age dependent. The reasons for their relative rarity under 6 months of age have been discussed in Chapter 4.

## Genetic influence

Individual susceptibility to febrile seizures appears to depend on the transmission of a specific trait by a single autosomal dominant gene of reduced penetrance (Ounsted, 1971). Rich *et al.* (1987) performed complex segregation analysis of 467 families ascertained through febrile convulsion probands. In families with multiple cases (i.e. more than three affected), the evidence was consistent with a single major locus model with nearly dominant seizure susceptibility. Further research in molecular biology may succeed in identifying genetically predisposed children more precisely. The proportion of patients whose family history shows the occurrence of febrile convulsions and/or epilepsy is high. Verity, Butler and Golding (1985a) reported such a positive history in 26% of their patients. Monozygotic twins show an 80% concordance for febrile seizures (Lennox-Buchthal, 1971). The proportion of siblings who also experience febrile convulsions has ranged from 9 to 17% (Hauser, 1981). It is likely that genetic links exist between febrile convulsions and some of the primary generalized and partial epilepsies of later onset, including childhood absence epilepsy and benign partial epilepsy with centro-temporal (rolandic) spikes (Kajitani *et al.*, 1981).

## Sex

The sex of the individual plays an important role in the incidence of febrile seizures. Boys outnumber girls in most series. There are biological differences between the sexes with regard to incidence and age. Taylor and Ounsted (1971) showed that the decline in incidence in males is smooth over the first 4 years, whereas in girls the decline is sharp and sudden and occurs mainly in the latter part of the second year of life. They explained this phenomenon by the hypothesis of differential cerebral maturation. This theory was based on the fact that as a rule girls mature faster than boys and that this also applies to the process of cerebral maturation. Because the latter process reduces the liability to convulse in response to fever, and perhaps sustain damage thereby, females will be at an advantage by being exposed to this risk for a shorter period of time than boys. Paradoxically, however, those females who do convulse with fever are relatively more prone to serious sequelae because they convulse more frequently at a younger age.

The chronological age at the time of the first seizure is of critical importance as far as sustaining brain damage is concerned because the brain is more vulnerable in the young. Boys certainly experience more febrile seizures than girls but these are spread out over a longer period of time. It is pertinent also at this point to mention the usual unilaterality of brain damage after febrile seizures. Taylor and Ounsted (1971) stressed that complicated febrile seizures damage those territories which are most rapidly acquiring ordered learning. In the first 2 years the non-dominant (normally right) hemisphere is learning visuospatial skills and at the age of 2 years the emphasis shifts to the dominant (usually left) hemisphere for learning speech and language.

## Severity of attack

The severity of a febrile convulsion is its most important feature as far as causing death or permanent damage is concerned, and the duration of the convulsive attack is the main yardstick by which its severity should be measured. Where the convulsive movements last longer than 30 minutes the attack should certainly be judged as severe, and a duration beyond 15 minutes should probably be similarly judged. It should be realized that the term 'status epilepticus' is normally given to a convulsion lasting more than an hour or to a series of convulsions without return of consciousness for the same period of time. In the young, however, the term should probably be applied when the duration exceeds 30 minutes.

Status epilepticus in childhood was reviewed by Aicardi and Chevrie (1970), who studied 239 patients who were under 15 years of age at the time of the first status. They found that status was an early event in the history of childhood epilepsy with the first attack occurring before 3 years of age in 75% of their cases. In nearly half the cases a definite cause was implicated, such as meningitis, encephalitis or a severe electrolyte disturbance; but in just short of a third of the cases, where fever was present at the onset, the clinical picture was indistinguishable from a prolonged febrile seizure and the possibilities for permanent brain damage occurring as a consequence of the status were great. Nearly all the episodes of febrile status reported by these authors were in children of less than 18 months of age and were equally divided between those less than and more than 12 months old.

In the series of children with febrile convulsions studied by Lennox-Buchthal (1973) in Denmark, 29% of the fits occurring in children below 13 months were severe, 15% were severe in the 14–17 months age group, 12% were severe in the 18–36 months age group and of those occurring in children over 3 years of age only 9% were severe. Consequently, age is the crucial factor in determining the severity of a febrile convulsion. Girls with severe febrile convulsions usually outnumber boys in the younger age group because of the reasons already given, namely that the peak age of onset for febrile seizures occurs earlier in girls. Multiple convulsions in the same febrile illness, which are also potentially brain damaging, are also commoner in the younger patient.

Severe, i.e. prolonged, febrile seizures are particularly likely to be unilateral. Gastaut et al. (1960) drew special attention to this fact and Aicardi and Chevrie

(1970), in their study of status epilepticus, confirmed that severe seizures are unilateral and made the point that the trained observer in hospital was more likely than the parents to note the predominant unilaterality of the attack.

Gastaut *et al.* (1960) described a syndrome associated with febrile status epilepticus which they called the *HHE syndrome* (i.e. a condition of hemiconvulsions, hemiplegia and later epilepsy). They reviewed 150 cases that had severe prolonged and mainly unilateral convulsions in a setting of fever, mainly occurring in children under 2 years of age. The condition was frequently followed by a permanent hemiplegia and by evidence of more extensive brain damage which manifested itself as mental handicap and later epilepsy. They also described acute pathological findings of venous congestion, vascular thrombosis and massive cerebral oedema with later evidence of cortical atrophy which was demonstrated by pneumoencephalography. There is evidence that these severe sequelae, such as postconvulsive hemiplegias, have become much rarer in subsequent decades (Roger *et al.*, 1982).

The exact micropathology is still far from clear. Presumably in the milder benign and transitory postictal hemiparesis (*Todd's paralysis*) vasospasm or neurological exhaustion may be mainly responsible, while in the irreversible postictal hemiplegic cases compression and occlusion of cerebral arteries by cerebral oedema occur. Once again the duration of the seizure seems to be a crucial factor. The severe febrile seizure is distinguished from the 'benign' febrile seizure by its duration and the consequent brain damage. The evidence is now overwhelming that severe febrile convulsions cause brain damage and various chronic brain syndromes including later epilepsy (Aicardi and Chevrie, 1976). The importance of febrile convulsions in the natural history of childhood epilepsy is evident once this point is grasped. It should be possible to make a major contribution to the prevention of later epilepsy by the effective treatment and prevention of severe febrile convulsions. The problem is, however, that the most severe febrile convulsions occur in the very young and the great majority are first convulsions which occur even before the infant is recognized as being febrile (Chevrie and Aicardi, 1975). As has already been mentioned, convulsions lasting longer than 30 minutes occurred in nearly 30% of Lennox–Buchthal's seizures when the children were aged 13 months or less.

## Classification

Livingston (1954) distinguished between what he called 'simple febrile convulsions' (by which he meant brief generalized seizures with no clinical or laboratory evidence of cerebral infection or intoxication) and what he termed 'epileptic seizures precipitated by fever' or 'atypical febrile convulsions', which were usually prolonged and often focal or lateralized and were frequently followed by later epilepsy. Livingston (1972) agreed that children with simple febrile convulsions showed strong hereditary tendencies to convulse with fever and cited a family history of 'simple febrile convulsions' in 58% of his series. He also stated that a hereditary factor was found in only 3% of cases of 'epileptic seizures precipitated by fever'. The implication was that the latter group of children had already sustained some brain injury producing an epileptogenic lesion and that they were, in fact, epileptics from the start. Furthermore, in his series, 93% of the atypical febrile seizure patients later developed spontaneous epilepsy while in the benign or simple group the incidence was only 3%. Similarly, of those who developed afebrile seizures later,

97% did so by the age of 5 years. Hauser *et al.* (1977) found that, in children with febrile seizures who had severe neurological handicaps, 36% developed epilepsy later, as compared with 3% in children without such neurological deficits.

Lennox-Buchthal (1973) considered that the major difference between febrile convulsions that remain benign and those that presage later epilepsy is related to the severity and the number of convulsions, to the age of onset and antecedent brain injury and possibly to the sex of the patient. Antecedent brain injury, usually perinatal, increases the likelihood of febrile convulsions occurring and also makes severe convulsions more probable and later epilepsy more frequent.

The great majority of febrile convulsions are single, brief, bilateral, tonic–clonic seizures occurring in infants or children of normal development. These are described as *simple* febrile convulsions and they are not followed by transient or permanent neurological sequelae. A minority of febrile convulsions are of longer duration (more than 15–20 minutes), occur repeatedly within 24 hours, may show partial or unilateral features, and may be followed by transient or permanent neurological sequelae. These are described as *complex* or complicated. The critical difference between the two types is one of duration of the seizure.

The reported incidence of simple and complex febrile convulsions has varied depending on whether the studies have been hospital or community based and also on whether or not they have included febrile convulsions occurring in association with infections of the central nervous system. Wallace (1975), in a hospital based study, identified up to a third of cases as complex. Nelson and Ellenberg (1976, 1978) in the National Collaborative Perinatal Project in the United States, found that up to a quarter of the cases had complex features (i.e. duration greater than 15 minutes, more than one seizure within 24 hours, focal features) and that the great majority of these were first attacks.

Wallace (1976) suggested that the syndrome of febrile convulsions should include more than age, fever, and individual susceptibility. She presented evidence that some children who convulse with fever have an increased incidence of factors associated with suboptimal neurological development, and proposed that a convulsion in a febrile child may draw attention to a developmental defect. She considered that minor alterations in brain structure are inseparable predisposing factors to some febrile seizures, especially those which are prolonged and potentially damaging in the very young.

There are arguments, therefore, for distinguishing two separate populations of children with complex febrile convulsion. Chevrie and Aicardi (1975) showed that the proportion of genetic antecedents in children with prolonged febrile convulsions was only half that in those who suffer the usual simple type of febrile seizure and who comprise the great majority of those affected. It may be proposed, therefore, that a proportion of children with complex febrile convulsions have a distinct epileptic syndrome which is different from the simple or prolonged febrile convulsion occurring in a normal child with a genetic predisposition to convulse with high fever. Such a proposal has prognostic implications. Maytal and Shinnar (1990) studied prospectively a group of children with febrile convulsions lasting longer than 30 minutes, 20% of whom had prior neurological deficits. They concluded that febrile status epilepticus in an otherwise normal child did not significantly increase the risk for subsequent febrile (brief or prolonged) or afebrile seizures in the first few years after the episode whereas febrile status epilepticus in a neurologically impaired child was a risk factor for subsequent febrile and afebrile seizures.

# Prognosis

What then is the prognosis for children who suffer febrile convulsions? They can certainly convulse to death in a febrile status epilepticus but this is relatively rare today. Serious and widespread neurological damage may follow prolonged seizures as in the HHE syndrome. The possibilities for damage to the medial areas of the temporal lobes will be discussed in Chapter 10. The cerebellum and thalamus may also be damaged. The prognosis depends very much on the severity of the individual attack, on the age when it occurs and on the possibility of recurrent seizures. The child's age, sex and family history can be clues to the possibility of recurrence. The overall risk of recurrence is about 33%. Young age of onset (1 year or less) and a family history of febrile convulsions increase the risk to 50% (Berg *et al.*, 1990). Recurrences are more likely in a female aged 1 year or less at the time of the initial attack. A family history of epilepsy is not consistently associated with an increased risk of recurrences. Half of all recurrences take place within 6 months of the initial episode and the majority occur by one year. Complex febrile seizures are associated with a small increased risk of recurrences. The risk of a severe recurrence is low, after either a simple or complex initial episode. Overall, the frequency of non-febrile seizures later is twice as high in those who have recurrences as among those who do not. The doubling of risk comes with the second febrile seizure, and there is no further increase with a greater number of febrile convulsions (Nelson and Ellenberg, 1981).

Most parents will want to know what are the chances of their child developing *later epilepsy*. There are no completely reliable criteria for answering this question. The duration of this seizure is important: long (i.e. over 30 minutes) or focal convulsions increase the risk of later epilepsy considerably, and repeated febrile convulsions are also significant in this respect. A history of antecedent brain injury is also pertinent. An earlier age of onset is important because the chance of a severe seizure is greater the younger the child.

The difficulty in assessing prognosis with respect to later epilepsy is due to the fact that any study which purports to do so must include all the cases of seizures, both mild and severe, occurring at home and in children admitted to hospital, that is, it must be population-based and attempt to follow all affected persons (Ellenberg and Nelson, 1980). Van den Berg and Yerushalmy (1969), who attempted to do this in California, found a rate of subsequent epilepsy of only 3% of the patients. Frantzen (1971) followed up 208 children for several years and found an incidence of later epilepsy of less than 2%, but she commented that about a third of the children had behavioural problems, difficulties in concentration and some degree of mental handicap or delayed speech development. Wallace (1977) reported a series of consecutive hospital admissions of children aged between 2 months and 7 years at the time of the initial seizure (a febrile convulsion was defined as any convulsion occurring with any febrile illness). Among the 112 patients successfully followed up, 55 were aged less than 19 months at the time of the first seizure and 75 had had a complicated initial seizure, that is a prolonged or repeated generalized convulsion or one with focal features. At least one spontaneous seizure occurred in 17% of those followed up for several years and 12% of the patients had recurrent afebrile seizures or epilepsy. Persistent major epilepsy, usually generalized epilepsy of the grand mal type, was commoner in those who had had perinatal problems or a preceding neurodevelopmental abnormality and in those of a lower social class, while prolonged unilateral seizures were more likely to be followed by temporal lobe epilepsy. The National Child Development Study in Great Britain also emphasised the contrasting outlooks for children observed at home or in hospital after their initial febrile convulsion. Of the former group, 12% later developed unprovoked seizures, while a diagnosis of epilepsy was made later in only 0.5% of the latter group (Ross et al., 1980).

Therefore, while all are agreed that children who have had one or more febrile seizures are more likely to become epileptic later, there is disagreement concerning the magnitude of the risk. Perhaps the most important attempt to resolve these apparent differences of opinion has been the prospective study of Nelson and Ellenberg (1976) based on the National Collaborative Perinatal Project (NCPP) of the National Institute of Neurological and Communicative Disorders and Stroke in the USA. Out of a total sample of 54 000 children, 1706 had had febrile convulsions and were examined for risk factors leading to the development of non-febrile seizures, both isolated or recurrent, by the age of 7 years (by this time the great majority of the children who were going to develop epilepsy as a consequence of earlier febrile seizures would have done so). In this study a child was considered to have had a febrile convulsion if the first seizure experienced was accompanied by fever, occurred between the ages of 1 month and 7 years and was not symptomatic of a recognized acute neurological illness such as meningitis, encephalitis or encephalopathy. They divided febrile seizures into those that were uncomplicated and those that had complex features. Characteristics referred to as complex features were a seizure of greater duration than 15 minutes, the occurrence of more than a single seizure within 24 hours and focal features. They also compared those children with febrile seizures whose developmental status had been normal prior to the time of the first seizure with those where it had been suspect or definitely abnormal. Later epilepsy was defined as the occurrence of recurrent non-febrile seizures, not symptomatic of an acute neurological illness, of which at least one attack occurred after 4 years of age.

Nelson and Ellenberg (1976) found that of 39 179 children in the Collaborative Perinatal Project who had never had a febrile seizure and were followed up until 7 years of age, epilepsy developed in 0.5%. Among those children in the series with febrile seizures, 34% had recurrences. The occurrence of later non-febrile seizures was twice as high among those who did have recurrences as among those who did not. Certain characteristics, recognizable after the first seizure, identified children who were at special risk of developing later epilepsy (Nelson and Ellenberg, 1978; Ellenberg and Nelson, 1981). These consisted of suspect or abnormal neurological or developmental status prior to the first seizure, a history of epilepsy of genetic origin in a parent or sibling and a first febrile seizure that lasted longer than 15 minutes, was focal or followed by transient neurological sequelae or was repeated in series on the same day. Sixty per cent of the children studied had no risk factors, and in these, the risk of later epilepsy was 1%. Of 34% with one risk factor, 2% were liable to develop later epilepsy. Two or more risk factors were present in 6% and the risk of later epilepsy in these rose to 10%. Wolf and Forsythe (1989), in a similar study, found a frequency of subsequent non-febrile seizures of 3–5% and three-quarters of their children developed these by 3 years and all by 5 years after the initial convulsion. Annegers et al. (1987), in their extended follow-up of children with febrile convulsions, found a five-fold increase of later unprovoked seizures compared with the general population. The cumulative risk was 4.5% by the age of 10 years and 7% by 25 years. The majority of their cases were in the low risk category, as defined in the NCPP study, and in those the risk of later epilepsy was 2.5% compared with 1.4% in the general population aged 2–25 years.

All who have studied the problem agree that the features associated with the likely development of later epilepsy include prolonged febrile convulsions especially when lateralized, repeated convulsions in the same illness, onset before 1 year, antecedent cerebral injury, associated mental handicap, female sex and a family history of epilepsy of genetic origin in first-degree relatives. Protracted and potentially damaging febrile convulsions are commoner under 1 year and are, more often than not, first seizures. Febrile convulsions with focal features, repeated convulsions in the same illness and long duration are strongly associated with the later development of unprovoked partial seizures, whereas the total number of febrile convulsions experienced and a positive family history of epilepsy are significantly associated with later generalized epilepsies (Annegers *et al.*, 1987). The absolute number of febrile convulsions is not associated with an increased risk of later epilepsy once prior neurodevelopmental abnormalities have been excluded. The risk doubles after the second febrile convulsion but does not increase with a greater number of febrile convulsions, the absolute risk remaining below 5% according to Nelson and Ellenberg (1981). The same authors reported a three fold increase in later epilepsy in the presence of a family history of a genetically-determined epilepsy in first-degree relatives but others have found family history to be a weak predictor of later epilepsy. Finally, Pavone *et al.* (1989) made the interesting observation in their study that, while the incidence of later epilepsy was 3.5% in children experiencing febrile convulsions in the early years of life, it rose to 15.8% in those having their first fever-provoked seizure after the age of 6 years.

Chevrie and Aicardi (1979) have drawn attention to the fact that, quite apart from infantile spasms and severe febrile convulsion, many serious and continuing epilepsies begin in infancy with recurring generalized or partial seizures. These were conveniently divided into cryptogenic or primary and symptomatic or secondary subgroups, the former with a strong genetic component and the latter with anteced-ent pre-or perinatal abnormalities. The cryptogenic cases in their series had a better prognosis, especially when the onset was later than 6 months, but 44% were still having seizures at 5 years. In the symptomatic group, the presentation was more often before 6 months and 73% were still epileptic at 5 years. It is clearly important to distinguish these infants with seizures from those with initial or recurring febrile convulsions, and the distinction is not always straight-forward. The detailed study by Cavazzuti, Farrari and Lalla (1984) showed that the outcome was more favour-able when the seizures were cryptogenic or febrile, were isolated, had their onset in the second 6 months, were generalized, and when the EEG was normal between seizures.

Apart from the development of later epilepsy, the child with febrile convulsions may have other neurological handicaps such as mental retardation. It seems likely that such deficits antedate the onset of febrile seizures. Wolf and Forsythe (1989) found an incidence of mental retardation of 1% in their prospectively studied cohort. However, half of these children had histories of developmental delay prior to the initial febrile convulsion and no child with mental retardation had a febrile convulsion of longer duration than 5 minutes. In a British national cohort studied up to 5 years of age (Verity, Butler and Golding, 1985b), no difference in intellectual performance was found in those with febrile convulsions compared with controls.

## Diagnosis and investigation

The diagnosis of a febrile seizure is relatively easy. The importance of not overlooking the possibility of meningitis as a cause does not require emphasis, especially under the age of 1 year. Occasionally, at least in the author's experience, Reye's syndrome or encephalopathy with fatty degeneration of the viscera can mislead when a convulsion is the presenting feature. The rapid development of coma, hyperpnoea and hyperpyrexia should suggest the correct diagnosis, and laboratory evidence of hypoglycaemia, hyperammonaemia and rising liver enzyme levels in the serum will usually help to confirm the diagnosis. Rigors occurring during acute febrile illnesses and reflex anoxic convulsive syncope (see Chapter 22) should also be considered in the differential diagnosis.

The question of which patients presenting with a febrile convulsion should have a lumbar puncture has been much debated. A lumbar puncture should be performed in selected cases and should probably be done in those under 18 months and certainly in those under 12 months (Rutter and Smales, 1977). The decision should preferably be made by an experienced doctor but should always be done if there is any doubt. A complex febrile convulsion is also an indication and a drowsy or comatose child should have one, bearing in mind the risk of coning (Horwitz *et al.*, 1980). Prior intravenous administration of mannitol is recommended in this latter situation. Routine blood glucose, calcium and electrolyte assays are usually unhelpful. Urinalysis and culture are important because urinary tract infection is a well-documented but unusual cause of a febrile seizure (Rutter and Smales, 1977). Bacterial infections and occult bacteraemia may also be responsible for the pyrexial illness and the indications for blood culture are those pertaining to any febrile child in this age-group (McIntyre *et al.*, 1983).

EEG examination is of very limited value in the diagnosis and assessment of the child with a febrile seizure and should not be performed as a routine investigation. Bilateral slow wave activity is found in the majority of records immediately after the attack and may persist for some days. Focal or asymmetrical slowing may identify the focal or lateralized nature of the attacks. Persistent focal slow waves may be followed by the appearance of a persistent spike focus later indicating the possibility, but not the certainty, of later epilepsy, because even these later abnormalities may disappear from the record with time. Spike-wave paroxysms may be found in older children with a history of febrile convulsions but should be regarded as an expression of a genetic predisposition to epilepsy and not as an indication that epilepsy will develop in the individual patient. Aicardi (1986) considers that prospective EEG studies in children with febrile convulsions have not shown a correlation between the presence of EEG discharges and the later development of non-febrile seizures.

## Treatment and prevention

The majority of febrile convulsions are brief and uncomplicated and have ceased long before medical help arrives. Repeated convulsions within the same illness are unusual. Despite their benign nature, febrile convulsions arouse great anxiety in families unfamiliar with them and many parents believe that their child is about to die, or that, if he survives, he will succumb in a subsequent attack (Baumer *et al.*, 1981). It is consoling to know that no deaths were reported in the American NCPP study. Most young parents are quite unprepared for seizures and do not know what

**Table 6.1 Advice for parents about febrile convulsions**

- Febrile convulsions are not as serious as they look
- The convulsion is due to fever in a child usually aged between 6 months and 4–5 years
- In the convulsion the child becomes unconscious and stiff, with jerking of arms and legs. It is caused by a storm of electrical activity in the brain
- During a convulsion, you should lie the child on his/her side, with the head level or slightly lower than the body
- Note the time when the convulsion starts
- Do not try to force anything into the mouth
- Wait for the convulsion to stop
- The hospital may give you medicine to inject into the child's rectum (rectal diazepam). If the convulsion continues for more than 5 minutes, give one 5 mg dose
- This should stop the convulsion within 10 minutes. If it does not, take the child immediately to the hospital or to your own doctor (dial 999 if necessary)

*Further information about febrile convulsions*
- About 1 child in 30 will have one by the age of 5 years
- Their occurrence does not mean that a child has epilepsy
- 99 out of 100 children with febrile convulsions never have further convulsions (with or without fever) after they reach school age
- Febrile convulsions almost never cause brain damage
- Any illness causing high temperature may bring on a febrile convulsion, usually a cold or other virus infection
- Febrile convulsions may recur in 3 out of 10 children but the risk is much less after 3 years of age
- During the febrile convulsion a child is unconscious and does not suffer pain

*What should I do if my child has a fever?*
- Take his/her temperature
- Keep him/her cool
- Do not overclothe the child or overheat the room
- Give plenty of fluids to drink
- Give a children's paracetamol medicine as follows:
  Up to 1 year — 120 mg (one 5 ml spoonful)
  1 year to 3 years — 240 mg (two 5 ml spoonfuls)
  4 years and over — 360 mg (three 5 ml spoonfuls)
- Repeat the dose 4 hourly until the temperature is normal and then 6 hourly for a further 24 hours
- If he or she seems ill, or has earache or sore throat, ask your doctor to see him/her

(Adapted from: Guidelines for the management of convulsions with fever. Produced by Joint Working Group of the Royal College of Physicians and the British Paediatric Association. British Medical Journal, 1991, 303, 634–636.)

to do when they occur (Rutter and Metcalfe, 1978). Therefore, the most important single item of medical management should be explanation and counselling for the parents with, in addition, appropriate reassurance. Explanatory leaflets should be available from both family doctors and paediatric departments.(Table 6.1)

Parents need to know about first aid treatment in the event of a seizure. Sudden vomiting may follow any seizure, however brief, with a consequent risk of inhalation of vomitus, and so the child should be positioned either prone and with the head to one side or on one side in the recovery position, with the head slightly lower than the trunk. No attempt should be made to force anything between the teeth or gums because damage may be caused to teeth, lips and oral cavity by this well-intentioned procedure.

Advice should be given about the management of future febrile illnesses. Fever is part of the body's response to infection. Excessive defervescence makes excessive metabolic demands on the body to maintain and increase body temperature in response to infection (Hull, 1989). However, reducing body temperature in the febrile child may help to prevent a convulsion and will also make the child feel more comfortable. Measures which may be employed are to remove excessive clothing and avoid too many bed coverings. At the same time, the child should be kept comfortably warm. Drinks should be encouraged to prevent dehydration. Tepid sponging is of doubtful value and cold or icy fluids should never be used. Gentle sponging with lukewarm water may be used and repeated every 2 hours if necessary. Drugs such as paracetamol (10 mg/kg, repeated 4 hourly) or one of the non-steroidal anti-inflammatory agents may be given to reduce fever and alleviate pains and aches. Aspirin is no longer recommended for use in childhood. Antibiotics may be required for bacterial infections.

A significant advance in treatment in the past decade has been the increasing use of diazepam solution rectally to treat a recurrent febrile seizure and shorten its duration (Knudsen, 1979). Diazepam is rapidly absorbed from the rectum and produces effective blood levels within a few minutes. Suppositories of diazepam may take up to 30 minutes to achieve the same blood level. Diazepam is most unlikely to cause respiratory depression when given in this way unless the patient is already on antiepileptic drugs, especially phenobarbitone. The parents are instructed in the method of administration of rectal diazepam, following the child's first febrile convulsion. They are advised to give the drug as soon as possible after the onset of a seizure. In practice, most febrile convulsions will have ceased by the time the parent is ready to give the drug. The recommended dosage is 0.5 mg/kg, repeated after 15 minutes if the child is still convulsing. However, it should be emphasized that if the convulsion lasts longer than a few minutes despite giving rectal diazepam, they should call their doctor, or take the child immediately to hospital. Diazepam for rectal use is produced in disposable plastic tubes (Stesolid) and there are two strengths available containing 5 mg and 10 mg, respectively. If this preparation is not available, diazepam for intravenous use may be given rectally via a short piece of plastic tubing such as an infant's nasogastric feeding tube.

There has been controversy for many years about the need to prevent recurrent febrile convulsions by means of daily antiepileptic drug therapy in doses sufficient to produce effective blood levels. This controversy has now been largely resolved and the use of antiepileptic drugs in this manner has virtually ceased, except possibly in certain exceptional circumstances. The large epidemiological studies of the past 2 decades have demonstrated convincingly that the prognosis for children with febrile convulsions is excellent and that the long-term use of prophylactic antiepileptic drugs does not reduce the incidence of later epilepsy, small though that is anyway. The use of these drugs in adequate daily dosage will undoubtedly reduce the incidence of recurrent febrile seizures (Wolf *et al.*, 1977). It was argued in the past that daily treatment, by reducing the risk of recurrences, thereby reduced the risk of having a severe prolonged febrile seizure. There is little substantial evidence, however, that recurrent febrile convulsions are likely to be more severe than the initial attack (Nelson and Ellenberg, 1978).

The two drugs which have been found to be most effective in reducing the incidence of febrile convulsions when given in adequate daily doses are phenobarbitone and sodium valproate. The definitive study with phenobarbitone was performed by Faerø et al. (1972), using a dosage schedule of 6 mg/kg per day for 2 days, followed by 3–4 mg/kg per day in divided doses. The intermittent use of phenobarbitone orally is quite ineffective, since the attainment of adequate blood levels by this route requires several days. The alternative drug for prophylactic daily use is sodium valproate, which is at least as effective as phenobarbitone in preventing febrile convulsions (Ngwane and Bower, 1980). Neither phenytoin (Melchior, Buchthal, and Lennox-Buchthal, 1971) nor carbamazepine (Camfield, Camfield and Tibbles, 1982) are effective in preventing febrile convulsions although they may make recurrences less frequent.

Although a cheap and effective drug, phenobarbitone unfortunately causes side-effects in over 40% of young children who take it regularly (Wolf and Forsythe, 1978). These include irritability, hyperactivity, aggressiveness and sleeplessness. Similar effects may be seen with primidone. Slow introduction of phenobarbitone and the use of a single dose (5 mg/kg) at bedtime, may reduce the incidence of side effects. Phenobarbitone may interfere with the learning process during critical periods of rapid learning. Farwell *et al.* (1990), in a study of children taking phenobarbitone prophylaxis for febrile convulsion, concluded that the drug depressed cognitive performance and that this disadvantage, which may outlast the administration of the drug by several months, was not offset by the benefit of seizure prevention.

The use of continuous sodium valproate therapy to prevent febrile convulsions is not really an option under 2 years of age because the danger of fatal hepatotoxicity is greatest then (Brown, 1988). When the drug has to be used in this age group, the precautions detailed in Chapter 26 should be observed.

Intermittent prophylaxis with diazepam may be employed successfully using the rectal solution 12-hourly in a febrile child who has previously had a febrile convulsion (Knudsen, 1985). The dose consists of 5 mg 12-hourly under 3 years and 7.5 mg 12-hourly over 3 years of age. Similar benefits have been claimed for oral diazepam administered 12-hourly in a dose of 0.5 mg/kg (Dianese, 1979). Both methods have the disadvantages that parental anxiety may lead to frequent unnecessary treatment and that excessive drug-induced drowsiness may mask the development of important clinical signs in a febrile sick child. Neither method is in wide clinical use, nor is recommended by the writer.

There is no doubt, therefore, that the therapeutic pendulum has swung strongly against the pharmacological prophylaxis of febrile convulsions during the past decade (Addy, 1990). Intermittent therapy with diazepam or no drug treatment are now preferred. Nevertheless, there may be occasions then consideration may need to be given to the need for continuous prophylactic therapy. The National Institutes of Health Consensus Development Panel (1980) recommended consideration of such treatment only in children with known high-risk factors, i.e. neurodevelopmental abnormality, complex and atypical seizures, and a history of epilepsy of genetic origin in parents or siblings. Other possible indications include multiple febrile convulsions, the occurrence of febrile convulsions at or under 1 year, especially in girls, and excessive parental anxiety about the risks of further febrile convulsions. As already indicated, the effective drugs for prophylaxis are phenobarbitone, primidone, and sodium valproate. Treatment, if employed, should be for the shortest period to time, not greater than 2 years in all, for 1 year after the last seizure, and taking care to withdraw treatment gradually.

It should be realized that the problem of febrile convulsions is central to the whole question of epilepsy in early childhood and that it has important implications for the problems of epilepsy in later childhood, adolescence and adult life. A major issue still is whether prolonged and potentially damaging febrile seizures are really the same condition as the common brief uncomplicated attacks. There is also the difficult problem that, in the majority of cases, the most severe convulsion is the initial one, occurring without warning, and it may be asked whether, in the future, it will become possible to investigate children at risk on the basis of a positive family history. Most important, however, is the need to educate family doctors, paramedical staff, accident and emergency staff, and others in proper first aid treatment of a seizure and of the urgent need to stop a continuing seizure as quickly as possible by means of rectal or intravenous diazepam.

There have been significant advances in the understanding of this complex and difficult problem since the first edition of this book was published and it is now possible to answer parents' questions with more assurance than in the past. There will be continuing interest in the problem worldwide. Wallace's (1988) monograph on the subject is strongly recommended to the reader. The report of the Joint Working Group the Research Unit of the Royal College of Physicians and the British Paediatric Association (1991) on this topic should also be consulted (see Table 6.1). The author has also reviewed the subject elsewhere (O'Donohoe, 1992).

## References

ADDY, D. P. (1990) Phenobarbitone and febrile convulsions. *Archives of Disease in Childhood*, **65**, 921

AICARDI, J. (1986) *Epilepsy in Children*, Raven Press, New York

AICARDI, J. and CHEVRIE, J. J. (1970) Convulsive status epilepticus in infants and children. A study of 239 cases. *Epilepsia*, **11**, 187–197

AICARDI, J. and CHEVRIE, J. J. (1976) Febrile convulsions: neurological sequelae and mental retardation. In *Brain Dysfunction in Infantile Febrile Convulsions. International Brain Research Monograph Series* (eds. M. A. B. Brazier and C. Cocceani), Raven Press, New York, pp. 247–257

ANDERSON, A. B., DESISTO, M. H., MARSHALL, P. C. and DEVITT, T. G. (1989) Duration of fever prior to onset of a simple febrile seizure. A predictor of significant illness and neurologic course. *Pediatric Emergency Care*, **5**, 12–15

ANNEGERS, J. F., HAUSER, W. A., SHIRTS, S. B. and KURLAND, L. T. (1987) Factors prognostic of unprovoked seizures after febrile convulsions. *New England Journal of Medicine*, **316**, 493–498

BAUMER, J. H., DAVID, T. J., VALENTINE, S. J., *et al.* (1981) Many parents think their child is dying when having a first febrile convulsion. *Developmental Medicine and Child Neurology*, **23**, 462–464

BERG, A. T., SHINNAR, S., HAUSER, W. A. and LEVENTHAL, J. M. (1990) Predictors of recurrent febrile seizures. A meta-analytic review. *Journal of Pediatrics*, **116**, 329–337

BROWN, J. K. (1988) Valproate toxicity. *Developmental Medicine and Child Neurology*, **30**, 121–125

CAMFIELD, P. R., CAMFIELD, C. S. and TIBBLES, J. A. R. (1982) Carbamazepine does not prevent febrile seizures in phenobarbital failures. *Neurology*, **32**, 288–289

CAVAZZUTI, G. B., FERRARI, P. and LALLA, M. (1984) Follow-up study of 482 cases with convulsive disorders in the first year of life. *Developmental Medicine and Child Neurology*, **26**, 425–437

CHEVRIE, J. J. and AICARDI, J. (1975) Duration and lateralization of febrile convulsions. Aetiological factors. *Epilepsia*, **16**, 781–789

CHEVRIE, J. J. and AICARDI, J. (1979) Convulsive disorders in the first year of life: persistence of epileptic seizures. *Epilepsia*, **20**, 643–649

DIANESE, G. (1979) Prophylactic diazepam in febrile convulsions. *Archives of Disease in Childhood*, **54**, 244–245

ELLENBERG, J. H. and NELSON, K. B. (1980) Sample selection and the natural history of disease. Studies of febrile seizures. *Journal of the American Medical Association*, **243**, 1337–1340

FAERØ, O., KARSTRUP, K. W., LYKKEGAARD NIELSEN, E. *et al.* (1972) Successful prophylaxis of febrile convulsions with phenobarbital. *Epilepsia*, **13**, 279–285

FARWELL, J. R., LEE, Y. J., HIRTZ, D. G. *et al.* (1990) Phenobarbital for febrile seizures: effects on intelligence and or seizure recurrence. *New England Journal of Medicine*, **322**, 364–369

FRANTZEN, E. (1971) The prognosis of febrile convulsions. *Epilepsia*, **12**, 192

GASTAUT, H., POIRIER, F., PAYAN, H. *et al.* (1960) HHE syndrome, hemiconvulsions, hemiplegia, epilepsy. *Epilepsia*, **1**, 418–447

HAUSER, W. A. (1981) The natural history of febrile seizures. In: *Febrile Seizures* (eds K. B. Nelson and J. H. Ellenberg), Raven Press, New York, pp. 5–17

HAUSER, W. A., ANNEGERS, J. F. and KURLAND, J. T. (1977) Febrile convulsions: prognosis for subsequent seizures. *Neurology*, **27**, 341

HIRTZ, D. G., NELSON, K. B. and ELLENBERG, J. H. (1983) Seizures following childhood immunizations. *Journal of Pediatrics*, **102**, 14–18

HORWITZ, S. J., BOXENBAUM, B. and O'BELL, J. (1980) Cerebral herniation in bacterial meningitis in childhood. *Annals of Neurology*, **7**, 524–528

HULL, D. (1989) Fever – the fire of life. *Archieves of Disease in Childhood*, **64**, 1741–1748

JOINT WORKING GROUP OF THE ROYAL COLLEGE OF PHYSICIANS AND THE BRITISH PAEDIATRIC ASSOCIATION (1991) Guidelines for the management of convulsions with fever. *British Medical Journal*, **303**, 634–636

KAJITANI, T., UEOKA, K., NAKAMURA, M. and KUMANOMIDOU, Y. (1981) Febrile convulsions and rolandic discharges. *Brain and Development*, **3**, 351–359

KNUDSEN, F. U. (1979) Rectal administration of diazepam in the acute treatment of convulsions in infants and children. *Archives of Disease in Childhood*, **54**, 855–857

KNUDSEN, F. U. (1985) Effective short-term diazepam prophylaxis in febrile convulsions. *Journal of Pediatrics*, **106**, 487–490

LENNOX-BUCHTHAL, M. A. (1971) Febrile and nocturnal convulsions in monozygotic twins. *Epilepsia*, **12**, 147–156

LENNOX-BUCHTHAL, M. A. (1973) Febrile convulsions: a reappraisal. *Electroencephalography and Clinical Neurophysiology*, Supplement 32

LEWIS, H. M., PARRY, J. V., PARRY. R. P. *et al.* (1979) Role of viruses in febrile convulsions. *Archives of Disease in Childhood*, **54**, 869–876

LIVINGSTON, S. (1954) *The Diagnosis and Treatment of Convulsive Disorders in Children*. Charles C. Thomas, Springfield, Illinois

LIVINGSTON, S. (1972) *Comprehensive Management of Epilepsy in Infancy, Childhood and Adolescence*. Charles C. Thomas, Springfield, Illinois

MCINTYRE, P., KENNEDY, R. and HARRIS, F. (1983) Occult bacteraemia and febrile convulsions. *British Medical Journal*, **286**, 203–206

MAYTAL, J., and SHINNAR, S. (1990) Febrile status epilepticus. *Pediatrics*, **86**, 611–616

MELCHIOR, J. C., BUCHTHAL, F. and LENNOX-BUCHTHAL, M. A. (1971) The ineffectiveness of diphenylhydantoin in preventing febrile convulsions in the age of greatest risk, under three years. *Epilepsia*, **12**, 55–62

MILLICHAP, J. G. (1968) *Febrile Convulsions*. Macmillan, New York

NATIONAL INSTITUTES OF HEALTH CONSENSUS DEVELOPMENT PANEL (1980) Febrile seizures: long-term management of children with fever-associated seizures. *British Medical Journal*, **281**, 277–279

NELSON, K. B. and ELLENBERG, J. H. (1976) Predictors of epilepsy in children who have experienced febrile convulsions. *New England Journal of Medicine*, **295**, 1029–1033

NELSON, K. B. and ELLENBERG, J. H. (1978) Prognosis in children with febrile seizures. *Pediatrics*, **61**, 720–727

NELSON, K. B. and ELLENBERG, J. H. (1981) The role of recurrences in determining outcome of children with febrile seizures. In *Febrile Seizures* (eds. K. B. Nelson and J. H. Ellenberg), Raven Press, New York, pp. 18–25

NGWANE, E. and BOWER, B. (1980) Continuous sodium valproate or phenobarbitone in the prevention of 'simple' febrile convulsions. Comparison by a double-blind trial. *Archives of Disease in Childhood*, **55**, 171–174

O'DONOHOE, N. V.(1992) Febrile convulsions. In: *Epileptic Syndromes in Infancy, Childhood and Adolescence*, 2nd edn (eds J. Roger, M. Bureau, C. Dravet *et al.*), John Libbey, London, pp.45–52

OUNSTED, C. (1971) Some aspects of seizure disorders. In *Recent Advances in Paediatrics* (eds D. Gairdner and D. Hull), J. and R. Churchill, London, pp. 363–400

PAVONE, L., CAVAZZUTI, G. B., INCORPORA, G., *et al.* (1989) Late febrile convulsions: a clinical follow-up. *Brain and Development*, **11**, 183–185

RICH, S. S., ANNEGERS, J. F., HAUSER, W. A. and ANDERSON, V. E. (1987) Complex segregation analysis of febrile convulsions. *American Journal of Human Genetics*, **41**, 249–257

ROGER, J., DRAVET, C. and BUREAU, M. (1982) Unilateral seizures (hemiconvulsion-hemiplegia syndrome and hemiconvulsion-hemiplegia-epilepsy syndrome). *Electroencephalography and Clinical Neurophysiology*, **Supplement 35**, S211–S221

ROSS, E. M., PECKHAM, C. S., WEST, P. B. and BUTLER, N. R. (1980) Epilepsy in childhood: findings from the National Child Development Study. *British Medical Journal*, **280**, 207–210

RUTTER, N. and SMALES, O. R. C. (1977) Role of routine investigations in children presenting with their first febrile convulsion. *Archives of Disease in Childhood*, **52**, 188–191

RUTTER, N. and METCALFE, D. H. (1978) Febrile convulsions – what do parents do? *British Medical Journal*, **277**, 1345–1346

TAYLOR, D. C. and OUNSTED, C. (1971) Biological mechanisms influencing the outcome of seizures in response to fever. *Epilepsia*, **12**, 33–45

VAN DEN BERG, B. J. and YERUSHALMY, J. (1969) Studies on convulsive disorders in young children. 1. Incidence of febrile and non-febrile convulsions by age and other factors. *Pediatric Research*, **3**, 198–304

VERITY, C. M., BUTLER, N. R. and GOLDING, J. (1985a) Febrile convulsions in a national cohort followed up from birth. I. Prevalence and recurrence. *British Medical Journal*, **290**, 1307–1310

VERITY, C. M., BUTLER, N. R. and GOLDING, J. (1985b) Febrile convulsions in a national cohort followed up from birth. II. Medical history and intellectual ability at 5 years of age. *British Medical Journal*, **290**, 1311–1315

WALLACE, S. J. (1975) Factors predisposing to a complicated initial febrile convulsion. *Archives of Disease in Childhood*, **50**, 943–947

WALLACE, S. J. (1976) Neurological and intellectual deficits: convulsions with fever reviewed as acute indications of life-long developmental defects. In *Brain Dysfunction in Infantile Febrile Convulsions* (eds M. A. B. Brazier and F. Coceani), Raven Press, New York, pp. 259–277

WALLACE, S. J. (1977) Spontaneous fits after convulsions with fever. *Archives of Disease in Childhood*, **52**, 192–196

WALLACE, S. J. (1988) *The Child with Febrile Seizures*. Wright, London, Boston

WALLACE, S. J. and ZEALLEY, H. (1970) Neurological, electroencephalographic and virological findings in febrile children. *Archives of Disease in Childhood*, **45**, 611–623

WOLF, S. M., CARR, A., DAVIS, D. C. *et al.* (1977) The value of phenobarbital in a child who has had a single febrile seizure. A controlled prospective study. *Pediatrics*, **59**, 378–385

WOLF, S. M. and FORSYTHE, A. (1978) Behaviour disturbance, phenobarbital and febrile seizures. *Pediatrics*, **61**, 728–731

WOLF, S. M. and FORSYTHE, A. (1989) Epilepsy and mental retardation following febrile seizures in childhood. *Acta Paediatrica Scandinavica*, **78**, 291–295

# Chapter 7

# Primary generalized epilepsy (childhood absence epilepsy)

In 1969, the Commission on Classification of Seizures (Gastaut, 1969) recognized primary generalized seizures as being generalized clinically from the start of each individual attack, as usually making their initial appearance during childhood or early adolescence and as not usually being associated with neurological or psychological evidence of cerebral pathology between attacks. The most important epilepsies causing such seizures are primary major tonic–clonic epilepsy (grand mal), childhood absence epilepsy (petit mal) and myoclonic epilepsy of the primary type. In all of these there is usually a lack of a clear-cut aetiology, suggesting that they are essentially dependent upon a hereditary predisposition which is sufficiently pronounced perhaps to render slight metabolic problems or slight acquired cerebral lesions epileptogenic.

## Terminology

The term 'petit mal' is perhaps the most misused in epileptology. Historically this is understandable because it was originally used as a general term and it was only later that it became condensed into a unitary concept of a particular type of attack. Hughlings Jackson, in his many papers on epilepsy written in the last quarter of the nineteenth century, introduced distinguishing terminology for automatisms and seizures of temporal lobe origin, and gradually the term petit mal came to refer to a particular kind of seizure occurring predominantly in children. In recent years the old term 'absence' has regained popularity as a more vivid and precise description of the attack than 'petit mal'. The word 'absence' was used originally to describe brief attacks of intellectual eclipse. 'Childhood absence epilepsy' is now the favoured term for this epileptic syndrome (Loiseau, 1992).

## Characteristics of the petit mal absence

This is usually associated with an interruption of consciousness, it is of sudden onset and termination, and is commonest in females between 5 and 12 years of age. The attacks are frequent, are usually precipitated by hyperventilation and are rarely associated with mental retardation or structural brain damage. Petit mal is likely to respond to certain specific drugs and the prognosis is good. As a rule there is a typical EEG pattern.

It is important to realize, however, that the diagnosis of the petit mal absence and its differentiation from other types of absence attacks are not always easy. The absences of the secondary generalized epilepsies of the myoclonic type have been mentioned in Chapter 5, and temporal lobe attacks, which give rise to dreamy states or absences of complex symptomatology, are often preceded by unusual or bizarre auras and will be described in Chapter 10. Temporal lobe absences are often associated with or terminate in gestural and oral automatisms including plucking at clothes, chewing, lip smacking and swallowing, and it is a common clinical observation that children having true petit mal absences may have similar motor and oral automatisms. They may, incidentally, also have incontinence of urine which can be extremely embarrassing when attacks are frequent.

## EEG patterns

In order to try to understand the reasons for the similarities between the various types of absence attack, it is necessary to say something about both the EEG patterns and the suggested pathophysiology of absences.

Petit mal attacks are associated with bilaterally synchronous and symmetrical paroxysmal activity in the EEG. The paroxysmal activity occurs bilaterally and begins and ends synchronously over both hemispheres. It is symmetrical, that is the discharges have the same shape and amplitude at homologous points in the two hemispheres. The generalized discharges of petit mal [*Figure 7.1*] consist of regular spike and wave complexes occurring at a rate of 3 per second (3 Hz). The spike lasts about 100 ms and precedes the wave, but it may only be seen as a small projection on the ascending segment of the wave. During an attack the frequency of the complexes is 3 Hz at the beginning of the discharge and slows to 2.5 – 2 Hz towards the end. This type of synchronous, symmetrical and rhythmic paroxysmal activity in the EEG is termed primary bilateral synchrony. In petit mal there is usually a direct temporal relationship between the EEG discharges and the clinical attack, although, of course, the discharges can also occur interictally. It is considered that bursts of spikewave activity should last at least 3 seconds to produce some degree of impairment of consciousness or errors in performance, and that automatisms do not usually appear unless the absences are prolonged (Penry and Dreifuss, 1969). Marked photosensitivity in the EEG is considered an unfavourable prognostic sign, while posterior slow rhythms are considered favourable (Loiseau *et al.*, 1983).

## Theoretical background

The pathogenetic mechanism of the bilaterally synchronous discharges is one of the major problems of epileptology. The classic theory is that of Penfield and Jasper (1954), who proposed that primary bilateral synchrony was produced by a 'pacemaker' situated in the 'centrencephalic system' (by which they meant the central integrating system of the upper part of the brain-stem) which is symmetrically connected with both cerebral hemispheres and serves to coordinate their function. The alternative hypothesis was that of Gibbs and Gibbs (1952), who proposed that the synchronous discharges primarily arose from the cortex.

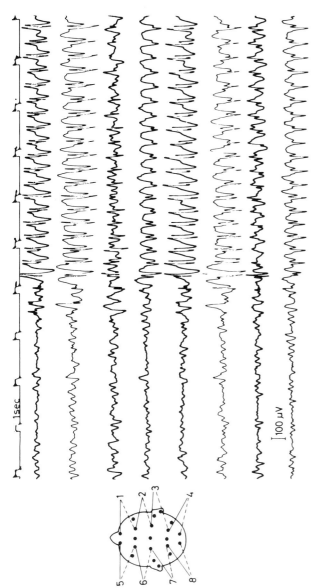

*Figure 7.1* Boy aged 11 years and awake with eyes open. EEG shows generalized bilaterally synchronous spike–wave complexes at 3 Hz occurring during hyperventilation

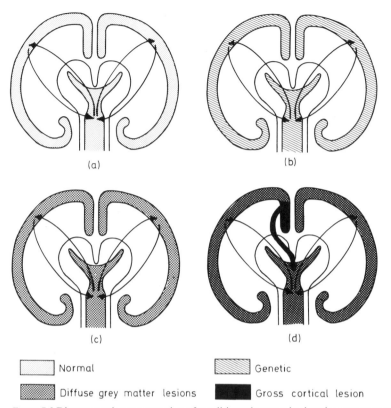

*Figure 7.2* Diagrammatic representation of conditions that may lead to the appearance of generalized bilaterally synchronous spike and wave discharge.

(a) Normal condition. Stippled areas: the cerebral cortex and the reticular systems of the upper brain-stem and thalamus which are mutually interconnected as indicated by the arrows. It is postulated that under normal conditions controls are operative to prevent the occurrence of generalized paroxysmal discharge within this system.

(b) Genetic form of generalized corticoreticular epilepsy. The hatching of cortex and reticular systems indicates a genetically determined disturbance in these areas giving rise to generalized spike and wave discharge.

(c) Diffuse organic grey matter disease giving rise to paroxysmal bilaterally synchronous spike and wave discharges. The coarse dots in the cortex and reticular systems signify diffuse lesions of cortical and subcortical grey matter.

(d) 'Secondary bilateral synchrony': a focal cortical lesion in the parasagittal cortex indicated in solid black, present in brain predisposed to produce paroxysmal bilaterally synchronous discharges, either due to genetic factors (hatching) or due to the presence of diffuse cortical and subcortical grey matter lesions (course dots) may serve as a pacemaker triggering generalized bilaterally synchronous spike and wave discharges. (From Prof. P. Gloor, *Epilepsia*, 1968, by courtesy of Charles C. Thomas, Publishers, Springfield, Illinois)

The generally accepted theory today derives from the work of Gloor (1968), and in a way it is a composite of the two classic theories described above [*Figure 7.2*]. He postulated that the underlying pathophysiological disturbance involved both the cortex and the reticular projection systems of the brain-stem and thalamus, and he avoided stressing a primary role for either. He used the term 'disturbance of the corticoreticular system'. Paroxysmal instability of this system may be genetically

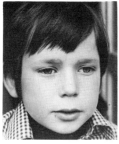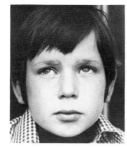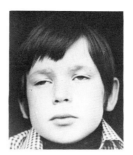

*Figure 7.3* Phases of a petit mal attack

determined or result from biochemical upset or may result from diffuse pathological processes involving either the cortex or the brain stem. In pure petit mal absences hereditary factors and biochemical changes (e.g. with hyperventilation) are paramount in causing discharges in the system with primary bilateral synchrony. In diffuse pathological processes involving grey matter in cortical and subcortical structures, Gloor (1968) suggested that a marked focal accentuation of the disease in some area of the cortex, combined perhaps with a hereditary predisposition, may trigger the system leading to what is called 'secondary bilateral synchrony'. Areas of focal disease in the brain may thus assume the role of pacemaker for the system, causing secondary generalized epilepsies as a result. Secondary bilateral synchrony may be suspected in the EEG when the paroxysmal activity demonstrates irregular morphology, imperfect symmetry, irregularities of form and synchronization, inconsistencies of frequency and also when the generalized discharges coexist with a focal epileptic abnormality.

The concept of diffuse and/or focal disease triggering the corticoreticular system (described above) offers an explanation for the similarities and differences that exist between the absences of true petit mal, the absences of the myoclonic epilepsies and the absences with complex symptomatology which occur in temporal lobe epilepsy.

## The petit mal attack

In the petit mal absence there is a suppression of or a decrease in mental functioning which starts and ends abruptly. The duration of the attack is usually 5 – 15 seconds and occasionally they are longer, but they are rarely longer than 30 seconds. Occasionally, a very prolonged absence or petit mal status may occur. Attacks are usually very frequent throughout the day. The patient is seen to stare, the eyes may drift upwards and the eyelids flicker (*Figure 7.3*). The term 'pyknolepsy' is used sometimes to describe very frequent absences. It is derived from a Greek word meaning 'close together'.

The original 'centrencephalic' theory of Penfield and Jasper (1954) postulated that the discharges arose in those parts of the brain regulating consciousness, i.e. the upper brain stem. Consciousness is an awareness of self and environment and depends on more than just the normal functioning of the brain-stem, which is primarily concerned with wakefulness. The cortex must also be functioning if one is to be conscious. The mental activity involved in consciousness requires the proper functioning of the cerebral hemispheres. In absence attacks attentiveness, perception, cognition and voluntary motor processes are all impaired and these are all higher cortical functions. However, some automatic motor movements may continue. Children with petit mal attacks have been shown to be impaired on tests of sustained attention (Mirsky and van Buren, 1965), which is an essential part of the learning process. The implications of such impairment are clearly important where school performance is concerned, and will be discussed further in Chapter 21.

Gloor (1979) summarized his concept of the petit mal attack by saying that in this condition there is a state of increased excitability of cortical neurons which, for genetic and/or biochemical reasons, makes them, at times, respond to normal afferent thalamocortical volleys by producing spike-wave discharges. These generalized discharges reflect a widespread phase-locked oscillation between excitation (spike) and inhibition (wave) in mutually interconnected thalamo-cortical neuronal networks. This profoundly disrupts the normal pattern of cortical neuronal activity necessary for sustaining such aspects of mental activity as perception, cognition, memory, and voluntary motor activity. It is disruption of such components, rather than the disruption of the more fundamental mechanism of maintenance of consciousness related to the sleep-wakefulness cycle and dependent on upper brain-stem function, which characterizes the absence attack.

No excuses need to be made for dwelling so long on the pathophysiological theories concerning absence attacks. The author is of the opinion that a knowledge of the mechanisms involved is essential for the understanding of many aspects of childhood epilepsy and its problems.

## Genetics

The classic studies on the *genetics of petit mal* are those of Lennox (1951, 1960) on twins. Monozygotic twins showed an 84% concordance for spike-wave discharges at 3 Hz in their EEGs and a 75% concordance for petit mal seizures. No dizygotic twins were concordant for petit mal seizures. Approximately one-third of the patients with petit mal have a family history of petit mal or grand mal; the highest incidence occurs in siblings and parents. Febrile convulsions are also common among siblings. Doose *et al.* (1973) found spike-waves at rest or during hyperventilation in 20% of the siblings of a large series of patients with petit mal while in controls the incidence did not exceed 3%. They suggested, on the basis of their findings, that several genetic factors were responsible for spike-wave absences. Earlier authors, particularly Metrakos and Metrakos (1961), favoured an autosomal dominant gene with an age-dependent manifestation being responsible.

Andermann (1982) has suggested that other genetic or environmental factors must interact with whatever is producing the spike-wave EEG trait before clinical absences occur. For example, two gene loci may need to interact to produce the appropriate phenotype. An unknown proportion of cases may be sporadic or due to phenocopies, that is clinically similar disorders but with different genotypes. However, analogy with gene identification in conditions such as the muscular dystrophies make this unlikely, and it seems probable that different types of the same disease are probably due to an allelic series of mutations at the same gene locus (Rowland, 1988). Absence seizures occurring during late childhood and adolescence may represent such cases, with atypical clinical features, the occurrence of grand mal attacks, relative resistance to therapy and a tendency for the epilepsy to persist into adult life (Delgado-Escueta, Treiman and Walsh, 1983). Not infrequently, this epileptic syndrome is associated with other manifestations of primary generalized epilepsy occurring during adolescence, viz., juvenile myoclonic epilepsy of Janz and generalized tonic–clonic seizures occurring mainly on awakening (Wolf, 1992)., These subjects are dealt with in more detail in Chapter 13. Another rare and probably related syndrome is one which has been entitled, *epilepsy with myoclonic absences*. The age of onset is at about 7 years and frequent daily absences occur accompanied by severe bilateral rhythmic myoclonus, often associated with tonic contractions. There is a male preponderance, unlike childhood absence epilepsy. The EEGs are similar in the two conditions, however. The prognosis is much less favourable than in childhood absence epilepsy and resistance to treatment is common. Combined ethosuximide – sodium valproate therapy is probably the most effective medication but many cases undergo mental deterioration and also progressive deterioration of the seizure disorder (Tassinari and Bureau, 1992).

## Prognosis

One of the most controversial questions concerning petit mal is that of prognosis. Gastaut (1954) believed that petit mal epilepsy is seen almost exclusively in children, more rarely in adolescents, and that it should be regarded as a curiosity in both the adult and the aged. Neurologists who study adults tend to disagree with this point of view, and Currier, Kooi and Saidman (1963) maintained that 56% of their patients continued to have attacks beyond the age of 21 years. Most physicians dealing with childhood epilepsy would very strongly disagree with this view. Probably the differences of opinion arise out of the problem of defining what various authors mean by petit mal. True or pure petit mal is rare.

In the series of Livingston *et al.* (1965) over 15 000 children with epilepsy were studied at the Johns Hopkins Hospital and only 354 or 2.3% fulfilled the true criteria for petit mal. These they defined as paroxysmal periodic attacks of altered consciousness, usually lasting 5–30 seconds, with associated vacant staring. Less frequently they occurred with slight clonic movements of the head and/or upper extremities, and even less often they were associated with automatisms such as smacking of the lips, chewing and swallowing movements and, occasionally, mumbling speech. All of their patients commenced symptoms before 15 years of age. Among the 354 patients 117 were followed up for periods ranging from 5 to 28 years. Ninety-two patients became free and remained free of both the petit mal attacks and the typical EEG abnormalities, and in 89 of these the attacks stopped before the age of 20 years. In 17 children, who had experienced other forms of epilepsy before petit mal started, epileptic fits continued. Of the 100 patients who started with pure petit mal 54 developed grand mal (major generalized epilepsy) later. Livingston *et al.* (1965) concluded that although petit mal itself has a good prognosis the later development of major seizures is common. They believed that the incidence of later major epilepsy could be significantly reduced by giving a drug such as phenobarbitone in combination with a specific petit mal drug such as troxidone or ethosuximide. They conceded that the later the onset of petit mal epilepsy the more likely was the patient to develop other types of seizures, particularly when the onset occurred after 10 years of age. Lennox (1960) shared this opinion precisely and, in the author's view, this is really the kernel of the problem of prognosis and explains why paediatricians and neurologists who study adults differ on the question of prognosis.

Roger (1974) studied 213 patients with petit mal and found that the prognosis was favourable when the onset was from 5 to 9 years of age, when there was no other form of seizure and when the intelligence was normal. An unfavourable prognosis was seen when the condition developed before 5 years or after 10 years. The prognosis was good in 48% of the patients he studied. Lugaresi *et al.* (1974), in an interesting study involving 249 patients from Bologna and Marseilles, were also of the opinion that the condition could be considered benign in 48% of their cases and that it tended towards chronicity in the remaining 52%. However, many of their cases had atypical absences and also atypical EEG findings. They stressed that the late onset of petit mal, the presence of any mental or neurological deficit and the occurrence of other types of seizure were all indicators of a poor prognosis. Sato, Dreifuss and Penry (1976), in a prospective study, demonstrated a 90% remission rate in patients with a negative history of generalized tonic–clonic seizures, normal or above normal intelligence and a negative family history of seizure disorders. However, Loiseau *et al.* (1983) found a 15-year remission rate of only 57.5% in patients with simple absence seizures and 36% of their patients developed tonic–clonic seizures.

To sum up this very difficult problem of prognosis, the author considers, looking from the point of view of the paediatric neurologist or the paediatrician, that pure or true petit mal is a relatively uncommon type of childhood epilepsy (2–5% of most large series of children who had epilepsy) and that it is usually very responsive to modern drugs with complete remission occurring in about three-quarters of the cases. Early onset (before 10 years of age), a good initial response to drugs, the absence of other types of seizure, a typical EEG pattern and normal mental and neurological status all indicate an excellent prognosis.

## Therapy

The specific drug therapy of epilepsy first became possible with the successful use of troxidone by Lennox in 1945. Paramethadione is another member of the oxazolidinedione group of drugs and it should rarely, if ever, be necessary to use these drugs today. They can cause fatal aplastic anaemia, very often in the first 6 months of therapy, and the author has had such a tragic experience of this toxic effect in a young patient. This group of drugs was superseded by the succinimide group of drugs after 1958, and *ethosuximide* is by far the most beneficial of these. Ethosuximide can cause side effects such as nausea, hiccups, headaches, drowsiness, behavioural disturbances and a rash and should be introduced slowly. Toxic blood dyscrasias have been reported, but are rare. Complete control of petit mal may be expected in nearly half the patients and significant improvement in a large proportion of the remainder (O'Donohoe, 1964). The maximum dosage of ethosuximide is usually 500 mg per day in those aged 6 years and under, and 750–1000 mg per day in those over 6 years. It is possible to assay plasma levels of the drug, but these are not often needed because the clinical and EEG responses to the drug are so definite. Ethosuximide still holds its place as a primary drug for petit mal.

*Sodium valproate* has become the leading contender as the drug of choice in petit mal, although it is considerably more expensive than ethosuximide. Simon and Penry (1975) summarized the results of several studies on the efficacy of sodium valproate in petit mal and reported that, of 218 patients, approximately 60% achieved a reduction in seizures ranging from 75 to 100% and a further 25%

improved considerably. Jeavons and Clark (1974) claimed that sodium valproate was the most effective drug for typical or atypical absences and that it would control patients not previously controlled by ethosuximide. They emphasized the comparative rarity of side effects and toxic effects with this drug. Dosage is usually within the range 20–30 mg/kg per day but up to 50 mg/kg per day can be used in intractable cases. When doses of 50 mg/kg per day and over are used plasma levels of the drug should be monitored and platelet counts and bleeding-time tests performed. Thrombocytopenia has been reported with high doses and the drug may also interfere with blood platelet aggregation, thereby prolonging the bleeding times (Sutor and Jesdinsky-Buscher, 1974).

Sherwin (1983), reviewing drugs for absence seizures, considered valproic acid (used instead of sodium valproate in the USA) as the drug of choice, permitting practical control of seizures in the majority of cases. Its efficacy against tonic–clonic seizures, which may occur in over a third of all those affected by absences, is an advantage since ethosuximide is ineffective against such attacks. He considers valproic acid more likely to control prolonged absences culminating in automatisms and less likely to produce minor adverse effects. Santavuori (1983), on the other hand, found little to choose between the drugs in controlling absence seizures and has recommended trying a combination of the two in refractory cases. The author has, like Rowan *et al.* (1983), found valproate–ethosuximide combination therapy extremely useful and effective in cases of childhood absence epilepsy which have resisted control by either drug alone.

*Acetazolamide*, a carbonic anhydrase inhibitor and diuretic, was originally tried as an anticonvulsant in the belief that it would cause a metabolic acidosis and possibly produce beneficial effects similar to those of the ketogenic diet. However, it produced only transitory acidosis and dehydration, but it was shown to have anticonvulsant properties, apparently by inhibiting carbonic anhydrase in the brain and thereby interfering with neuronal conduction. Acetazolamide is always worth trying in the refractory case of petit mal, although its effect sometimes tends to be transient. It occasionally works well in combination with ethosuximide. An average daily dose of the former is 750 mg (10–20 mg per kg per day). Acetazolamide has also been used in females with major seizures who show an increase in the frequency of seizures around the time of menstruation, but the results have been disappointing. Its use is contraindicated in conjunction with the ketogenic diet because the combination can produce a severe metabolic acidosis. Its use in different kinds of epilepsy has been discussed by Forsyth, Owens and Toothill (1981) and by Woodbury and Kemp (1982).

*Clonazepam* has also been used for refractory petit mal. Lund and Trolle (1973) treated resistant cases with clonazepam and reported results comparable with those obtained when using ethosuximide, and other authors have confirmed these findings. The main problem of using clonazepam in this way is that drowsiness may be troublesome in some patients.

Whatever drug is employed, it is essential that treatment is continued for 2 years after the absences have been controlled. Some authors recommend combining the drugs used in major generalized epilepsy with the drugs used in petit mal, claiming that this prevents the later emergence of major convulsions (Loiseau *et al.*, 1983). The author does not usually follow this practice, preferring monotherapy with a drug specific for petit mal. It is important to realize that the drugs commonly used in major epilepsy, such as phenobarbitone, phenytoin and carbamazepine, have no beneficial effect on true petit mal. Sodium valproate, of course, is an exception to this rule and is effective against major seizures and absences. Carbamazepine may, in fact, cause an exacerbation of the epilepsy when used to treat absences (Snead and Hosey, 1985).

## References

ANDERMANN, E. (1982) Multifactorial inheritance of generalized and focal epilepsy. In *Genetic Basis of the Epilepsies* (eds V. E. Anderson, W. A. Hauser, J. K. Penry and C. F. Sing), Raven Press, New York, pp. 335–374

CURRIER, R. D., KOOI, K. A. and SAIDMAN, L. J. (1963) Prognosis of 'pure' petit mal. A follow-up study. *Neurology*, **13**, 959–967

DELGADO-ESCUETA, A. V., TREIMAN, D. M. and WALSH, G. O. (1983) The treatable epilepsies. I. *New England Journal of Medicine*, **308**, 1508–1514

DOOSE, H., GERKEN, H., HORSTMANN, T. and VÖLZKE, E. (1973) Genetic factors in spike-wave absences. *Epilepsia*, **14**, 57–75

FORSYTHE, W. I., OWENS, J. R. and TOOTHILL, C. (1981) Effectiveness of acetazolamide in the treatment of carbamazepine-resistant epilepsy in children. *Developmental Medicine and Child Neurology*, **23**, 761–769

GASTAUT, H. (1954) *The Epilepsies: Electro-Clinical Correlations*, Charles C. Thomas, Springfield, Illinois, p. 86

GASTAUT, H. (1969) Clinical and electroencephalographical classification of epileptic seizures. *Epilepsia*, **10**, Supplement, pp. 2–21

GIBBS, F. A. and GIBBS, E. L. (1952) *Atlas of Electroencephalography*, Vol. 2. Epilepsy, Addison-Wesley, Cambridge, Mass

GLOOR, P. (1968) Generalized cortico-reticular epilepsies. Some considerations of the pathophysiology of generalized bilaterally synchronous spike and wave discharge. *Epilepsia*, **9**, 249–263

GLOOR, P. (1979) Generalized epilepsy with spike-and-wave discharge: a reinterpretation of its electrographic and clinical manifestations. *Epilepsia*, **20**, 571–588

JEAVONS, P. M. and CLARK, J. E. (1974) Sodium valproate in the treatment of epilepsy. *British Medical Journal*, **2**, 584–586

LENNOX, W. G. (1945) The petit mal epilepsies: their treatment with Tridione. *Journal of the American Medical Association*, **129**, 1069–1073

LENNOX, W. G. (1951) The heredity of epilepsy as told by relatives and twins. *Journal of the American Medical Association*, **146**, 529–536

LENNOX, W. G. (1960) *Epilepsy and Related Disorders*, J. and A. Churchill, London, Little, Brown, Boston

LIVINGSTON, S., TORRES, I., PAULI, L. L. and RIDER, R. V. (1965) Petit mal epilepsy: results of a prolonged follow-up of 117 patients. *Journal of the American Medical Association*, **194**, 227–232

LOISEAU, P. (1992) Childhood absence epilepsy. In. *Epileptic Syndromes in Infancy, Childhood and Adolescence*, 2nd Edition (eds J. Roger, M. Bureau, C. Dravet, *et al.*), John Libbey, London, Paris, pp. 135–150

LOISEAU, P., PESTRE, M., DARTIGUES, J. F., *et al.* (1983) Long-term prognosis in two forms of childhood epilepsy: typical absence seizures and epilepsy with rolandic (centrotemporal) EEG foci. *Annals of Neurology*, **13**, 642–648

LUGARESI, E., PAZZAGLIA, P., ROGER, J. and TASSINARI, C. A. (1974) Evolution and prognosis of petit mal. In. *Epilepsy. Proceedings of the Hans Berger Centenary Symposium* (eds P. Harris and C. Mawdsley), Churchill Livingstone, Edinburgh, London, pp. 151–153

LUND, M. and TROLLE, E. (1973) Clonazepam (Ro5–4023) in the treatment of epilepsy. *Acta Neurologica Scandinavica*, **49**, Supplement 53, p. 82

METRAKOS, K. and METRAKOS, J. D. (1961) Genetics of convulsive disorders. 2. Genetic and electroencephalographic studies in centrencephalic epilepsy. *Neurology*, **11**, 464–483

MIRSKY, A. F. and VAN BUREN, J. (1965) On the nature of the 'absence' in centrencephalic epilepsy: a study of some behavioural, electroencephalographical and autonomic factors. *Electroencephalography and Clinical Neurophysiology*, **18**, 334–348

O'DONOHOE, N. V. (1964) Treatment of petit mal with ethosuximide. *Developmental Medicine and Child Neurology*, **6**, 498–501

PENFIELD, W. and JASPER, H. (1954) *Epilepsy and the Functional Anatomy of the Human Brain*. Little Brown, Boston

PENRY, J. K. and DREIFUSS, F. E. (1969) Automatisms associated with the absence of petit mal epilepsy. *Archives of Neurology*, **21**, 142–149

ROGER, J. (1974) Prognostic features of petit mal absence. *Epilepsia*, **15**, 433

ROWAN, A. J., MEIJER, J. W. A., DE-BEER PAWLIKOWSKI, N. *et al*. (1983) Valproate-ethosuximide combination therapy for refractory absence seizures. *Archives of Neurology*, **40**, 797–802

ROWLAND, L. P. (1988) Clinical features of Duchenne muscular dystrophy. The impact of molecular genetics. *Brain*, **111**, 479–495

SANTAVUORI, P. (1983) Absence seizures: valproate or ethosuximide? In *Current Therapy in Epilepsy* (ed. M. V. livanainen). *Acta Neurologica Scandinavica*, **68**, Supplement 97, 41–48

SATO, S., DREIFUSS, F. E. and PENRY, J. K. (1976) Prognosis factors in absence seizures. *Neurology*, **26**, 788–796

SHERWIN, A. L. (1983) Absence seizures. In *Antiepileptic Drug Therapy in Pediatrics* (eds P. L. Morselli, C. E. Pippenger and J. K. Penry), Raven Press, New York, pp. 153–163

SIMON, D. and PENRY, J. K. (1975) Sodium di-n-propylacetate (DPA) in the treatment of epilepsy. *Epilepsia*, **16**, 549–573

SNEAD, O. C. and HOSEY, L. C. (1985) Exacerbation of seizures in children by carbamazepine. *New England Journal of Medicine*, **313**, 916–921

SUTOR, A. H. and JESDINSKY-BUSCHER, C. (1974) Coagulation changes caused by dipropylacetic acid. *Medizinische Welt*, **25**, 447–449

TASSINARI, C. A., BUREAU, M. and THOMAS, P. (1992) Epilepsy with myoclonic absences. In *Epileptic Syndromes in Infancy, Childhood and Adolescence*, 2nd Edition (eds J. Roger, M. Bureau, C. Dravet *et al*.), John Libbey, London, Paris, pp. 151–160

WOLF, P. (1992) Juvenile absence epilepsy. In: *Epileptic Syndromes in Infancy, Childhood and Adolescence*, 2nd edn (eds J. Roger, M. Bureau, C. Dravet *et al*.), John Libbey, London, Paris, pp. 307–312

WOODBURY, D. M. and KEMP, J. W. (1982) Other antiepileptic drugs. Sulphonamides and derivatives: acetazolamide. In: *Antiepileptic Drugs*, 2nd Edition (eds D. M. Woodbury, J. K. Penry and C. E. Pippinger), Raven Press, New York, pp. 771–789

# Chapter 8

# Major generalized epilepsy (grand mal)

At this point it is important to state that, despite the many unusual types of seizure which have already been described, the major tonic-clonic convulsion or grand mal attack is the commonest epileptic manifestation of childhood. Approximately 75–80% of children with epilepsy have this type of seizure as the only evidence of their epilepsy or in combination with other types of seizures. It is this particular type of attack which is associated in the lay mind and, to a lesser extent, in the medical mind with the word 'epilepsy'. This is the archetypal seizure which means total loss of control. Taylor (1973) eloquently described it as an excursion through madness into death. Indeed, as noted already in connection with the first febrile seizure, many parents think that their child has died in the seizure. The individual in a major attack appears totally out of control and this frequently fills the observer with fear and revulsion. A great deal of the prejudice about epilepsy arises from this unfortunate feature.

## Typical attack

A major seizure may occur without warning or may be preceded by an aura. Sometimes the child may be irritable or show other unusual behaviour for hours or even days before an attack. At the beginning of the ictal phase there is sudden loss of consciousness and if standing the patient may fall. Generalized rigidity (tonic phase) is soon followed by very rapid generalized jerking movements (the clonic phase). During this stage the patient may bite his tongue, although this is unusual in children. Similarly, urinary or faecal incontinence are also less frequent in children during this stage than in adults. Children rarely 'cry out' at the onset of a major attack. In the tonic phase the face is cyanosed when respiration ceases briefly. Breathing becomes jerky and stertorous in the clonic phase and the cyanosis lessens. The clonic movements gradually die away and the patient is left limp and relaxed. The patient may recover swiftly after a short seizure, but after any sort of protracted attack he will usually pass into a deep postictal sleep. When he recovers from this, he may feel weak, complain of headache and fatigue, demonstrate irritability and confusion or vomit persistently. Altered speech and transient paralyses or ataxia may occur. Plantar responses may be extensor for a time. Postictal phenomena may be brief or last for hours or even for days. When a series of tonic–clonic seizures takes place without recovery of consciousness between attacks it constitutes status epilepticus, a serious medical emergency. Generalized tonic–clonic seizures occurring in relation to the sleeping-waking cycle are discussed in Chapter 17.

## Classification and diagnosis

Generalized seizures may be subdivided into *primary and secondary generalized attacks*. Primary generalized seizures are generalized from the start and may take the form of convulsive tonic–clonic attacks (grand mal), non-convulsive absences or massive bilateral myoclonic jerks. The EEG patterns during the petit mal absence and the myoclonic attack have already been described. During a major generalized convulsive attack there are diffuse bursts of multiple spikes which continue during the entire period of the active phase of the convulsion and are followed by diffuse high-voltage slow waves in the postconvulsive phase. In the interictal EEGs of patients with major tonic–clonic attacks, one may see a normal background activity on which are superimposed at intervals polyspike and wave discharges or spike and slow-wave discharges without any regular pattern of frequency. One may also see classic spikewave complexes occurring at 3 Hz.

This type of primary grand mal may begin at any time of life but, when it starts in childhood, the onset is usually after the age of 5 years. There is a strong genetic influence. The patient, as a rule, does not show any neurological or psychiatric evidence of central nervous system disease. There is usually an excellent response to the antiepileptic drugs in general use (barbiturates, phenytoin, carbamazepine, sodium valproate). The prognosis for this type of epilepsy (so-called pure grand mal) is excellent, with remission rates of over 90% reported. When absence attacks are also present or when primary grand mal begins in adolescence, the prognosis is not as good (Oller-Daurella and Oller, 1992). Generalized tonic–clonic seizures of the primary type may also occur as part of the syndrome of reflex epilepsy (see Chapter 12).

In general, secondary generalized tonic–clonic seizures are a much commoner manifestation of childhood epilepsy than are grand mal attacks due to primary generalized epilepsy and are encountered as symptoms of many of the secondary or symptomatic epileptic syndromes from infancy onwards. They are often difficult to differentiate precisely from primary generalized convulsive seizures. An accurate history may be helpful. An aura or focal onset indicates that the attack is secondary in type but children may not be able to describe auras. A family history of primary grand mal or of petit mal absences is more likely to be obtained when the patient's epilepsy is primary in type. The patient with primary epilepsy is usually normal physically and intellectually and investigations such as CT scan are negative. EEG abnormalities in patients with primary tonic–clonic seizures are either normal or show generalized discharges, especially those of the 3 Hz spike-wave type. In contrast, patients with secondary generalized tonic–clonic seizures may additionally have a history of partial seizures, either simple or complex, and the family history is often negative for epilepsy. There may be associated neurological or neuropsychiatric findings and neuroimaging is more likely to show evidence of structural brain disease, either localized or diffuse. EEG findings often show focal or multifocal epileptiform discharges. The response to treatment is less predictable and the prognosis is uncertain.

However, it is not always easy to make this sharp differentiation between the two types of generalized epilepsy presenting with generalized convulsive seizures. These epilepsies may be regarded as representing a spectrum of disease (Berkovic *et al.*, 1987). One extreme constitutes pure primary generalized epilepsy, where the major aetiological factor is an inherited trait that is expressed in the EEG as generalized spike-wave discharges at 3 Hz or faster. The other extreme is constituted by secondary generalized epilepsy with a diffuse grey matter disease, usually due to acquired causes. In between, there are a considerable number of patients with a heterogeneous mixture of features of both types. Attempts to categorize the patient's epilepsy as precisely as possible and to construct what has been termed an 'epileptic phenotype' for the patient need to be based on clinical, electrophysiological, radiological, and neuropsychological data.

## Theoretical background

Theories concerning the pathophysiology of primary generalized epilepsy have already been discussed in the preceding chapter. Experimental studies suggest that the primary disturbance is a moderate hyperexcitability of cortical neurons which causes them to respond to thalamocortical volleys by inducing spike-wave discharges. The thalamus constitutes an essential component of the neuronal system which sustains the spike-wave discharges (Gloor, 1979). Generalized spike-wave discharges reflect a widespread phase-locked oscillation between excitation (spike) and inhibition (wave) in mutually interconnected thalamo-cortical neuronal networks. Both levels, cortex and thalamus, are essential for the maintenance of the spike-wave rhythms. Other subcortical structures, for example the substantia nigra, may have a moderating influence on the process (Moshé *et al.*, 1989).

If diffuse cortical hyperexcitability is the dominant neurophysiological disturbance in generalized epilepsy, what is the underlying cause? In primary generalized epilepsy, it seems most likely that genetic and maturational factors are most important in determining whether epilepsy develops or not. Indeed, in some primary generalized epilepsies, such as juvenile myoclonic epilepsy of Janz, a genetic linkage has been confirmed (Delgado-Escueta *et al.*, 1989). Although it is usually assumed that the brain is structurally normal in primary generalized epilepsy, studies have revealed minor morphological changes which have been called 'microdysgenesis' (Meencke and Janz, 1985). The significance of these changes is debatable but they may represent the gross morphological correlate of abnormal synaptic connectivity due to genetic or acquired intrauterine factors, that underlies diffuse cortical hyperexcitability (Berkovic *et al.*, 1987). The mystery of microdysgenesis is further complicated, however, by the fact that these changes have also been described in secondary generalized epilepsy, in addition to the focal or diffuse changes which may be present due to inherited or acquired disease. The implications of this finding have already been discussed in the section dealing with infantile spasms (Chapter 4).

Diffuse cortical hyperexcitability must also have a neurochemical basis. It could be due to decreases in the activity of inhibitory neurotransmitters such as GABA or to increases in the level of excitatory neurotransmitters such as glutamic acid. Changes in the activity of other neurotransmitters might also be present. Firm evidence for such changes is still lacking (Chapman, 1988).

The paramount importance of cortical hyperexcitability in epileptogenesis is borne out by the fact that epileptic activity is rarely, if ever, initiated at the brain-stem or subcortical level (Williams, 1965). Studies of patients with tumours of the central nervous system have shown that while tumours of certain parts of the cortex are particularly likely to be associated with the occurrence of epilepsy, tumours of the diencephelon and mesencephalon are rarely complicated by epilepsy. The cerebellum is known to have a natural inhibitory effect on epileptogenesis and, some years ago, electrical stimulation of the cerebellum by implanted electrodes was used in an attempt to control intractable major generalized seizures. Diffuse degenerative diseases of the upper brain-stem structures are unassociated with epilepsy.

Whatever the site of initiation of the discharges in primary generalized epilepsy, it seems reasonably certain that a central pacemaker system is involved and this is presumably situated in the upper brain-stem or the thalamus. The spike and wave complex in the EEG during an absence seizure is due to reverberating discharges in the corticoreticular and corticothalamic systems, during which inhibition, represented by the slow wave, prevents recruitment of excitation, represented by the spike, and so prevents the development of a tonic-clonic seizure. The hallmark of absence is loss of consciousness due to involvement of the reticular system while there is relative uninvolvement of the motor, sensory and limbic systems. In primary grand mal attacks, however, although the initiation is the same as in an absence, excitatory forces predominate and/or there is a failure of the inhibitory process. Primary generalized grand mal is the genuine, essential or idiopathic epilepsy of the older writers and is historically the first type of epilepsy to be recognized as a separate entity, i.e. the original sacred disease or falling sickness.

As has already been described, a generalized tonic–clonic seizure is frequently a clinical manifestation of secondary generalized epilepsy in the presence of diffuse cerebral disease or of multifocal cerebral lesions. Another common phenomenon is for a partial seizure to become secondarily generalized. This may happen so rapidly that the focal features may not be obvious to an observer and simultaneous video and EEG monitoring may be required for elucidation. In the case of partial or focal seizures due to cortical pathology, activation of the focus is associated with the spread of abnormal brain activity (slow wave and spiking that is asynchronous and asymmetrical). As this activity develops, secondary, bilaterally equal and synchronous discharges appear and involve all cortical areas diffusely. This synchronous discharge has been shown to be the result of corticofugal discharge and involvement of the ascending reticular activating system. In many instances, activation of homologous secondary foci, contralateral to the primary foci, also occurs (Aird, Masland and Woodbury, 1989). Whether or not a partial seizure, either simple or complex, becomes secondarily generalized, depends on the capacity of the inhibitory systems to block the spread of discharge. Some antiepileptic drugs, for example phenytoin, act by blocking the spread of focal discharge and also stimulate the cortico-cerebellar inhibitory systems.

## Prognosis

The prognosis and treatment of grand mal vary depending on the category to which it belongs. In general, grand mal epilepsy is the type most likely to remit in childhood and the one least likely to relapse; pure absence epilepsy is another. Primary generalized epilepsies have an excellent prognosis as a rule but the secondary generalized epilepsies, as emphasized in this and in previous chapters, show a poor response to anticonvulsant medication and generally have a poor prognosis. The prognosis for partial seizures will be considered later but, apart from those of complex symptomatology such as temporal lobe attacks, they respond well to modern therapy. The time of onset of grand mal is also an important prognostic index. By and large, the later the onset in childhood, the better the outlook for seizure control. Major generalized seizures developing in the first 3 years of life, apart from uncomplicated febrile convulsions, do not have a favourable outlook. They are often associated with other seizure types in this age group and are due to serious prenatal, perinatal or postnatal pathology. In contrast, major epilepsy beginning after the age of 5 years and before puberty has a good prognosis (Ellenberg, Hirtz and Nelson, 1984).

The initial response to therapy is important in the prognosis of this condition. Prompt control by medication usually implies a good prognosis and less chance of later relapse. To put this another way, the greater the duration of epilepsy after diagnosis and commencement of therapy, the less likely the prospect of permanent remission (Holowach, Thurston and O'Leary, 1972; Thurston et al., 1982). Livingston (1972) stressed the possibility of relapse during puberty, particularly in females, but Holowach and her colleagues were unable to confirm this observation.

## Therapy

There is now a wide range of drugs available for treating grand mal. These drugs are mainly effective in primary generalized tonic–clonic seizures and partial seizures with secondary generalization. They include phenobarbitone, phenytoin, primidone, carbamazepine and sodium valproate. The relative advantages and disadvantages of these various drugs and of others such as the benzodiazepines will be discussed in detail in the later chapters on drug therapy (see Chapters 25 and 26).

A controlled comparative study of the major drugs available for treating generalized tonic-clonic seizures in children, i.e. the barbiturates, phenytoin, carbamazepine, and sodium valproate, failed to detect any differences in efficacy between the various drugs with reference to seizure type (de Silva et al., 1989). Clinicians will be influenced in their choice by the relative safety of the various drugs, by their tendency or otherwise to cause side-effects, particularly effects on cognition and behaviour, and in some countries, by their relative costs. Sodium valproate is effective across a wide range of seizure types but is particularly successful in controlling the seizures of primary generalized epilepsies, especially those seizures characterized by generalized spike and wave abnormalities in the EEG. These include both absences and tonic-clonic seizures (Collaborative Study Group, 1987). The seizures of secondary generalized epilepsy also show a good response to this drug. Sodium valproate may also be effective in partial seizures which are complicated by secondary generalization (Dean and Penry, 1988), although in those circumstances carbamazepine or phenytoin will generally be preferred as initial treatment.

The optimal duration of therapy with major generalized seizures is also a debatable issue. There is no doubt in the author's mind that the aetiology of the epilepsy is all-important in determining the response to and the duration of treatment and also the likelihood of a long-term permanent remission. In these respects, primary generalized seizures usually present less of a problem than do secondary generalized seizures or partial seizures with secondary generalization. Formerly, 4 asymptomatic years were considered necessary before withdrawing therapy, but the general opinion nowadays is that, in children with epilepsy of whatever kind who have been seizure free for 2–3 years, antiepileptic medications may safely be withdrawn with the expectation that 75% of cases will remain free of seizures (Robinson, 1984; Shinnar et al., 1985). Treatment should always be discontinued gradually over a period of several months, and if the child is receiving more than one antiepileptic drug, they should be withdrawn independently. It is wise to exercise caution in stopping treatment where the seizures had resisted initial control for a period of years, where different kinds of attack were occurring in the same patient, where there are associated neurological and psychological deficits and where the EEG continues to show frequent paroxysmal abnormalities, was severely abnormal initially or has changed little over a prolonged period of observation (Holowach, Thurston and O'Leary, 1972). However, although the EEG is a valuable diagnostic tool, particularly during the initial evaluation, it is usually imprudent to prolong daily administration of antiepileptic medication on the basis of the EEG alone, in the absence of other risk factors.

## The single attack

It is appropriate at this point to consider the child with the isolated epileptic seizure, i.e. the convulsion which occurs only once. These are usually generalized tonic–clonic attacks, and since epilepsy is a chronic recurrent condition these individuals should not be regarded as epileptic.

Any person in untoward circumstances may be liable to a convulsion, and it is only when attacks are habitual that a diagnosis of epilepsy should be made. When any convulsion has occurred, and this is particularly true of the single attack, a very careful history should be obtained, including a full account of the physical and psychological circumstances surrounding the attack. The more potent the immediate cause the less serious is the convulsion's significance. This is as true in childhood is it is in adult life. The patient who has had a single major seizure is in need of careful examination and investigation and does not necessarily need treatment. Indeed, if all investigations are negative prescribing antiepileptic drugs may not help the patient because it may never be known whether or not he would have had another attack. Isolated seizures are not uncommon and treating them may imply a diagnosis of epilepsy without justification. Subsequently, the 'undiagnosis of epilepsy' [a term coined by Jeavons (1983)] may be difficult. It may well be that the child with a single major seizure is suffering from primary generalized epilepsy even though all investigations are entirely negative but, in this particular context, it is better to withhold drugs until further attacks occur, if they ever do. However, it is dangerous to generalize about the problem of the single seizure and each case must be judged on its merits. Livingston (1960) argued that anticonvulsant treatment was mandatory in the child with the single seizure. His reasons were that parents were frightened by the dramatic events of a convulsion and were afraid that injury, prolonged unconsciousness or death might occur in another one. Parents also feared the social stigma attached to their child having a convulsion in public. He felt that parents were happier and more confident about the future when their child was on therapy, and he considered that prevention of recurrent seizures was important because of the known association between prolonged attacks and irreversible organic brain damage. This must now be considered on extreme view of the problem.

The best way to reconcile these two opposing views about the problem of the single seizure is to look at each case individually and, particularly, to examine the circumstances in which the convulsion takes place. In the first place the clinician must be sure that an actual epileptic attack has occurred. This matter will be dealt with in detail later in the differential diagnosis of epilepsy (see Chapter 22), but, at this point, it should be emphasized that the brief tonic stiffening which so often occurs in a syncopal attack should not be misdiagnosed as epilepsy. It must be realized that anybody can have a seizure given the right precipitating circumstances. Convulsions occurring in a setting of intercurrent illness and high fever have been described already and, indeed, severe illness and fever at any time may lead to some degree of encephalopathy and be associated with a seizure. Biochemical and metabolic upset may lead to a single seizure occurring; for instance, this may be seen when renal function is compromised either temporarily or permanently. Certainly severe emotional upset can bring about a seizure in an individual with an increased susceptibility to epilepsy (for genetic reasons) and the attack may be an isolated one. For example, the author remembers an 11-year-old boy who witnessed the sudden unexpected death of his father from coronary thrombosis and 1 week later, while suffering considerable emotional anguish, he had a generalized tonic–clonic seizure which subsequently never recurred. Sometimes, emotional upset and severe fatigue may combine to precipitate a single seizure and, particularly in adolescents with epilepsy, chronic fatigue is a well-known precipitating cause of habitual epileptic attacks. Similarly, the frustrations and irritations which beset the individual with epilepsy in his daily life may make his epilepsy worse. Occasional generalized tonic–clonic seizures may occur, often in a setting of intercurrent infection, in patients with a previous history of febrile convulsions in early childhood. Such recurrences are rare after the age of 10 years.

There have been several studies in recent years of large groups of children having their first single unprovoked afebrile seizure. Reviewing these, Robinson (1984) concluded that the risk of a recurrence was of the order of 50% or less. Shinnar et al. (1990), in a prospective study of 288 patients, aged 1 month to 19 years, who presented in the emergency room with their first unprovoked afebrile seizure, found that the cumulative risk of recurrence was 26% at 12 months, 36% at 24 months, 40% at 36 months and 42% at 48 months. A total of 84% were untreated with drugs and only 9% were treated for longer than 3 months. The key risk factors for recurrence were the aetiology of the seizures (idiopathic versus a remote symptomatic cause) and the EEG. Using these two variables, the authors were able to identify a large group with a low risk of recurrence, i.e. those having an idiopathic first seizure with a normal EEG. Those with an idiopathic first seizure combined with an abnormal EEG and a history of epilepsy in a first-degree relative had a much higher recurrence risk. In those patients with a possible remote symptomatic cause, a previous history of a febrile seizure or the occurrence of a partial seizure as the presenting symptom were significant predictors of recurrence. It is worth noting, however, that in benign partial epilepsy with centro-temporal spike discharges (see Chapter 9), 20% or more of those affected experience a single seizure only (Loiseau and Duché, 1989).

## Counselling and advising parents

Parents of children who suffer from major epileptic seizures are naturally apprehensive about the attacks and fear that their child may die in one of them. It is important to reassure them that this seldom occurs, provided the attacks are not prolonged. The dangers of sustained and repeated attacks (status epilepticus) will be discussed in Chapter 11. It is also important to remember that seizures which are atypical for a particular individual or which last longer than usual may, in fact, sometimes be symptomatic of some other acute disorder, e.g. meningitis.

### What to do for a major attack

The parents should be instructed in what they should do during a grand mal attack. If possible, the patient should be allowed to remain where he is, ensuring at the same time that he cannot injure himself by knocking against some immovable object or falling off a bed or chair, and he should be prevented from burning himself if he collapses near a fire. The danger of drowning in a bath should be remembered and bathroom doors should never be locked. Moreover, if convulsions are frequent, showering is preferable. Tight clothing around the neck should be loosened, and the patient should be turned on his side so that mucus and saliva can flow easily from the mouth. Furthermore, this is a safe posture if vomiting occurs and avoids the danger of aspiration of vomitus. It is not necessary to insert an object between the teeth in children, as a rule, unless the individual habitually bites his tongue or cheeks during the seizure. If something must be inserted, then hard metal objects should be eschewed as they may break the teeth. Firm blunt non-damaging objects such as a well-padded tongue depressor or a piece of leather may be used, inserting it anteriorly and then moving it sideways to lie between the posterior teeth. The tongue may fall back and cause respiratory obstruction. With the patient on his side the tongue may be brought forwards by slightly extending the head and neck, inserting one's fingers behind the ramus of the mandible on both sides and drawing the mandible, and with it the tongue, forwards.

If the parents wish to have medication available at home for use in the event of a generalized seizure becoming prolonged, then it is reasonable to prescribe diazepam for rectal use (0.5 mg per kg) in such an emergency. However, there is an increased risk of respiratory depression occurring when diazepam is given to patients who are already on long-term treatment of their epilepsy with barbiturates.

*The postictal symptoms* vary in duration depending on the severity of the actual seizure. The postictal period of unconsciousness is something which alarms many parents, and they should be told that this is a recovery phase, that no interference is necessary and that the patient should be allowed to 'sleep off' the attack in a comfortable position. This should preferably be on a bed from which the pillows have been removed in order to maintain a horizontal position, thus avoiding the risk of respiratory obstruction. It is important that teachers, who may be involved in the care of a child with epilepsy, should also be familiar with the ordinary management of a major convulsion. Hospitalization is rarely necessary unless the particular episode is prolonged or complicated in some way.

# References

AIRD, R. B., MASLAND, R. L. and WOODBURY, D. M. (1989) Hypothesis: the classification of epileptic seizures according to systems of the CNS. *Epilepsy Research*, 3, 77–81

BERKOVIC, S. F., ANDERMANN, F., ANDERMANN, E. and GLOOR, P. (1987) Concepts of absence epilepsies. Discrete syndromes or biologic continuum? *Neurology*, 27, 993–100

CHAPMAN, A. G. (1988) Amino acid abnormalities in plasma, CSF and brain in epilepsy. In

*Recent Advances in Epilepsy*, No. 4. (eds. T. A. Pedley and B. S. Meldrum), Churchill Livingstone, Edinburgh, London, pp. 45–62

COLLABORATIVE STUDY GROUP (1987) Monotherapy with valproate in primary generalized epilepsies. *Epilepsia*, 28, Supplement 2, S8–S11

DE SILVA, M., MCARDLE, B., MCGOWAN, M. *et al.* (1989) Monotherapy for newly diagnosed childhood epilepsy. A comparative trial and prognostic evaluation. *Epilepsia*, 30, 662

DEAN, J. C. and PENRY, J. K. (1988) Valproate monotherapy in 30 patients with partial seizures. *Epilepsia*, 29, 140–144.

DELGADO-ESCUETA, A. V., GREENBERG, D. A., TREIMAN, L. *et al.* (1989) Mapping the gene for juvenile myoclonic epilepsy. *Epilepsia*, 30, Supplement 4, S8–S18

ELLENBERG, J. H., HIRTZ, D. G., and NELSON, K. B. (1984) Age of onset of seizures in young children. *Annals of Neurology*, 15, 127–134

GLOOR, P. (1979) Generalized epilepsy with spike-and-wave discharge: a reinterpretation of its electrographic and clinical manifestations. *Epilepsia*, 20, 571–588

HOLOWACH, J., THURSTON, D. L. and O'LEARY, J. (1972) Prognosis in childhood epilepsy. Follow-up study of 148 cases in which therapy had been suspended after prolonged anti-convulsant control. *New England Journal of Medicine*, 286, 169–174

JEAVONS, P. M. (1983) Non-epileptic attacks in childhood. In *Research Progress in Epilepsy* (ed. F. C. Rose), London, Pitman, pp. 224–230.

LIVINGSTON, S. (1960) Management of the child with one epileptic seizure. *Journal of the American Medical Association*, 174, 135–139.

LIVINGSTON, S. (1972) *Comprehensive Management of Epilepsy in Infancy, Childhood and Adolescence*. Charles C. Thomas, Springfield, Illinois, p. 585.

LOISEAU, P. and DUCHÉ, B. (1989) Benign childhood epilepsy with centrotemporal spikes. *Cleveland Clinic Journal of Medicine*, 56, Supplement Part 1, S17–S22

MEENCKE, H. J. and JANZ, D. (1984) Neuropathological findings in primary generalized epilepsy: a study of eight cases. *Epilepsia*, 25, 8–21.

MOSHÉ, S. L., SPERBER, E. F., BROWN, L. L. *et al.* (1989) Experimental epilepsy: developmental aspects. *Cleveland Clinic Journal of Medicine*, 56, Supplement Part 1, S92–S99

OLLER-DAURELLA, L., and OLLER, F.-V. (1992) Epilepsy with generalized tonic-clonic seizures in childhood. Does a childhood 'grand mal' syndrome exist?. In: *Epileptic Syndromes in Infancy, Childhood and Adolescence* (eds. J. Roger, M. Bureau, C. Dravet, *et al.*) John Libbey, London, Paris, pp. 161–172

ROBINSON, R. (1984) When to start and stop anticonvulsants. In *Recent Advances in Paediatrics*, No. 7 (ed. R. Meadow), Churchill Livingstone, Edinburgh, London, pp. 155–174

SHINNAR, S., VINING, E. P. G., MELLITS, E. D. *et al.* (1985) Discontinuing antiepileptic medication in children with epilepsy after two years without seizures. *New England Journal of Medicine*, 313, 976–980

SHINNAR, S., BERG, A. T., MOSHÉ, S. L. *et al.* (1990) Risk of seizure recurrence following a first unprovoked seizure in childhood. A prospective study. *Pediatrics*, 85, 1076–1085.

THURSTON, J. H., THURSTON, D. L., HIXON, B. B. and KELLER, A. J. (1982) Prognosis of childhood epilepsy: additional follow-up of 148 children 15 to 23 years after withdrawal of anticonvulsant therapy. *New England Journal of Medicine*, 306, 831–836

TAYLOR, D. C. (1973) Aspects of seizure disorders. II. On prejudice. *Developmental Medicine and Child Neurology*, 15, 91–94

WILLIAMS, D. (1965) The thalamus and epilepsy. *Brain*, 88, 539–556.

# Chapter 9

# Partial or localization-related epilepsies I

## Definitions

Partial epilepsies are disturbances which apparently originate in more or less well defined areas of the brain and produce a variety of symptoms depending on the site of the epileptic focus. The hallmark of a partial epilepsy is the presence of an epileptiform EEG discharge localized to a portion of one cerebral hemisphere. At the onset, the epileptic episode seems to involve only particular regions of the body, but the attack may spread and become generalized, thereby becoming a secondarily generalized seizure. The word 'focal' may be used synonymously with 'partial' in this context. The partial seizures are further subdivided into those of simple or elementary symptomatology and those of complex symptomatology. In the former, where the attack remains localized, consciousness is usually retained but in the latter it is impaired or lost. Partial seizures, as already discussed (Chapter 3), are common in the neonate but, excluding benign partial epilepsy with centro-temporal spike discharges, simple partial seizures are relatively uncommon in childhood. The symptomatology is motor in type in the great majority although a proportion experience somatosensory symptoms (Blume, 1989). Although motor or somatosensory symptoms may precede the onset of a complex partial seizure and then represent the aura (See Chapter 10), disturbances of affect or memory, autonomic or special sensory sensations are more commonly experienced as antecedent auras in these attacks. Some generalized motor seizures (grand mal) begin as partial or focal attacks in one part of the cortex, but generalization occurs so rapidly that the initial features may not be apparent to the observer, even though the child may experience a brief motor or sensory aura.

The term *Jacksonian or Rolandic convulsion*, 'a marching spasm or sensation' to quote Lennox (1960), is used to describe an attack which begins in a distal part of a limb and travels proximally. The patient or an observer may see clonic movements beginning, say, in a toe and then travelling to the foot, the knees and to the ipsilateral upper limb. Consciousness is usually lost when the head and neck are reached. In a corresponding sensory attack, feelings of pins and needles or tingling spread proximally and there may be indescribable sensations of heat or cold or other bizarre feelings in the limbs. Mixtures of motor and sensory phenomena may occur. Sometimes, an older patient can abort or limit an attack by applying strong stimuli to the affected limb by the contralateral hand, for example by grasping it firmly, but most patients feel helpless in the face of a 'marching' seizure. As already stated, loss of consciousness occurs when the head and neck are reached and this is usually followed by generalization of the attack. The period of unconsciousness is usually shorter than in a primary generalized major attack but postictal confusion, sleep and transient paralysis (Todd's paralysis) do occur and the period of paralysis may be brief or last up to 12 or even 14 hours. Its resolution may be followed by the persistence of minimal neurological signs on the affected side.

Unfortunately, the term 'Jacksonian', as with so much of the terminology of epilepsy, is used very loosely in the medical literature and is often applied to any attack with a focal motor component. Livingston (1972) strongly emphasized that, in his experience, true Jacksonian seizures, with the characteristic march, were comparatively rare in childhood and this is certainly the author's experience also. A more common type of partial seizure which is seen in children, including young children, is what is known as an adversive attack. There may or may not be prodromal symptoms followed by turning of the eyes and head, and later rotation of the body away from the side of the epileptogenic focus. There is usually a gradual loss of posture and consciousness and the patient may fall to the ground. As he does so the limbs towards which he faces extend and the contralateral limbs flex, much as in the posture associated with the asymmetrical tonic neck reflex in early infancy. Sometimes, partial motor clonic seizures involving face, arm, hand or leg may follow the adversive turning and provide evidence of lateralization to the contralateral hemisphere. Adversive turning is usually associated with the presence of a frontal lobe lesion and occurs as an initial ictal manifestation. There is an associated loss of consciousness in the majority of cases. Such unconscious head turning may, however, sometimes be observed in seizures arising in the temporal, parietal and occipital lobes, presumably as a result of spread to the frontal areas. Conscious head turning, on the other hand, although it is less common than unconscious turning, is usually of frontal lobe origin only. Some frontal lesions may be associated with ipsilateral eye deviation and head turning (Quesney, 1986). Complex partial seizures of frontal lobe origin are described in the following chapter.

## Pathophysiology

The pathophysiology of focal seizures is fairly well understood. Local changes occurring in groups of cortical neurons produce spontaneous and repetitive neuronal discharges. Such discharges are usually recorded as localized spike foci in the EEG.

Periodically, the epileptic discharges may propagate to the corresponding point in the opposite hemisphere via the corpus callosum, forming a 'mirror focus' but without any clinical change. However, continuous electrical bombardment initiated at the primary site may permanently alter the excitability of the secondary site. As a result of this kindling-like phenomenon, the secondary site may begin independently to generate epileptiform activity and, eventually, even clinical seizures (Moshé and Ludvig, 1988). Alternatively, the discharge may spread locally in the brain through short association fibres and involve progressively wider areas of the cortex or they may extend to the appropriate segment of the thalamus establishing a thalamocortical circuit of impulses. In this case, the patient experiences a focal seizure which may constitute the complete ictal event or may appear as an aura before a secondarily generalized seizure develops.

The discharges may be confined to one area of the cortex only, so that jerking of a limb or one side of the body continues for hours or days. This is called *epilepsia partialis continua* and is rare in childhood except in association with serious brain disease (see page 103). The discharges may advance over the cortex, producing a Jacksonian march of symptoms, and they may extend to the medial thalamic nuclei bilaterally and thence to the reticular activating system in the brain stem. When this happens consciousness is lost and the discharges then spread upwards and symmetrically to involve both hemispheres diffusely. At this stage the EEG will show bilateral high voltage high-frequency discharges and the pyramidal and extrapyramidal systems then conduct the discharges downwards again to the spinal cord, producing the tonic stage of the grand mal attack. After some seconds of tonic contraction, during which the high-frequency discharges continue, the patient relaxes intermittently, producing the clonic stage of the seizure. This stage is due to a periodic interruption of the tonic stage and at this point in the EEG the cortical spikes are followed by surface-negative slow waves due to the development of inhibitory postsynaptic potentials acting as a 'brake' on the excitatory postsynaptic potentials characterized by the surface negative spike discharges. The EEG record then enters a silent or isoelectric flat stage as the convulsive movements cease and this is followed by the appearance of generalized high-voltage irregular slow waves and a gradual return to the resting interseizure EEG pattern with the reappearance of the original focal abnormality. Focal postictal or Todd's paralysis, when it occurs, may be the result of enhanced focal inhibitory activity rather than the result of neuronal exhaustion (Efron, 1961). This suggestion appears to be supported by the observation that some of the most severe Todd's paralyses occur in patients who have had sensory seizures only.

## Aetiology

The International Classification (Gastaut, 1970) defines the aetiology of partial seizures as follows: 'usually related to a wide variety of local brain lesions (cause known, suspected or unknown); constitutional factors may be important.' Constitutional or genetic factors certainly play a much less significant role than in the primary generalized epilepsies but there are exceptions, for example where an inherited predisposition to convulse with fever is complicated by a prolonged febrile seizure and subsequent focal damage and also in benign partial epilepsy (see page 103).

Furthermore, it should be remembered that in the genesis of any focal epilepsy, exogenous environmental factors and also maturational factors must interact with the genotype to produce the final clinical and EEG phenotype with respect to epilepsy (Andermann, 1982).

Although perinatal brain lesions, particularly those due to hypoxia–ischaemia, are frequently thought to be implicated in the genesis of partial epilepsies, it seems unlikely that they are common aetiological factors and experience shows that the epilepsies that result from perinatal factors are usually of a diffuse rather than a localized type and are associated with grave mental and neurological deficits (Hauser and Nelson, 1989). However, even an uneventful birth history does not exclude the possibility of minor brain injury occurring at that time and leaving slight gliotic scarring in its wake. Very often in the past the exact aetiological cause of a partial epilepsy could not be identified, but, with the increasing use of computed tomography (CT) and magnetic resonance imaging (MRI) to study such cases, structural causes are being identified provided they are of sufficient size to be visualized by these techniques. Cortical developmental abnormalities, including areas of pachygyria, microgyria and heterotopias, are responsible more often than was realized and slow-growing tumours are also being identified more frequently nowadays (Blume, 1989; Lee *et al.*, 1989). Neurocutaneous syndromes, arteriovenous malformations, and old infarctions (sometimes prenatal and followed by the development of a porencephalic cyst) are less common but well recognized causes. The severe infections of childhood, such as meningitis or encephalitis, may cause focal seizures, usually within 2 years (Pomeroy *et al.*, 1990). Metabolic disturbances in the dehydrated infant, especially hypernatraemia, may be responsible. Prolonged febrile seizures predominently damage the temporal lobes, but may also cause cortical damage elsewhere. Head injury as a cause of post-traumatic epilepsy is an important aetiological factor at all stages of life (see Chapter 14).

Partial or focal motor seizures are frequent in children with *cerebral palsy*, as are also generalized convulsions. The incidence of epilepsy in cerebral palsy has been variously reported as being from 20 to 50%. Up to 50% of children with hemiplegia may suffer from epilepsy, often partial in type, and fits are also common in severely tetraplegic children. Some cases of spastic diplegia are associated with epilepsy but it is rare in the athetoid or dystonic variety of cerebral palsy and in ataxic cerebral palsy. Babies with cerebral palsy may develop infantile spasms or one of the myoclonic epilepsies. Epilepsy is a most important complication of cerebral palsy and may be as handicapping as mental retardation as far as the patient's chances of obtaining employment later are concerned. There is a close relationship between cerebral palsy, mental handicap, and the occurrence of epilepsy. When cerebral palsy is complicated by the presence of mental handicap, epilepsy may develop in up to half of the affected children. The risk of epilepsy is increased the greater the degree of intellectual deficit and the more severe the motor handicap (Hauser and Nelson, 1989).

Partial and secondarily generalized seizures may occur in children in whom *hydrocephalus* has been treated by ventriculoatrial shunt procedures. Hosking (1974) studied 200 randomly selected children with hydrocephalus and in half of the cases the condition was associated with spina bifida and in half the hydrocephalus was either primary or secondary to cerebral haemorrhage in the neonate or meningitis in infancy. Children who did not survive for more than 6 months were not included. Of the 200 cases 197 were treated early by a shunting procedure incorporating a Spitz–Holter valve, and follow-up in the majority exceeded 5 years. The overall frequency of seizures, either single or recurrent, in the whole group was approximately 30%, 26% in the hydrocephalus–spina bifida group and 35% in the group with hydrocephalus alone. The incidence of seizures was 27% in primary or congenital hydrocephalus, 35% of the posthaemorrhage group and 54% in the postmeningitis group. A small number of patients had seizures in relation to valve blockage and two children in the hydrocephalus–spina bifida group developed infantile spasms. Frequent valve revisions appeared to increase the tendency to have seizures subsequently.

More recent studies suggest that the incidence of epilepsy following shunting procedures is still very high – of the order of 20% (Dan and Wade, 1986). This is related to the high level of epileptogenicity of the anatomical areas in which shunts are placed and to the fact that children requiring shunting procedures usually have other pathology which may also be associated with an increased propensity for seizures.

Epilepsia partialis continua is also known as Kojewnikow's syndrome after the author of the original description in 1895. The condition is a form of partial status epilepticus, persisting for prolonged periods of time and characterized by rhythmically repeated twitching of a group of muscles, usually involving a distal part of a limb. It is caused by structural lesions involving the motor cortex or a closely adjacent area. It is now accepted that there are two distinct groups of patients who develop this syndrome in childhood (Bancaud, 1992). In the first group, the onset is early and usually before the age of 2 years. Generalized and unilateral convulsions occur and there may be episodes of status epilepticus. The condition is non-progressive in this group and is usually caused by a stable brain lesion of central location and of prenatal, perinatal or postnatal origin. These patients do not demonstrate a progressive course.

In the second group, the onset is later but usually before the age of 10 years. The median age of onset is 5 years and it may sometimes occur as early as the second year of life (Rasmussen and Andermann, 1989). Rasmussen and his colleagues first described this particular syndrome of progressive epilepsy in 1958 and it is now often called by his name. He has observed that, in the majority of patients, there is an infectious or inflammatory episode involving the patient or the immediate family at or just before the onset of the seizures. A variety of seizure types occurs and there are repeated episodes of epilepsia partialis continua. The occurrence of a slowly progressive neurological deterioration, particularly some combination of hemiparesis, gradual reduction in mental capacity, dysphasia and hemianopsia, is a pathognomonic feature of the syndrome. The disease process is, however very gradual and insidious.

Lateralized EEG abnormalities become more prominent as the disease progresses and neuroradiological investigations show progressive unilateral atrophy of the involved hemisphere. The cerebrospinal fluid is usually normal. Rasmussen and Andermann (1989) consider that the relatively stereotyped clinical features and the consistency of the pathological changes found in the brain tissue removed at operation (perivascular cupping by round cells, scattered glial nodules and diffuse proliferation of microglia, mainly in the cortex but to a lesser degree in white matter) suggest that patients with this disease share a common pathogenic basis. A chronic viral encephalitis has been proposed as a cause but no virus has thus far been identified. The treatment is by total or subtotal hemispherectomy and, in the Montreal series, this operation has resulted in complete or nearly complete abolition of seizures in 13 of 18 patients. The operation is discussed further in Chapter 27.

## Benign partial epilepsy of childhood with centro-temporal (rolandic) spike discharges

The commonest partial epilepsy in childhood is that first described by Nayrac and Beaussart in 1958 and known by various titles including benign focal epilepsy, benign centrotemporal epilepsy, Rolandic or Sylvian epilepsy. The reader might be forgiven for thinking that this must be an ill-defined entity, but in fact it is now a well established and specific epileptic syndrome of childhood.

The main characteristics are as follows:

1   It is age related, beginning between 2 and 12 years, with about 80% of cases

beginning between 5 and 10 years. The peak time of onset is 9 years and it rarely begins after 12 years of age.

2   It occurs in both sexes with males predominating.

3   It occurs in otherwise normal children without any neurological or intellectual deficit.

4   In the majority of cases, the seizures are partial with motor signs predominating although these are frequently combined with somatosensory symptoms.

5   A spontaneous remission occurs during adolescence.

Benign partial epilepsy of this type is a sleep-related disorder and attacks occur only during sleep, whether nocturnal or diurnal, in 70–80% of cases. In approximately 15%, seizures occur both during sleep and while awake and, in the remainder, attacks occur in the waking state only (Lerman and Kivity, 1986). The nocturnal seizures usually occur in the middle of the night or towards morning and the distinction as to whether they have generalized or partial characteristics is difficult since they are often unobserved. However, attacks which have occurred during sleep recordings of the EEG have indicated that the seizure begins as a partial seizure which rapidly undergoes secondary generalization (Ambrosetto and Gobbi, 1975).

The diurnal attacks, when they occur, are quite remarkable. The patient may show clonic jerking of one side of his face (hemifacial seizures), occasionally with jerking of an ipsilateral limb. Oropharyngeal signs are frequently associated with the hemifacial attack consisting of salivation, gurgling noises, contractions of the jaws and peculiar subjective sensations involving the tongue. One of the author's patients complained that his tongue felt too large and felt as it if was moving in an odd way. Some children may have feelings of suffocation and an inability to swallow, and inability to speak has also been reported in up to 40% of diurnal attacks (Loiseau and Beaussart, 1973). Although these children could not speak, consciousness was retained, as it usually is in this type of simple partial seizure, and children have said 'I heard my parents speak, I could see them move but I could not answer.' Such arrest of speech may occur irrespective of whether the EEG lesion is located in the speech area or not, and it has been suggested that it is really due to a peripheral aphonia caused by involvement of the articulatory muscles in the seizure movements.

The frequency of seizures in this epileptic syndrome is usually low, about 20% or more of patients experiencing a single seizure only, even without medication. Seizures are infrequent in about two-thirds of patients and clusters of attacks over a short period of time are not unusual, separated by long seizure-free intervals. About 20% of patients have frequent seizures, sometimes occurring even daily, and occasionally with episodes of status epilepticus (Lerman and Kivity, 1986). A transient hemiplegia (Todd's paralysis) occurs occasionally after a partial seizure in this syndrome, but the immediate and long-term prognosis remains excellent.

The typical EEG pattern consists of the presence of spike discharges or localized spike-wave discharges situated unilaterally or bilaterally in the lower central or rolandic area with maximal expression in the central-midtemporal leads of the conventional 10–20 EEG placement. The discharges should be distinguished from the interictal discharges of predominantly temporal lobe origin in children having complex partial seizures. In those, the discharges usually have a temporal emphasis with little or no suprasylvian extension and they frequently occur in conjunction with focal slowing and disorganization of the background rhythm (Drury, 1989). In benign partial epilepsy, the spike discharges are typically slow, disphasic, of high voltage, and often followed by a slow wave. The rate of spike discharges is increased in drowsiness and in all stages of sleep and, in about a third of cases, spikes appear only in sleep. A sleep record is mandatory if the diagnosis is suspected on clinical evidence and even if the waking EEG is normal (Loiseau and Duché, 1989). It is important to note that similar EEG discharges may occur in normal children without epilepsy in this age group.

Genetic factors appear to play an important role in the causation of this variety of epilepsy. Heijbel, Blom and Rasmuson (1975), in their study of inheritance in this condition, favoured an autosomal dominant manner of inheritance with an age dependent penetrance which reaches its maximum between the ages of 5 and 15 years. A previous history of cerebral insult, either at birth or subsequently, is unusual, whereas a positive family history of epilepsy is frequently found. Perhaps the most remarkable statistic given by Heijbel, Blom and Bergfors (1975), based on the Swedish studies, was that this type of epilepsy might account for some 16% of children with epilepsy and that its incidence was nearly four times greater than that of true petit mal in the normal child population. Other findings (Heijbel and Bohman, 1975) were that children with this type of epilepsy were no different from the general population of children with regard to intelligence, behaviour and school adjustment. Furthermore, all those who have studied this condition have emphasized its ready response to therapy and the excellent prognosis for cure of the epilepsy (O'Donohoe, 1983). Most of the children affected become completely free of epilepsy, usually soon after puberty and nearly always by their middle teens (Beaussart and Faou, 1978). About 2% of patients experience seizures after apparent recovery from this type of epilepsy. These seizures are usually isolated or infrequent generalized tonic–clonic convulsions and further partial seizures seldom occur (Loiseau and Duché, 1989).

There has been speculation about the aetiology of this particular convulsive disorder, particularly in view of the strong genetic influences present and the excellent prognosis. Beaussart (1972) suggested that this is a functional disorder of the brain in which both strong genetic factors and minimal cerebral damage may play a part, and that it gradually disappears as maturation of the brain takes place. There are some analogies with the situation in true petit mal. Other, and much rarer, types of benign partial epilepsy have been described in recent years (see Roger et al., 1992). The best known of these is *benign occipital epilepsy with occipital spike-waves* (Gastaut, 1982). Onset is usually around 6 years of age and transient loss of vision, scotomata, visual hallucinations, and visual illusions (macropsia, micropsia) may be experienced. These visual symptoms may be followed by a partial or generalized motor seizure. Headaches closely resembling migraine may follow the seizure and cause problems in differential diagnosis. The condition is rather more resistant to drugs than is the previous disorder but usually remits fully during adolescence. The reader's attention is also drawn to so called 'atypical benign partial epilepsy of childhood', discussed in Chapter 5.

*The clear definition of benign partial epilepsy in childhood has been a most important advance.* There are many reasons why children with epilepsy develop behavioural disturbances and not least because of the effect their epilepsy has on both their parents and family. Seizures cause considerable anguish to parents and they may react either by overprotection or rejection of the patient. Their attitudes lead in turn to emotional disturbance in the child. When the parents of children with benign partial epilepsy are given early, exact and repeated information about the nature of the disorder, particularly about its good prognosis, and when this is coupled with the fact that the children usually become seizure free fairly rapidly after initiation of treatment, there is usually a diminution or disappearance of the parents' anxieties and a happier and more optimistic emotional atmosphere is generally created from which the child benefits immeasurably.

## Investigation

This must include an EEG examination. Because they occur far more commonly than EEG-recorded clinical seizures, interictal EEG abnormalities play a major part in the diagnosis of a partial epilepsy. In the common benign partial epilepsy with centro-temporal spike discharges, the characteristic discharges may be absent in the waking state and a sleep recording is necessary for diagnosis. Cavazzuti, Cappella and Nalin (1980) found focal spike discharges in 3.5% of their normal children without epilepsy and the majority of these were centro-temporal in situation. Therefore, the correlation between epileptic activity and the EEG and a clinical seizure disorder in children is imperfect. Furthermore, if all partial seizures in children are examined, including complex partial seizures, then EEG discharges may be absent in as many as one-third of the cases (Deonna et al; 1986). Therefore, it is quite possible to have focal spikes in the EEG of a child without an associated clinical epilepsy and the opposite is also true.

Radiological investigations may provide relevant information in partial epilepsies other than benign partial epilepsies. Plain skull X-ray is of little value, although it may show evidence of calcification in a tumour or in a neuroectodermal disorder such as tuberose sclerosis or Sturge–Weber syndrome. The revolutionary impact of neuroimaging by CT and MRI on neurology continues and these investigations are more likely to show abnormalities in partial than in generalized epilepsies. Although neoplasm is a rare cause of partial seizures in childhood, it should be remembered in any child who shows progressive neurological symptoms and/or signs or when a partial epilepsy is unexpectedly resistant to drug treatment. A CT scan at least is mandatory in such circumstances. In general, partial seizures commencing during adolescence are more likely to be linked to structural abnormality demonstrable by neuroimaging than are partial seizures starting in childhood.

## Therapy

The question of whether to treat partial seizures of simple symptomatology with antiepileptic drugs at all is relevant because in the very common syndrome of benign partial epilepsy with centro-temporal spike discharges, seizures are infrequent in two-thirds of the patients. Therefore, treatment should not be started after the first seizure and may even be delayed after the second. However, when a second attack follows quickly on the first (within a month or less) early institution of treatment is mandatory. The early onset of this type of epilepsy is also considered to be an indicator of repeated seizures subsequently (Loiseau and Duché, 1989). Nocturnal seizures may frighten parents who worry about the possibility of death during sleep. The prescription of an antiepileptic drug in such a situation is reassuring.

The main drugs used for partial seizures of simple symptomatology have been phenobarbitone, primidone, phenytoin and carbamazepine. Each of these drugs has similar efficacy for controlling such seizures but they differ in their ability to produce side effects and in their effects of cognition and behaviour. For this reason, carbamazepine has become the drug of first choice for treating partial seizures (Gamstorp, 1983). It has a marked anticonvulsant action, a possible psychotropic effect and infrequent and mild side-effects (see Chapter 25). The psychotropic effects have been described as improved behaviour with a relaxation of tension and calming of aggression. Phenytoin is equally as effective as carbamazepine, and sometimes more so, in treating partial seizures, but produces rather more side effects. Sodium valproate may also be effective in this situation (Dean and Penry, 1987) although its main use is in treating generalized epilepsies. The two new antiepileptic drugs, vigabatrin and lamotrigine, are also being used as adjunctive or 'add-on' therapy in the treatment of patients with intractable partial seizures.

Carbamazepine is particularly valuable in the treatment of benign partial epilepsy with centro-temporal spike discharges. It may be effective in apparently sub-therapeutic doses, given at bedtime only (O'Donohoe, 1983). However, if attacks are frequent, full therapeutic doses are needed. Treatment may be stopped after 1–2 years but early withdrawal of treatment can be followed by relapse because, in this age-related syndrome, natural remission may not begin to occur until about the age of 14 years. One should therefore be cautious about withdrawing treatment too soon in a patient whose seizures have been frequent and drug withdrawal should always be slow. The EEG is not helpful in deciding about withdrawal of therapy, since EEG discharges may persist long after clinical epilepsy has ceased to be a problem. If the seizures are solely diurnal and consist of hemifacial twitching, the careful distinction of this epileptic syndrome from childhood absence epilepsy (petit mal) is important because treatment with carbamazepine may make absence seizures of various kinds worse (Snead and Hosey, 1985).

The use of surgical treatment for the partial epilepsies is considered in Chapter 27.

### References

AMBROSETTO, G. and GOBBI, G. (1975) Benign epilepsy of childhood with Rolandic spikes, or a lesion? EEG during a seizure. *Epilepsia*, **16**, 793–796

ANDERMANN, E. (1982) Multifactorial inheritance of generalized and focal epilepsy. In *Genetic Basis of the Epilepsies* (eds V. E. Anderson, W. A. Hauser, J. K. Penry and C. F. Sing), Raven Press, New York; pp. 353–374

BANCAUD, J. (1992) Kojewnikow's syndrome (epilepsia partialis continua) in children. In *Epileptic Syndromes in Infancy, Childhood and Adolescence*. 2nd Edition (eds J. Roger, M. Bureau, C. Dravet, *et al.*), John Libbey, London, Paris, pp. 363–379

BEAUSSART, M. (1972) Benign epilepsy of children with Rolandic (centro-temporal) paroxysmal foci: a clinical entity. Study of 221 cases. *Epilepsia*, **13** 795–811

BEAUSSART, M. and FAOU, R. (1978) Evolution of epilepsy with Rolandic paroxysmal foci: a study of 324 cases. *Epilepsia*, **19**, 337–342

BLUME, W. T. (1989) Clinical profile of partial seizures beginning at less than four years of age. *Epilepsia*, **30**, 813–819

CAVAZZUTI, G. B. (1980) Epidemiology of different types of epilepsy in school age children of Modena, Italy. *Epilepsia*, **21**, 57–62

DAN, N. G. and WADE, M. J. (1986) The incidence of epilepsy after ventricular shunting procedures. *Journal of Neurosurgery*, **65**, 19–21

DEAN, J. C. and PENRY, J. K. (1987) Valproate monotherapy for partial seizures. *Epilepsia*, **28**, 605

DEONNA, T., ZIEGLER, A-L., DESPLAND, P-A. and VAN MELLE, G. (1986) Partial epilepsy in neurologically normal children. Clinical syndromes and prognosis. *Epilepsia*, **27**, 241–247

DRURY, I. (1989) Epileptiform patterns of children. *Journal of Clinical Neurophysiology*, **6**, 1–39

EFRON, R. (1961) Post epileptic paralysis: theoretical critique and report of a case. *Brain*, **84**, 381–394

GAMSTORP, I. (1983) Partial seizures. In *Antiepileptic Drug Therapy in Paediatrics* (eds P. L. Morselli, C. E. Pippenger and J. K. Penry), Raven Press, New York pp. 163–171

GASTAUT. H. (1970) Clinical and electroencephalographical classification of epileptic seizures. *Epilepsia*, **11**, 102–113

GASTAUT, H. (1982) A new type of epilepsy: benign partial epilepsy of children with occipital spike-waves. *Clinical Electroencephalography*, **13**, 13–22

HAUSER, W. A. and NELSON, K. B. (1989) Epidemiology of epilepsy in children. *Cleveland Clinic Journal of Medicine*, **56**, Supplement Part 2. S185–S194

HEIJBEL, J. and BOHMAN, M. (1975) Benign epilepsy of children with centrotemporal EEG foci: intelligence, behavior and school adjustment. *Epilepsia*, **16**, 679–687

HEIJBEL, J., BLOM S., and BERGFORS, P. G. (1975) Benign epilepsy of children with centrotemporal foci: a study of the incidence rate in outpatient care. *Epilepsia*, **16**, 657–664

HEIJBEL, J., BLOM, S. and RASMUSON, M. (1975) Benign epilepsy of childhood with centrotemporal foci: a genetic study. *Epilepsia*, **16**, 285–293

HOSKING, G. P. (1974) Fits in hydrocephalic children. *Archives of Disease in Childhood*, **49**, 633–635

KOJEWNIKOW, A. Y. (1895) Eine besondere form von corticaler Epilepsie. *Neurologisches Zentralblatt*, **14**, 47–48

LEE, T. K. Y., NAKASU, Y., JEFFREE, M. A., et al. (1989) Indolent glioma a cause of epilepsy. *Archives of Disease in childhood*, **64**, 1666–1671

LENNOX, W. G. (1960) *Epilepsy and Related Disorders*, J. and A. Churchill, London, Little Brown, Boston, pp. 212–220

LERMAN, P. and KIVITY, S. (1986) Benign focal epilepsies of childhood. In *Recent Advances in Epilepsy*, No. 3 (eds. T. A. Pedley and B. S. Meldrum), Churchill Livingstone, Edinburgh, London, pp. 137–156

LIVINGSTON, S. (1970) *Comprehensive Management of Epilepsy in Infancy, Childhood and Adolescence*. Charles C. Thomas, Springfield, Illinois, p. 49.

LOISEAU, P. and BEAUSSART, M. (1975) The seizures of benign childhood epilepsy with Rolandic paroxysmal discharges. *Epilepsia*, **14**, 381–389

LOISEAU, P. and DUCHÉ, B. (1989) Benign childhood epilepsy with centrotemporal spikes. *Cleveland Clinic Journal of Medicine*, **56**, Supplement Part I, S17–S22

MOSHÉ, S. L. and LUDVIG, N. (1988) Kindling. In *Recent Advances in Epilepsy*, No. 4 (eds T. A. Pedley and B. S. Meldrum), Churchill Livingstone, Edinburgh, London, pp. 21–44

NAYRAC, P. and BEAUSSART, M. (1958) Les pointes-ondes prérolandiques: expression EEG très particulière. Étude electroclinique de 21 cas. *Revue Neurologique*, **99**, 201–206

O'DONOHOE, N. V. (1983) Benign focal epilepsy of childhood. In *Research Progress in Epilepsy* (ed. F. C. Rose), Pitman, London, pp. 240–243

POMEROY, S. L., HOLMES, S. J., DODGE, P. R. and FEIGIN, R. D. (1990) Seizures and other neurologic sequelae of bacterial meningitis in children. *New England Journal of Medicine*, **323**, 1651–1657

QUESNEY, L. F. (1986) Seizures of frontal lobe origin. In *Recent Advances in Epilepsy*. No. 3 (eds. A. Pedley and B. S. Meldrum) Churchill Livingstone, Edinburgh, London. pp. 81–110

RASMUSSEN, T., OLSWESKI, J. and LLOYD-SMITH, D. (1958) Focal seizures due to a chronic localized encephalitis. *Neurology*, **8**, 435–455

RASMUSSEN, T. and ANDERMANN, F. (1989) Update on the syndrome of 'chronic encephalitis' and epilepsy. *Cleveland Clinic Journal of Medicine*, **56**, Supplement Part 2. S181–S184

ROGER, J., BUREAU, M., DRAVET, C., et al. (1992) *Epileptic Syndromes in Infancy, Childhood and Adolescence*. 2nd Edition, John Libbey, London, Paris

SNEAD, O. C. and HOSEY, L. C. (1985) Exacerbation of seizures in children by carbamazepine. *New England Journal of Medicine*, **313**, 916–921

# Chapter 10

# Partial or localization-related epilepsies II

Partial seizures of complex symptomatology are the result of a partial or localization-related epilepsy and are usually secondary to and symptomatic of the presence of an identifiable brain lesion. The term psychomotor was introduced to describe them and to encompass their psychic and motor manifestations (Gibbs, Gibbs and Lennox, 1937), but this is now obsolete. They are among the commonest and most intractable seizures encountered in all age groups. The majority of adults with complex partial seizures begin their epilepsy before 20 years of age. Such seizures occur in up to 25% of children with epilepsy and can begin as early as under 2 years of age (Harbord and Manson, 1987). Complex partial seizures present considerable diagnostic problems, are often intractable to medication, yet the focal cause may sometimes be amenable to surgery. For all these reasons, they represent one of the most interesting and challenging problems in paediatric epileptology.

Localization-related epilepsies which cause complex partial seizures may be subdivided into those which arise in the temporal lobe area and those which arise extratemporally. Children with temporal lobe epilepsy typically have complex partial seizures, but not all children with complex partial seizures have temporal lobe epilepsy. Seizures arising in the frontal regions may have the same clinical characteristics and will be considered separately.

## Aetiology

Temporal lobe epilepsy, as it continues to be called, is of particular interest to paediatricians because of controversy about its causation, whether due to birth injury or to subsequent brain-damaging illnesses. Ounsted, Lindsay and Norman (1966), in their classic monograph, described three aetiological groups of which each formed approximately a third of their series of 100 children with temporal lobe epilepsy. The first group consisted of children who had a known brain-damaging illness or a chronic neurological disease. The conditions included birth injury, head injury, meningitis, encephalitis, tuberose sclerosis and phenylketonuria. The second group consisted of those children who had had an episode of status epilepticus in early life. In the remaining group no definite cause could be identified.

Those who argue in favour of birth injury as an important cause of temporal lobe epilepsy postulate that moulding of the head during birth may lead to herniation of the medial and inferior parts of a temporal lobe into the tentorial opening with consequent occlusion of blood vessels in the area (Earle, Baldwin and Penfield, 1953). It is suggested that the infant may show little or no evidence of damage at the time but that there is later development of an epileptogenic focus. Others have suggested that birth injury is only an indirect cause of temporal lobe epilepsy which acts by producing an epileptogenic focus or foci in the brain which themselves cause prolonged major seizures in early childhood, perhaps triggered by high fever, and resulting in temporal lobe damage due to the status epilepticus (Wallace, 1976). The history of birth injury in temporal lobe epilepsy, however, does not necessarily imply that the presumed temporal lobe lesions occurred at birth.

As will be emphasized in Chapter 11, status epilepticus, is an early event in the history of childhood epilepsy with three-quarters of the cases occurring in children under 3 years of age (Aicardi and Chevrie, 1970). Brain swelling, hypoxia, circulatory and metabolic disturbances consequent on status epilepticus lead to neuronal damage and death (particularly in the hippocampal areas of the temporal lobes), and the injurious effects are usually predominantly unilateral. Moreover, apart from epilepsy, diffuse damage may also result in later neurological abnormality and mental retardation. Permanent hemiplegia associated with hemispheric atrophy and later intractable epilepsy and also cerebellar atrophy may follow severe status epilepticus. The role of acute potentially brain-damaging illness, such as meningitis, in causing later epilepsy is also quite complex. Apart from the possibility of the infection itself producing neuronal damage, the prevalence of seizures in children with meningitis aged less than 4 years is much higher than it is in children above that age (Ounsted, 1951) and, if the seizures are prolonged, they may produce the serious sequelae of status epilepticus, including mesial temporal sclerosis (Ounsted *et al.*, 1985).

Ounsted, Lindsay and Norman (1966) also examined the role of genetic factors in the causation of temporal lobe epilepsy in childhood. Inheritance seemed to play a major role only in children whose epilepsy had followed status epilepticus. In those, the overall risk for any convulsive disorder occurring in brothers and sisters was nearly 30%, and in most cases the particular convulsive disorder was a febrile seizure. In other words, both the patients and their siblings were prone to febrile seizures in early childhood, the difference being that the patient unfortunately had a prolonged and severe attack while his affected siblings had short and mild ones. The genetic factor in temporal lobe epilepsy therefore seems to consist in part of a predisposition to febrile convulsions and, if the convulsion happens to be prolonged and severe, temporal lobe damage results and an epileptogenic lesion follows later.

Temporal lobe epilepsy may have a very early onset. Ounsted, Lindsay and Norman (1966) reported the ages of onset in their series as being widely scattered around a median age of 5 years 4 months. Where the epilepsy was related to previous status epilepticus the median age of onset was earlier than this, and where no definite cause could be identified the median age was 9 years. Aird, Venturini and Spielman (1967), in a large retrospective survey, noted that 42% of patients with temporal lobe epilepsy reported an onset of some form of convulsive phenomena in the first decade of life. Harbord and Manson (1987) studied 63 children with complex partial seizures and found that 16% had an onset of seizures before the age of 2 years, even though most were not diagnosed until several years later. Diagnosis is much more difficult in infants and very young children because impairment of consciousness is more difficult to assess and the often bizarre subjective sensations which may be experienced are difficult for children to describe.

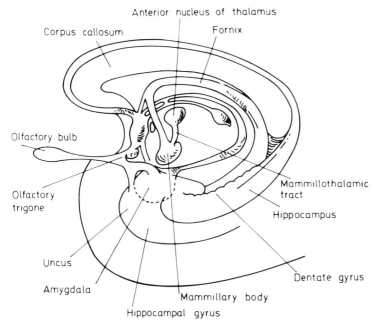

*Figure 10.1* The hippocampus and amygdala in the depths of the temporal lobe (After J. R. Daube and B. A. Sandok, 1978, *Medical Neurosciences*. Boston: Little, Brown and Co.)

## Anatomy

In order to understand the phenomena of temporal lobe epilepsy it is necessary to know something of the anatomical and pathological substrates of the condition. To anatomists the temporal lobe is that part of the brain below the lateral or Sylvian fissure which extends posteriorly to blend with the occipital lobe. In clinical practice the temporal lobe area is taken to include the hippocampal gyrus lying medially on the undersurface of the cortex and extending forwards as the uncus, and the hippocampus which is a cylindrical grey mass lying in the floor of the inferior horn of the lateral ventricle which extends forwards to fuse with the tail of the caudate nucleus to form the amygdaloid nucleus or amygdala at the tip of the inferior horn. The hippocampus continues posteriorly as the fornix and the hippocampus-fornix complex lies eccentrically round the thalamus in such a way that the hippocampus lies below and lateral to it, while the fornix continues forwards over the dorsal aspect of the thalamus and then extends to lie medial to it, finally ending in the mammillary bodies of the hypothalamus. The anterior thalamic nuclei receive afferents from the fornix and the mammillary bodies are also connected by the mammillothalamic tract. The anterior thalamic nuclei also project to the cingulate gyrus, lying above and parallel to the corpus callosum, and to the frontal cortex, and there are returning afferent fibres to the hippocampus via the hippocampal gyrus. There are also connections to the insula and to the homologous areas on the opposite side of the brain. This whole interconnecting system is now usually known as the '*limbic system*' or the 'visceral brain'. Phylogenetically it represents an old part of the forebrain which has been overlain and surrounded by the larger and more highly differentiated neocortex (*Figure 10.1*).

Functionally, it is now considered that the limbic system is a complex and highly integrated mechanism responsible for the autonomic functions of the individual and the one which is also concerned with emotional expression. The cardiovascular, respiratory and alimentary systems have their higher cortical representation in this region. The limbic system influences brain-stem function through the reticular system and pituitary function through the hypothalamus, and it is thought to be concerned with consciousness, with the regulation of sleep and with memory. The olfactory input terminates in the uncus and hippocampal gyrus, thereby intimately connecting the sense organs of smell to those parts of the brain which are concerned with memory and also with the hypothalamus. From the evolutionary standpoint, the first parts of the cerebral hemispheres to develop were those connected with olfactory input, and these were evolved to deal with the world of smells and to store the memory of what had been smelt.

## Pathology

Our knowledge of the pathology of temporal lobe epilepsy began in the early nineteenth century when at postmortem induration and other changes were observed macroscopically in the hippocampus of affected patients, and this lesion became known as Ammon's horn sclerosis. Renewed interest in this particular finding has been greatly stimulated in the recent past by the examination of material obtained at postmortem and following the operation of temporal lobectomy. Falconer and his coworkers at the Maudsley Hospital, London, made outstanding contributions in this regard and coined the term 'mesial temporal sclerosis' (Falconer, Serafetinides and Corsellis, 1964) to include the classic Ammon's horn sclerosis and also the more widespread sclerosis extending into neighbouring structures such as the amygdala and the uncus (*Figure 10.2*). The term is used to embrace both gliosis and neuronal loss. Margerison and Corsellis (1966), in autopsy studies of epileptics, showed that mesial temporal sclerosis was the most common single lesion found in the brains they examined and it occurred in more than half the cases. Furthermore, the lesion was unilateral in 80% of the patients. Taylor and Ounsted (1971) explained this finding on the basis of differential rates of cerebral maturation between the hemispheres and between sexes, the right hemisphere suffering damage up to the age of 2 years and the left hemisphere subsequently. Falconer (1970) cited mesial temporal sclerosis as the example *par excellence* of a lesion of the limbic system and believed that the two most important factors in its causation are prolonged febrile convulsions in early childhood and a genetic predisposition to epilepsy.

Among the other lesions found in resected material from Falconer's (1970) patients were hamartomas, which constituted about 20%. These are benign indolent lesions which are mainly congenital malformations. They include glial malformations, vascular malformations and occasionally areas of tuberose sclerosis. They tend to cluster around the amygdala and in the hippocampal gyrus and so involve the limbic system. Miscellaneous lesions constituted just over 10% of the material and included scars and old infarcts. Some of these may have been secondary to head injury and others may have been consequent on infection. The final 20% of the material included equivocal or non-specific lesions, and Falconer pointed out that in these cases surgery was not so effective therapeutically as it would be when a definite lesion was found. Davidson and Falconer (1975) reviewed their case material with particular reference to children; 24 out of 40 children operated on had

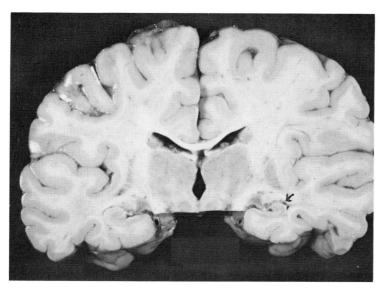

*Figure 10.2* Sclerosis and atrophy of the hippocampus on the left side compared with the right, in an adult with a history of a prolonged febrile convulsion in early childhood and subsequent temporal lobe epilepsy (*Courtesy of Dr S. Murphy*)

mesial temporal sclerosis, including 2 with hamartomas, and of those with mesial temporal sclerosis only nearly 80% had a history of a prolonged febrile seizure. Falconer and his coworkers stressed that, taking all age groups together, not only do those with mesial temporal sclerosis form the largest pathological group, but also they constitute a group of patients in which the onset of habitual epilepsy occurs in the first decade of life in nearly 60%.

The precise relationship between febrile convulsions and temporal lobe epilepsy is debatable. Much of the evidence identifying complex febrile convulsions as the most important aetiological cause has come from highly selected surgical series. Epidemiological studies have suggested that febrile convulsions could not account for more than 10% of cases of temporal lobe epilepsy (Leviton and Cowan, 1981). Annegers *et al.* (1987) have suggested that the tendency to develop complex febrile convulsions reflects the existence of pre-existing brain disease which is also responsible for the subsequent development of a partial or localization-related epilepsy. However, Rocca *et al.* (1987), in their population-based study of risk factors for complex partial seizures, did not find a significant association between a wide range of prenatal and perinatal risk factors and the later development of complex partial seizures. The debate continues. Meanwhile, the incidence of prolonged and potentially damaging febrile convulsions may be declining and treatment to terminate them is more effective nowadays. The devastating HHE syndrome, for example, has become very uncommon (Aicardi, 1986).

Using modern neuroimaging methods, especially magnetic resonance imaging, it is now possible to demonstrate a structural cause for temporal lobe epilepsy in the majority of cases (Kuzniecky *et al.*, 1987). In children, a most important and potentially curable cause of intractable complex partial seizures arising from the temporal or frontal lobes is the presence of an indolent glioma (Lee *et al.*, 1989).

## Clinical manifestations related to pathology

The description of temporal lobe seizures in the International Classification as partial seizures of complex symptomatology is extremely apt. Epilepsy usually mimics the normal function of the part of the brain involved in the seizure, although it may distort it. The more uncomplicated the function of the area of cortex involved, the more accurately will the epileptic event mimic that function. In an area with the elaborate functions of the temporal lobe the epileptic event will necessarily be complex and is more likely to be a travesty of normal activity. Leaving aside its place in the physiology of hearing and speech, the most important function of the temporal lobe is the integration of sensations of all kinds. Williams (1966) argued that the temporal lobe and limbic system enable an individual to appreciate himself as a unified being because they receive information from the special senses, the viscera and the higher centres. When a person with temporal lobe epilepsy is bombarded with autonomic and indescribable auras he loses this sense of himself, and this leads to emotional disturbance and even terror. Flor Henry (1969) wrote of temporal lobe epilepsy that the epileptic patient may experience his aura as 'weird, terrifying or ominous in its inexplicable foreignness to his personality'. What the patient with a temporal lobe attack feels is unnatural and beyond his or her normal experience and, in consequence, it is often impossible to describe to relatives or to the physician.

## Symptomatology

Excessive local neuronal discharges in one or other temporal lobe can give rise to a remarkable variety of seizure patterns, many of them associated with bizarre sensory phenomena. The hallmark of a complex partial seizure as compared with a simple partial seizure is impairment of consciousness. The impairment of consciousness may occur at the onset of the attack or after an initial simple partial seizure with preserved consciousness. When the preceding simple partial seizure is sensory, it is usually called an aura. An aura may be further defined as an event which occurs before consciousness is lost and for which memory is retained afterwards. The diversity of auras is remarkable and includes somatosensory, auditory, visual, olfactory, and gustatory sensations; visceral sensations such as oropharyngeal, epigastric, abdominal, genital or retrosternal; and experiences such as fear, strangeness, embarrassment, dizziness, vertigo, déjà vu or jamais vu. It is important to realize that the aura is an ictal phenomenon, preceding impairment of consciousness, and warning the patient of an impending loss of consciousness. Although auras are reported in the majority of adults with complex partial seizures, they are reported in less than 50% of children (Holmes, 1986). This is probably related to a child's inability to describe such symptoms. Sometimes an initial aura may be suspected if the child runs to a parent for help before consciousness is impaired. Where fear is the aura (and many of the indescribable and bizarre sensations induce a feeling of fear), the child may drop down wherever he or she happens to be, or may run to a parent in terror. Later, children may avoid the room in which they experienced the frightening sensation.

Impairment of consciousness is more difficult to assess in infants and children than in adults and may manifest itself as an arrest of activity, decreased responsiveness, or a blank stare. Such absences must be carefully distinguished from the absences of childhood absence epilepsy (petit mal) because the treatment and prognosis are quite different for the two conditions. Petit mal is usually age-related and occurs in otherwise normal children whereas complex partial seizures may occur at any age and there are often other associated problems. Penry, Porter and Dreifuss (1975), in a study of 48 children with absences, in which the clinical seizures and EEGs were videotaped, showed that simple absences (petit mal) with impaired consciousness only were relatively infrequent and usually lasted less than 10 seconds and rarely longer than 45 seconds. They were not preceded by an aura and mental clarity returned abruptly at the end of the attack. On the other hand, temporal lobe absences were rarely less than 30 seconds in duration, frequently lasted from 1 to 2 minutes and were not uncommonly prolonged for several minutes. A proportion of the attacks were preceded by an aura and full consciousness returned slowly rather than abruptly.

Automatisms frequently occur after consciousness has been impaired in a complex partial seizure. They may also be seen, but to a lesser extent, in the absences of childhood absence epilepsy. They vary widely in type but tend to be stereotyped from one seizure to another in the individual patient. They include chewing, swallowing or lip-smacking, especially in infants and young children (Duchowny, 1987), gestural automatisms such as fumbling at clothes or objects, verbal automatisms such as screaming, repeating phrases, or laughing, and also many other activities (Holmes, 1986). Autonomic symptoms may also occur during a complex partial seizure, and include colicky abdominal pain and vomiting associated with impairment of consciousness. Complex partial seizures may present with brief periods of apnoea, especially in infancy. In a personal case, an infant who had a deep-seated hamartoma in one temporal lobe presented with brief episodes of apnoea in early infancy.

If the seizure discharge spreads to produce general cortical involvement, a generalized tonic-clonic seizure ensues and, indeed, this type of epilepsy may present initially with grand mal attacks which are the result of partial seizures evolving rapidly into secondary generalized seizures. During the process of spread of the ictal discharge from the original focus through the ipsilateral hemisphere, a variety of motor phenomena may be seen, including dystonic posturing of the contralateral limbs, clonic jerking of the contralateral limbs or face, versive turning of the face to the contralateral side and, in infancy, peculiar 'boxing' movements of the arms, loss of neck muscle tone, or posturing resembling the asymmetrical tonic neck reflex (Wyllie and Lüders, 1989).

During the postictal phase, the child is usually confused. Further automatic movements may be observed and the child may react aggressively if restrained. Tiredness is common but, in contrast to generalized tonic-clonic seizures, deep sleep is unusual. If the dominant hemisphere has been involved, there may be a short period of dysphasia. Crying is another common postictal event in children. Again, it is important to note that such postictal events are not seen following the absences of childhood absence epilepsy (petit mal).

## Diagnosis

The diagnosis of temporal lobe epilepsy is made easier if recognizable epileptic phenomena of a motor kind occur. Difficulties in diagnosis arise where sensory phenomena or automatisms occur, since these may be difficult to distinguish from behavioural aberrations of one sort or another. In this respect it is important to remember that complex partial seizures are generally paroxysmal episodes of relatively short duration, usually without any precipitating factor, and they start and end abruptly, while the reverse is characteristic of psychiatric disturbances. The latter are usually provoked by some disturbing situation. However, the distinction between the two can be blurred by the fact that temporal lobe epileptic attacks are more likely to happen when the subject is emotionally disturbed. Careful history taking should make it possible to recognize the repeated stereotyped epileptic events and distinguish them from the more continuous disturbance associated with a personality disorder. Lennox (1960) said: 'the burden of proof rests on anyone who contends that a given psychic episode, isolated from other evidence of epilepsy, is epileptic.'

When psychic symptoms, defined as disturbances of higher cerebral function, do occur in complex partial seizures, they usually precede the impairment of consciousness and serve as an aura for the patient. They comprise hallucinations (including special sensory hallucinations of smell and taste), affective symptoms (usually fearful but occasionally associated with mirthless laughter), disturbances of thought (with feelings of unreality), and rarely in children, disturbances of memory such as the well-known feeling of having seen or heard or never having seen or heard the event being experienced before (déjà vu and jamais vu).

There are certain *severe behavioural disturbances*, commonly associated with temporal lobe epilepsy in childhood and adolescence, which are described in detail in Chapter 20. The hyperkinetic syndrome occurred in 26% of the cases described by Ounsted, Lindsay and Norman (1966), and these children were most frequently those who had suffered an early brain insult or who had had status epilepticus, and many of them also showed a significant degree of mental handicap. Ounsted (1970) later postulated that the disruption of exploratory learning in these hyperkinetic children disbarred them from developing the basic mental structures which are the foundation of normal learning and intelligence. He emphasized the importance of remembering that phenobarbitone and related compounds can potentiate hyperkinetic behaviour, and conversely that such behaviour can be alleviated by withdrawing these drugs. Outbursts of catastrophic rage may also be seen in children and adolescents with temporal lobe epilepsy, which is interesting in view of the suggested relationship between limbic dysfunction and aggression. Behavioural disturbances with hyperkinesis or aggressive conduct are much more frequent in children with temporal lobe epilepsy than are the psychoses which are sometimes associated with the condition in adolescent and adult life. In fact, it is exceptionally rare to see a psychotic illness in an individual with mesial temporal sclerosis, probably the commonest single lesion in children with temporal lobe epilepsy. It seems likely that psychosis is a reaction to temporal lobe epilepsy of later onset and this is rarely due to mesial temporal sclerosis. This matter is further amplified in Chapter 20.

## Investigation

The investigation of a child presenting with a clinical history suggestive of complex partial seizures depends particularly on the EEG examination. When such seizures are arising from a temporal lobe, the causative lesion usually lies deep in that part of the brain or on its inferior or medial aspects. The presence of interictal spikes or sharp waves in the temporal region on one or other side is strong supportive evidence for a diagnosis of a secondary partial epilepsy of the temporal lobe type in such a patient. In the first decade of life, the discharges are most commonly seen in the posterior and midtemporal regions and, in older children and adults, in the anterior temporal region (Hughes and Olson, 1981). However, in children, there may be bilateral foci which do not crystallize into a clearly defined unilateral focus until adolescence. A normal interictal EEG cannot be relied upon to rule out a diagnosis of epilepsy in patients whose clinical episodes have the characteristics of complex partial seizures. This is especially true of infants and young children (Holmes, 1984). If the history is suggestive, then further EEG procedures such as prolonged recordings, sleep recordings and, if surgical treatment is being considered, the use of specially sited electrodes (sphenoidal, nasopharyngeal, extra scalp electrodes) may increase the yield of interictal discharges (*Figures 10.3 and 10.4*). The chance of actually obtaining an electrographic recording of a seizure may be increased by reducing gradually any antiepileptic medication or by sleep deprivation. Combined video and EEG recordings, if available, may be particularly valuable in such a situation. It is most important to distinguish the focal spikes arising from the temporal areas from the centrotemporal spikes of benign partial (Rolandic) epilepsy, discharges which may also be observed in the EEG of a proportion of normal children. The latter are usually maximal above the level of the Sylvian fissure and have a typical configuration whereas true temporal spikes are usually confined to the temporal areas.

As far as the diagnosis of a focal structural cerebral lesion is concerned, it is becoming increasingly clearer that magnetic resonance imaging (MRI) is superior to computed tomography (CT) in this respect and that, in some cases, MRI may reveal lesions which are not visible on CT (Kuzniecky *et al.*, 1987). If a focal structural lesion is found, then there will inevitably be concern about the possibility of a neoplasm, especially if the lesion is seen to expand in serial neuroimages. Furthermore, even apparently static lesions may turn out to be slow-growing gliomas (Lee *et al.*, 1989). The discovery of a focal structural lesion in a patient with complex partial seizures nowadays always leads to a consideration of surgical treatment.

## Chronicity and prognosis

Authorities are not agreed on the incidence of temporal lobe epilepsy in childhood. Exact incidence and age of onset are difficult to evaluate because the symptoms are so variable and diagnosis is difficult, particularly in young children. Ounsted, Lindsay and Norman (1966) put the incidence at 10% of all epileptic children referred for hospital consultation in the Oxford area, whereas others authors give an incidence ranging from 13 to 25% of patients, (Wyllie and Lüders, 1989). Glaser (1980) considered that complex partial seizures occurred in over half of all patients with epilepsy, often in addition to generalized tonic–clonic seizures. In at least half the cases, symptoms were already well established in early or late childhood and a treatment response was known by puberty. Chronicity is one of the most characteristic features and in this it contrasts with other forms of childhood epilepsy which tend to die out as the child gets older and so do not contribute to the adult epileptic population. The persistence of seizures, the occurrence of disturbing automatisms, the possible deterioration in cognitive–intellectual functioning, the

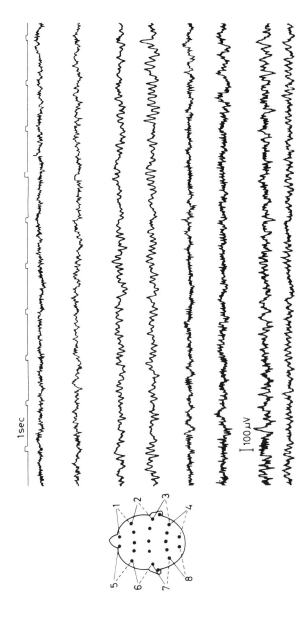

*Figure 10.3* Girl aged 11 years and awake with eyes open. EEG shows irregular slow-wave activity in the left temporal area

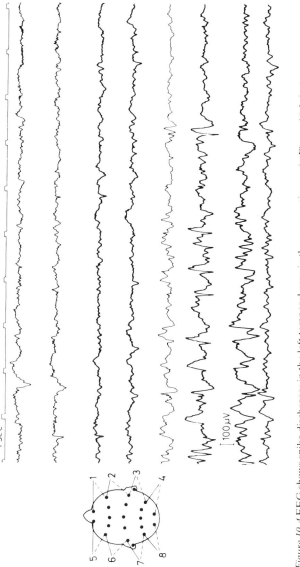

*Figure 10.4* EEG shows spike discharges in the left temporal area in the same patient as in Figure 10.3 during light sleep

increasingly disordered social behaviour and the personality changes all produce a situation in the growing child or adolescent with chronic temporal lobe epilepsy which leads to severe problems in family, school and vocational relationships.

It is important to realize that much psychopathology in temporal lobe epilepsy is due to the interaction of multiple factors. Patients with complex partial seizures, especially when this is associated with structural brain abnormality, tend to have more frequent attacks, take more drugs, and suffer more adverse psychosocial stresses than patients with generalized seizures (Reynolds, 1983). Early and more effective treatment is likely to prevent the development of chronic psychopathology.

Lindsay, Ounsted and Richards, in a series of papers published in 1979–80, have described the follow-up into adult life of 100 children with temporal lobe epilepsy who were first studied in 1966 by Ounsted, Lindsay and Norman. Of these, 33% were found to be seizure free and independent; 32% were socially and economically independent but were still receiving anticonvulsant treatment and were not necessarily seizure free; 30% were either dependent on their parents or in institutions; 5% died under 15 years of age. The aetiology was more likely to be unknown in those who did well than in those who did badly, where a known brain insult was more often identifiable. Other adverse factors included lower than average intelligence, early onset of seizures, associated frequent grand mal attacks, frequent temporal lobe seizures, a left-sided epileptic focus, severe behavioural disturbances and a need for special schooling. This classic prospective study is a milestone in the understanding of this serious epilepsy and should be read by all concerned with the problem.

More recent studies suggest that temporal lobe epilepsy is frequently as intractable in children as it is known to be in adults. In the study of Kotagal et al. (1987), remission was defined as being seizure free while on drugs. In a 5-year follow-up study, only 18% of their patients were fully controlled and none was seizure free off drugs. In all, the diagnosis had been confirmed by the demonstration of a temporal lobe EEG focus. Harbord and Manson (1987), in a study of 63 children followed for up to 15 years, noted a tendency for the seizures to reduce in frequency with time, but only 10% of those managed with drugs alone were free of seizures at an average of 6.6 years follow-up.

## Therapy

As Penry (1975) stated, the treatment of complex partial seizures is one of the greatest challenges in neurology today, and although many patients with these seizures live successful and happy lives with their attacks completely controlled the proportion is relatively small in comparison with those who are permanently afflicted by the condition. Furthermore, those who do become seizure free on medical treatment are frequently impaired in their vocational and social adjustments because of the side effects of medication, and such impairment is sometimes compounded by further neurological deficits resulting from the structural lesion of the region of the brain associated with the seizures.

The advent of phenobarbitone in 1912 and of phenytoin in 1938 significantly improved the situation but, because many patients proved refractory to these drugs, the search for new antiepileptic agents continued with the arrival of primidone in 1954, which brought further benefit to some patients. The availability of carbamazepine since 1963 has undoubtedly been the most significant development in the drug therapy of temporal lobe epilepsy so far. Parsonage (1975), reviewing its use in adults, concluded that it was the best drug available for the treatment of complex partial seizures, and that it should be used as the drug of choice for this type of epilepsy.

Gamstorp (1983) reviewed her experience with carbamazepine for complete partial seizures in children over many years and concluded that it was her drug of choice with phenytoin as an alternative therapeutic agent if carbamazepine failed. She reported complete control or almost complete control of seizures in 50% of cases on carbamazepine alone. The author's experience with carbamazepine has been similar (O'Donohoe, 1973). Side-effects and toxic effects are uncommon with this drug, apart from an annoying rash which necessitates stopping the drug, but it is important to introduce it gradually, taking several days or weeks to attain the final dose. By this means, initial side-effects such as drowsiness and ataxia are avoided. If the seizures remain uncontrolled on the maximum tolerated dose of carbamazepine, phenytoin should be substituted, again as monotherapy. If this drug is ineffective, then phenobarbitone or primidone may be used, accepting that these drugs may have undesirable effects on cognition and behaviour. However, it is important to remember that sodium valproate may be very successful in some cases and it should be tried (Dean and Penry, 1987). As a rule, two-drug combinations are not usually more effective than monotherapy but may be tried in resistant cases. Acetazolamide may work successfully as an adjunct to carbamazepine in refractory cases (Oles *et al.*, 1989). The dosage ranges from 3 to 22 mg/kg per day. Recently, two new antiepileptic drugs, vigabatrin and lamotrigine, have begun to be used as adjunctive therapy in resistant cases.

## Surgery

Surgical removal of part of one or other temporal lobe is playing an increasingly important part in the treatment of chronic and intractable temporal lobe epilepsy in childhood. The pioneering surgery in children was performed by Falconer (1972), who devised the operation of anterior temporal lobectomy in which major parts of the temporal cortex and also deeper structures were removed. The rationale of the operation is that the removal of the affected areas interrupts the neuronal circuits responsible for the propagation of seizure discharges. Falconer's criteria for operation were that the individual should have resistant epilepsy, should not have a gross space-occupying lesion, should have a unilaterally discharging EEG focus, and should be at least of average intelligence. Davidson and Falconer (1975), in a study of 40 children treated surgically, reported that over half of the cases had mesial temporal sclerosis and that the best long-term results of treatment were obtained when this lesion was present. Of 24 children with mesial temporal sclerosis, 14 (58%) became seizure-free in the long term, usually without medication, while eight out of ten (80%) with hamartomas achieved this goal. Corresponding improvement in behavioural difficulties, notably with regard to aggression, was also achieved.

Ounsted and his colleagues in Oxford have been following a series of 100 children with temporal lobe epilepsy since 1948 and their paper describing their reasons for referral for neurosurgery is required reading for those interested in the subject (Lindsay, Ounsted and Richards, 1984). Their group was studied contemporaneously with the development of neurosurgery for children and, although they were reluctant to refer patients in the early years, they became so impressed by the results of surgery that they advise as follows:

Analyses of the biographies in this series suggest that all children on drug treatment for temporal lobe epilepsy should be most scrupulously reviewed before leaving school. Some will be found to be in natural remission: they should be weaned from their drugs and have the label 'epileptic' taken off them. Others will not have remitted, and they should be carefully investigated by epileptologists and considered for neurosurgery

This author concurs wholeheartedly with this view. Indeed, many authors now believe that surgery should be considered early in the course of the disease if medical treatment is ineffective. Wyllie and Lüders (1989), analysing their experience at the Cleveland Clinic, point out that children have a special problem in coping with epilepsy while developing a sense of self. The unpredictable, recurrent nature of the attacks causes anxiety, depression, and poor self-esteem, leading to a sense of decreased competence and independence. Their parents tend to overprotect them and they are socially ostracized by their peers. In adolescence, their epilepsy limits educational, social, and vocational potential. The Cleveland group consider that if there is clear EEG and clinical evidence of localization-related epilepsy, with rigorous exclusion of childhood absence epilepsy and benign partial epilepsy with Rolandic or centrotemporal spikes, and if the seizures are truly intractable and disabling despite aggressive medication for 2–3 years, then it is appropriate to consider surgical treatment, even in young children. They agree with the Oxford group that surgery should certainly be considered before the patient leaves school, that is by mid- or late adolescence, in order to facilitate a more natural entry into adulthood. They do not consider mental retardation an absolute contraindication to surgery, pointing out that successful surgery will improve the quality of life of retarded children and obviate the need for constant medical supervision of such children.

In every surgical series reported, the favourable results have far outweighed the occasional complications. A satisfactory outcome with remission of seizures has been reported in about 75% of operated children overall (Meayer *et al.*, 1986). As Ounsted and others have emphasized, surgery can lead to a remarkable reversal of social, intellectual and personality handicaps, suggesting that the brain is capable of remarkable powers of recovery when the adverse effects of chronic epilepsy and continuous heavy medication are removed. The surgical treatment of epilepsy is considered further in Chapter 27.

## References

AICARDI, J. (1986) *Epilepsy in Children*. Raven Press, New York, pp. 163–166

AICARDI, J. and CHEVRIE, J. J. (1970) Convulsive status epilepticus in infants and children. A study of 239 cases. *Epilepsia*, 11, 187–197

AIRD, R. B., VENTURINI, A. M. and SPIELMAN, P. M. (1967) Antecedents of temporal lobe epilepsy. *Archives of Neurology*, 16, 67–73

ANNEGERS, J. F., HAUSER, W. A., SHIRTS, S. B. and KURKLAND, L. T. (1987) Factors prognostic of unprovoked febrile convulsions. *New England Journal of Medicine*, 316, 493–498

DAVIDSON, S. and FALCONER, M. A. (1975) Outcome of surgery in 40 children with temporal lobe epilepsy. *Lancet*, 1, 1260–1263

DEAN, J. C. and PENRY, J. K. (1987) Valproate monotherapy for partial seizures. *Epilepsia*, 28, 605

DUCHOWNY, M. S. (1987) Complex partial seizures of infancy. *Archives of Neurology*, 44, 911–914

EARLE, K. M., BALDWIN, M. and PENFIELD, W. (1953) Incisural sclerosis and temporal lobe seizures produced by hippocampal herniation at birth. *Archives of Neurology and Psychiatry*, 69, 27–42

FALCONER, M. A. (1970) Historical review: the pathological substrates of temporal lobe epilepsy. *Guy's Hospital Reports*, 119, 47–60

FALCONER, M. A. (1972) Place of surgery for temporal lobe epilepsy during childhood. *British Medical Journal*, 2, 631–635

FALCONER, M. A., SERAFEDINIDES, E. A. and CORSELLIS, J. A. N. (1964) Etiology and pathogenesis of temporal lobe epilepsy. *Archives of Neurology*, **10**, 233–248

FLOR HENRY, P. (1969) Psychosis and temporal lobe epilepsy. *Epilepsia*, **10**, 363–395

GAMSTORP, I. (1983) Partial seizures. In *Antiepileptic Drug Therapy in Pediatrics* (eds P. L. Morselli, C. E. Pippenger and J. K. Penry), Raven Press, New York, pp. 163–171

GIBBS, F. A., GIBBS, E. L. and LENNOX W. G. (1937) Epilepsy: a paroxysmal cerebral dysrhythmia. *Brain*, **60**, 377–388

GLASER, G. H. (1980) Treatment of intractable temporal lobe – limbic epilepsy (complex partial seizures) by temporal lobectomy. *Annals of Neurology*, **8**, 455–459

HARBORD, M. G. and MANSON, J. L. (1987) Temporal lobe epilepsy in childhood. A reappraisal of etiology and outcome. *Pediatric Neurology*, **3**, 263–268

HOLMES, G. L. (1984) Partial complex seizures in children. An analysis of 69 seizures in 24 patients using EEG FM telemetry and videotape recording. *Electroencephalography and Clinical Neurophysiology*, **57**, 13–20.

HOLMES, G. L. (1986) Partial seizures in children. *Pediatrics*, **77**, 725–731

HUGHES, J. R. and OLSON, S. F. (1981) An investigation of eight different types of temporal lobe discharges. *Epilepsia*, **22**, 421–435

KUZNIECKY, R., de la SAYETTE, V., ETHNIER, R. *et al.* (1987) Magnetic resonance imaging in temporal lobe epilepsy. Pathological correlations. *Annals of Neurology*, **22**, 341–347

LEE, T. K. Y., NAKUSA, Y., JEFFREE, M. A. *et al.* (1989) Indolent glioma: a cause of epilepsy. *Archives of Disease in Childhood*, **64**, 1666–1671

LENNOX, W. G. (1960) *Epilepsy and Related Disorders*. Little Brown, Boston, J. and A. Churchill, London

LEVITON, A. and COWAN, L. D. (1981) Do febrile seizures increase the risk of complex partial seizures? An epidemiologic assessment. In *Febrile Seizures* (eds K. B. Nelson and J. H. Ellenberg), Raven Press, New York, pp. 65–74

LINDSAY, J., OUNSTED, C. and RICHARDS, P. (1979) Long-term outcome in children with temporal lobe seizures. I Social outcome and childhood factors; II Marriage, parenthood and sexual indifference; III Psychiatric aspects in childhood and adult life. *Developmental Medicine and Child Neurology*, **21**, (I) 285–298; (II) 433–440; (III) 630–636

LINDSAY, J., OUNSTED, C. and RICHARDS, P. (1980) Long-term outcome in children with temporal lobe seizures. IV Genetic factors, febrile convulsions and remission of seizures. *Developmental Medicine and Child Neurology*, **22**, 429–439

LINDSAY, J., OUNSTED, C. and RICHARDS, P. (1984) Long-term outcome in children with temporal lobe seizures. V Indications and contra-indications for neurosurgery. *Developmental Medicine and Child Neurology*, **26**, 25–32

MARGERISON, J. H. and CORSELLIS, J. A. N. (1966) Epilepsy and the temporal lobes: a clinical, electroencephalographic and neuropathological study of the brain in epilepsy, with particular reference to the temporal lobes. *Brain*, **89**, 499–530

MEYER, F. B., MARSH, W. R., LAWS, E. R. and SHARBROUGH, F. W. (1986) Temporal lobectomy in children with epilepsy. *Journal of Neurosurgery*, **64**, 371–377

O'DONOHOE, N. V. (1973) A series of epileptic children treated with Tegretol. In *Tegretol in Epilepsy. Report of an International Clinical Symposium* (ed. C. A. S. Wink), Geigy Pharmaceuticals, Macclesfield, Cheshire pp. 25–29

OLES, K. S., PENRY, J. K., COLE, D. L. W. and HOWARD, G. (1989) Use of acetazolamide as an adjunct to carbamazepine in refractory partial seizures. *Epilepsia*, **30**, 74–78

OUNSTED, C. (1951) Significance of convulsions in children with purulent meningitis. *Lancet*, **1**, 1245–1248

OUNSTED, C. (1970) A biological approach to autistic and hyperkinetic syndromes. In *Modern Trends in Paediatrics* (ed J. Apley), Butterworths, London, pp. 286–316

OUNSTED, C., LINDSAY, J. and NORMAN, R. (1966) *Biological Factors in Temporal Lobe Epilepsy. Clinics in Developmental Medicine*, No. 22. Spastics International/Heinemann Medical, London

OUNSTED, C., GLASER, G. H., LINDSAY, J., and RICHARDS, P. (1985) Focal epilepsy with mesial temporal sclerosis after acute meningitis. *Archives of Neurology*, **42**, 1058–1060

PARSONAGE, M. (1975) Treatment with carbamazepine: adults. In *Advances in Neurology*, Vol II (eds J. K. Penry and D. D. Daly), Raven Press, New York, pp. 221–234

PENRY, J. K. (1975) Perspectives in complex partial seizures. In *Advances in Neurology*, Vol II (eds J. K. Penry and D. D. Daly), Raven Press, New York, pp. 1–11

PENRY, J. K., PORTER, R. J. and DREIFUSS, F. E. (1975) Simultaneous recording of absence seizures with video-tape and electroencephalography: a study of 374 seizures in 48 patients. *Brain*, **98**, 427–440

REYNOLDS, E. H. (1983) Interictal behaviour in temporal lobe epilepsy. *British Medical Journal*, **286**, 918–919

ROCCA, W. A., SHARBROUGH, F. W. and HAUSER, W. A. (1987) Risk factors for complex partial seizures. A population-based case-control study. *Annals of Neurology*, **21**, 22

TAYLOR, D. C. and OUNSTED, C. (1971) Biological factors influencing the outcome of seizures in response to fever. *Epilepsia*, **12**, 33–45

WALLACE, S. J. (1976) Neurological and intellectual deficits. Convulsions with fever viewed as acute indications of life-long developmental defects. In *Brain Dysfunction in Infantile Febrile Convulsions* (eds M. A. B. Brazier and F. Coceani), Raven Press, New York, pp. 259–277

WILLIAMS, D. (1966) Temporal lobe epilepsy. *British Medical Journal*, **1**, 1439–1442

WYLLIE, E. and LUDERS, H. (1989) Complex partial seizures in children: clinical manifestations, and identification of surgical candidates. *Cleveland Clinic Journal of Medicine*, **56**, Supplement Part 1, S43–S52

# Chapter 11

# Status epilepticus

Status epilepticus is a paediatric emergency requiring urgent and effective treatment. It has been defined as a condition in which there is a continuous epileptic seizure or in which seizures recur with such frequency that there is no return of consciousness between them. For practical purposes in childhood, seizures lasting more than 15–30 minutes fall into this definition. Series of seizures with recovery of consciousness between attacks are defined as serial epilepsy, a condition which often evolves into status epilepticus.

## Classification and terminology

Classifications of status epilepticus divide it into generalized and partial forms and into convulsive and non-convulsive types (Gastaut, 1983). In practice, it is the continuous or closely recurrent generalized convulsive status that represents the greatest threat to the integrity of the brain and to life itself. This convulsive status may have its onset with a brief tonic phase followed by a prolonged clonic phase of seizure activity, or the convulsive status may present as a series of discrete tonic–clonic events without intervening recovery of consciousness. Another and much rarer type of convulsive status is *tonic status epilepticus*, described by Gastaut *et al.* (1963). This occurs in children who have chronic epilepsy and are mentally retarded, particularly those with the Lennox–Gastaut syndrome. It consists of a rapid succession of tonic seizures with contractions of the facial and neck muscles, the thoracic and abdominal musculature and, to a much lesser extent, the limb muscles. Opisthotonos may result. Autonomic disturbances with sweating, tachycardia, excessive secretions and hypertension may be associated. Tonic status may be combined in some patients with non-convulsive status, to be described later. It may be precipitated in patients at risk by the intravenous administration of benzodiazepines (Bittencourt and Richens, 1981). *Myoclonic status epilepticus* is characterized by the occurrence of prolonged episodes of bilateral myoclonic jerks and occurs infrequently in juvenile myoclonic epilepsy (Asconape and Penry, 1984). Remarkably, in such cases consciousness is usually preserved despite continuous prolonged jerking but the status may culminate in a generalized tonic-clonic seizure and loss of consciousness.

## Incidence

Younger children are more susceptible to the development of convulsive status than are older children and adults, with the majority of cases occurring during the first 5 years of life (Aicardi and Chevrie, 1971) and more than 20% occurring during the first year of life (Maytal *et al.*, 1989). Mortality and all types of sequelae are significantly commoner in younger children and infants, although recent studies suggest that aggressive treatment by modern intensive care methods and adequate ventilatory procedures have lowered both mortality and morbidity in this age group (Maytal *et al.*, 1989).

## Pathophysiology

Clinicians have long been aware that the longer tonic-clonic status continues, the more difficult it is to control and the higher the incidence of mortality and morbidity. Experimental studies provide compelling arguments that convulsive status should be terminated as soon as possible (Meldrum and Brierley, 1973). Permanent neuronal damage in the hippocampus, amygdala, cerebellum, thalamus, and laminar destruction in the cortex have been reported after prolonged status in experimental animals and in man. Since vulnerable neurons can succumb in convulsive status in spite of adequate cerebral oxygenation and in the presence of sufficient supplies of glucose and after correction of metabolic side-effects, cell death is suspected to result from excessively increased metabolic demands made by continually firing neurons. The mechanisms of brain damage in prolonged status are complex and are excellently reviewed by Brown and Hussain (1991a). They include inability on the part of the cell to obtain enough energy from intracellular metabolic processes despite adequate oxygen supplies, impairment of mitochondrial function, intracellular acidosis, ATP depletion, rupture of lysosomes, calcium influx with resultant cytotoxicity, free radical toxicity, and the development of brain oedema. The increased body temperature, resulting from the generalized convulsive movements, and perhaps also due to a precipitating illness, leads to an increase in the body's metabolism and, in addition, the convulsing muscles require increased oxygen supplies. As these increased demands for oxygen generally outstrip the supply, some tissues commence anaerobic respiration. An initial rise in the blood glucose is followed by a fall, the arterial $pO_2$ drops, a systemic metabolic acidosis develops and the blood lactate concentration rises. Autonomic dysfunctions appear consisting of hyperthermia, excessive sweating, dehydration, hypertension followed by hypotension, and eventual shock. Excessive muscle activity may lead to myolysis and myoglobinuria. Cardiovascular, respiratory and renal failure may eventually result.

## Brain damage

Clinically, the effect of a prolonged seizure may be transient if the convulsion is terminated. The short-lived Todd's post-ictal hemiparesis after a prolonged febrile convulsion is an example of this. Parenthetically, it is worth noting that transient hemiparesis may sometimes occur as a post-ictal phenomenon, even though there has been little in the way of actual convulsive movements (Hanson and Chodos,

1978). A permanent hemiplegia may follow a prolonged episode of status epilepticus. However, both post-convulsive hemiplegia and also the disastrous HHE syndrome of hemiconvulsions, hemiplegia and later epilepsy are less common now than at the time Gastaut *et al.* (1960) described the latter, probably because effective treatment (and especially the introduction of intravenous diazepam in the early 1960s) is more widely available. Bilateral hemisphere damage may also result from prolonged convulsive status. Cerebral congestion and cerebral oedema produce raised intracranial pressure. The rise in intracranial pressure results in a fall in cerebral perfusion pressure and the cerebral ischaemia is particularly felt in the so-called watershed areas between the different vascular territories in the brain. This results in cell death and infarction. Acute brain shifts and coning may occur. Herniation through the tentorial opening may be clinically manifested by the development of decerebrate rigidity and progressive brainstem failure (Brown and Habel, 1975). Death usually follows or, if the child lives, cerebral atrophy develops and the survivors are mentally retarded, have cortical blindness, and show evidence of severe cerebral palsy.

## Long-term sequelae

Another important sequela of prolonged convulsive status which must be mentioned is the development of gliosis in one or both hippocampal areas as a result of cellular damage there (Corsellis and Burton, 1983). 'Mesial temporal sclerosis', the name coined by Falconer, Serafetinides and Corsellis (1964), to describe the hippocampal damage is a most important cause of secondary partial epilepsy with complex partial seizures later, better known as temporal lobe epilepsy. Lindsay *et al.* (1984) showed that, in patients with intractable epilepsy necessitating temporal lobectomy, those with histologically proven mesial temporal sclerosis showed a very high incidence (85%) of status epilepticus before the age of 3 years. There is usually a latent period between the episode of status and the development of temporal lobe seizures. Children need prolonged follow-up after a severe episode of status before one can be sure that they have escaped hippocampal neuronal damage. The use of MRI scanning has greatly improved our ability to visualize even small areas of abnormality deep in the brain (see Chapter 23).

## Aetiology

The response to treatment of status epilepticus and, consequently, its long-term outcome are very much determined by its underlying aetiology. The causes may be subdivided as follows:

1   Idiopathic or cryptogenic causes.
2   Acute symptomatic or remote symptomatic causes.

The description 'acute symptomatic' refers to cases of acute neurological or acute systemic disorder which may be responsible for or precipitate status, while remote symptomatic refers to cases associated with a chronic non-progressive or progressive disturbance of brain function (encephalopathy). It is most important to realize that status epilepticus if very often the first epileptic seizure in infants and young children (Aicardi and Chevrie, 1970). In a recent series (Maytal *et al.*, 1989) 90% of children whose status epilepticus occurred before 3 years of age had had no prior seizures. Even when those with febrile status epilepticus were excluded, 83% of those younger than 3 years had status epilepticus as their first seizure. In comparison, 57% of those who were older than 5 years at the time of their status epilepticus had had a history of prior afebrile seizures.

Febrile convulsions are the major cause of acute idiopathic or cryptogenic status, especially under the age of 3 years. Most febrile convulsions are brief; less than 10% last longer than 15 minutes and about 4% last longer than 30 minutes (Nelson and Ellenberg, 1978). Nevertheless, acute febrile status accounts for approximately a quarter of all episodes of status epilepticus in children (Aicardi and Chevrie, 1970; Maytal *et al.*, 1989). The occurrence of an apparently idiopathic status may sometimes herald the onset of a severe and progressive epileptic syndrome, for example, severe myoclonic epilepsy of infancy syndrome or Lennox–Gastaut syndrome. All studies of status epilepticus in childhood show that age correlates with aetiology. In the newborn, anoxic–ischaemic, infective or metabolic encephalopathies are important causes and, in infancy, acute meningitis or acute metabolic derangements (e.g. hyponatraemia) are significant causes. Status epilepticus may follow even relatively minor head trauma, especially in young children (Grand, 1975).

Brain tumours are very exceptional causes of status in children, mainly because cortical tumours, and especially the frontal lobe tumours which often cause status in adults, are uncommon in early childhood. Non-compliance with antiepileptic drugs only starts to become an important cause in adolescence. Important remote symptomatic causes include neonatal anoxic–ischaemic brain damage, and also other chronic encephalopathies. As is the case with chronic and intractable epilepsy generally, modern neuroimaging, especially MRI scanning, is now capable of detecting various developmental brain lesions whose presence may offer a reason for the sudden development of severe status epilepticus (Guerrini *et al.*, 1992).

## Treatment

### First-line treatment

It is mandatory to stop the seizures as soon as possible. There is no excuse for sending a still convulsing child to hospital by ambulance without instituting some treatment. Time is of the essence if brain damage or death are to be prevented. First-time treatment consists of the administration of diazepam, correct positioning of the patient, and attention to the airway. A problem arises when diazepam must be given at home by a doctor who, quite reasonably, may not wish to attempt intravenous injection in a small convulsing child. The drug should preferably not be given intramuscularly because of slow absorption, although injections of not less than 1 mg/kg will produce an effective blood level in 15–30 minutes. Rectal administration is the best alternative to intravenous injection and, using a dosage of 0.5 mg/kg will produce a blood concentration above the minimal anticonvulsant level within 2 minutes and peak levels after 6 minutes (Dulac *et al.*, 1978). It may be given either as the proprietary preparation (Stesolid), available in disposable rectal tubes in 5 mg and 10 mg doses, or, alternatively, the standard intravenous preparation may be employed, using a disposable syringe and a short piece of tubing such as an infant's nasogastric tube. In an emergency, the protective sheath which normally covers the needle of a disposable syringe may be used, after first removing the needle and then snipping off the end of the sheath which, after re-attachment to the syringe, is inserted into the rectum. Lubricating jelly may be used, if available, and the buttocks should be held together for 2 minutes to prevent expulsion of the solution. A Mantoux syringe may also be used (without a needle), inserting the whole syringe for at least 5 cm and then injecting the solution. Rectal diazepam may be repeated after 15–20 minutes if convulsions continue or re-start.

Paraldehyde may also be administered intramuscularly in an emergency, using 1 ml per year of age and not giving more than 5 ml into any one site. Injection into the buttock area should be avoided because of possible sciatic nerve damage, and care should be taken to prevent subcutaneous leakage which may cause tissue necrosis. Sterile abscess formation may also occur sometimes after intramuscular injection. When a plastic syringe is used, the drug must be given immediately after loading to prevent sticking of the plunger. Paraldehyde takes up to 20 minutes to produce any sort of effective blood level and, when given rectally, it achieves such levels very slowly indeed.

The child should be *transported* in a semi-prone position and, if possible, an anaesthetic airway should be inserted after first suctioning with a mucus extractor or mechanical sucker. If an airway is not available, extension of the neck and elevation of the jaw will suffice to prevent obstruction by the tongue.

**Second-line treatment**

On arrival at the hospital, further treatment should be started at once in the emergency room and subsequently, and ideally, in an intensive care unit where modern electronic monitoring equipment and special nursing care are available.

The insertion of an anaesthetic airway is essential. A secure intravenous line should be erected and blood should be withdrawn for urea, electrolytes, glucose, calcium and blood gases. Serum drug levels may be required if the patient is already taking antiepileptic drugs. A restricted intravenous fluid intake (60% of normal requirements) should be commenced, and half-normal glucose saline solution is preferred. Any acidosis present should be corrected, oxygen is administered, and it is essential to keep the patient cool since hyperthermia commonly develops if the convulsions continue. A bolus injection of hypertonic glucose may be given and some advise the intravenous injection of 200 mg pyridoxine for infants less than 2 years of age (Aicardi, 1985). Pyridoxine dependency may manifest itself at up to more than 1 year of age with any type of seizure, and status epilepticus seems to be the most common presentation (Goutières and Aicardi, 1985). The obtundation and coma which characteristically accompany and follow status epilepticus, and which are a consequence of *acute cerebral oedema and brain swelling*, may be rapidly relieved by the use of mannitol. It is given intravenously as a 20% solution in a dose of 0.5–1.5 g/kg over a period of 20–30 minutes, which may be repeated after 6–8 hours, although the state of hydration, serum osmolality and electrolytes should be monitored before using repeated doses. Mannitol may help to prevent or reduce the incidence and severity of brain damage and, by reducing cerebral oedema, it has an anticonvulsant action by interrupting the self-perpetuating convulsive mechanism produced by acute brain swelling. Cerebral oedema may also cause the Cushing effect, i.e. a rise in systemic blood pressure in an attempt to improve cerebral perfusion. Very high levels of systolic and diastolic blood pressure may be recorded and serious hypertensive changes may develop in the retinae, including haemorrhages. In prolonged status, hypotension may develop later as general deterioration occurs and dopamine and plasma volume expanders may be needed to support systemic blood pressure.

Reduction of intracranial pressure in the unconscious child is mandatory before performing a lumbar puncture, especially if intracranial pressure monitoring is not available, and mannitol and frusemide may be used for this purpose. Acute bacterial meningitis should always be considered in the convulsing child, especially since all common types of bacterial meningitis, including meningococcal infection, may present with status. In some cases, where meningitis is suspected but lumbar puncture is considered too dangerous, antibiotic therapy may have to be commenced without a proven diagnosis.

*EEG monitoring* can be useful in the management of status epilepticus. Intermittent recordings may be made using a conventional EEG machine or the so-called 'cerebral function monitor' may be used to provide information from one or two channels, thereby permitting moment-to-moment evaluation of the EEG.

## Antiepileptic drugs in the treatment of status epilepticus

There is considerable controversy about drug regimes to control seizures in convulsive status. In children, most clinicians prefer to use monotherapy via a single intravenous line. *Diazepam* is the most widely used first-line drug. However, its antiepileptic effect is temporary only, because it is dispersed quickly to various organs and tissues. Seizures may recur after 10–20 minutes when diazepam is used, although this is less likely to happen in children with acute febrile status. The initial bolus should not be less than 0.3 mg/kg (some use up to 0.5 mg/kg), which can be repeated after 15 minutes if seizures recur. If the child's weight cannot be measured easily, it is safe to give 1 mg per year of age plus 1 mg (e.g. at 2 years give 3 mg intravenously). The drug should be administered at a rate of 1 mg/min.

When seizures continue to recur despite the administration of two repeat bolus doses of diazepam, it is necessary to continue other treatment strategies. Diazepam may be given as a continuous infusion well diluted with dextrose saline (up to 10 mg diazepam per hour). However, the drug tends to bind to plastic in intravenous giving sets, which means that dosage can be uncertain by this method. Localized irritation of veins and other tissues is also a problem, which may be avoided by using the emulsion of diazepam (Diazemuls) intravenously instead of the standard preparation (Brown and Hussain 1991b). The main hazard with intravenous diazepam is the possibility of producing respiratory arrest. This is more likely to happen when the drug is used in combination with phenobarbitone or when the child has previously been on continuous phenobarbitone therapy. However, the risk of producing respiratory arrest in these situations is slight if caution is observed during the intravenous administration of diazepam and if overdosage is avoided. If apnoea does occur, it is usually transitory and oxygenation can be maintained by using an Ambu bag or similar device. Large doses of diazepam can cause a paradoxical reaction in which there is an increasing frequency of seizures (Livingston and Brown, 1988). Yet a further problem with the continued use of diazepam over some days is that, as with all benzodiazepines, tolerance to the drug may develop rapidly and diminish its anticonvulsant action.

Dissatisfaction with the use of diazepam for treating status epilepticus has led to increasing use of another benzodiazepine, *lorazepam* (Ativan), intravenously for this purpose. It acts as rapidly as diazepam, stopping seizures within 2–3 minutes in over 80% of cases, with a similar overall success rate (Crawford, Mitchell and Snodgrass, 1987). Unlike diazepam's brief period of action, it controls seizures for a much longer period of time. This allows clinicians more time to assess the patient and to arrange investigations including possibly neuroimaging, before deciding on further treatment. The need for additional drugs, such as phenytoin, may be avoided. However, the risk of respiratory depression also exists with lorazepam and measures to support breathing should be available. Lorazepam is given intravenously (0.05–0.1 mg/kg; maximum dose 4 mg) over 1–2 minutes. It may be repeated twice at 10–15 minute intervals. A third benzodiazepine drug, *clonazepam*, has also been used intravenously for status in a bolus dosage of 0.05 mg/kg and it may also be given as a continuous infusion. It probably has no significant advantages over diazepam. Because of the problems with continuous intravenous use of the benzodiazepines, it is recommended that, if the benzodiazepine chosen fails to control convulsive status quickly, *phenytoin* intravenously should be used. Phenytoin takes 20–30 minutes to achieve maximum anticonvulsant action and therefore its use in tandem with diazepam is recommended. Such a combination does not significantly increase the risk of respiratory depression. Brown and Hussain (1991b) recommend a 10 mg/kg bolus dose, followed by 5 mg/kg 1 hour later, followed by 10 mg/kg in divided doses over the remaining 23 hours, a total of 25 mg/kg per day. They prefer intermittent to continuous intravenous administration because of difficulties with precipitation of the drug. Administration is by slow injection into a saline-containing drip tube over 20–30 minutes and the vein should be well flushed afterwards with saline to avoid precipitation of the drug. The rate of injection should not exceed 25–50 mg per minute and should preferably be done under ECG monitoring (watching for bradycardia and prolongation of the QT interval) because the drug may cause arrhythmias.

The author has found phenytoin, used in conjunction with diazepam, a most satisfactory drug for treating status epilepticus. It is important, however, to have reliable drug level monitoring readily available because, in the case of phenytoin, what is called the 'therapeutic index' is low, i.e. therapeutic doses are close to toxic doses, and also because phenytoin works best within its narrow therapeutic band. Phenytoin may be continued orally (6 mg/kg per day) when consciousness has been regained. Phenytoin is infinitely preferable to the use of barbiturates particularly *phenobarbitone*, which is a potent cause of respiratory depression, delays the recovery of consciousness, and may also cause hypotension, thereby further diminishing cerebral perfusion. Used intramuscularly, it takes up to 4 hours to achieve a satisfactory serum level. It has been used in a dosage of 5 mg/kg, giving half the dose intravenously and the other half intramuscularly and repeating the intramuscular dose after 30 minutes (Weiner, Urion and Levitt, 1982). Higher doses are not recommended and the risk of respiratory depression with phenobarbitone should constantly be borne in mind. Browne and Hussain (1991b) advise that paediatricians without access to an intensive care unit or who are working in third world countries, should not embark on treatment régimes using high-dosage intravenous phenobarbitone. It is salutary to remember that more deaths have probably been caused by the overtreatment of convulsive status than by undertreatment, and constant re-evaluation should be made of the regimen being employed and its effects on the patient (see Table 11.1).

Various other drug regimens have been used for resistant status epilepticus. The use of *short-acting intravenous barbiturates* such as thiopentone sodium and

**Table 11.1 Antiepileptic drugs for treatment of status epilepticus**

| Drug | Mode | Dose |
|---|---|---|
| Diazepam | Intravenous | Initially 0.3–0.5 mg/kg repeat after 15 minutes if necessary, or 1 mg per year of age + 1 mg. |
| | Intramuscular | 1 mg/kg |
| | Per rectum | 0.5 mg/kg |
| Phenobarbitone (see text) | Intravenous/Intramuscular | 5 mg/kg. Give half i.v. and half i.m. Repeat i.m. dose in 30 minutes |
| Phenytoin (see text) | Intravenous | 10 mg/kg followed by 5 mg/kg after 1 hour and 10 mg/kg over remaining 23 hours, not exceeding 20–50 mg per minute given over 20–30 minutes. |
| Paraldehyde (see text) | Intramuscular or per rectum | 1 ml per year of age up to 5 ml. |
| Lorazepam | Intravenous | 0.05–0.1 mg/kg; maximum dose 4 mg; repeat after 15 minutes if necessary. |
| Clonazepam | Intravenous | 0.05 mg/kg. |
| Lidocaine (lignocaine) | Intravenous | 3.5 mg/kg per hour for 24–48 hours, then reduce dose. |
| Chlormethiazole | Intravenous | 0.8% solution; 5 mg/kg per hour, gradually increasing to 25 mg/kg per hour. |
| Sodium valproate | Per rectum | 10–20 mg/kg initially, then 10–15 mg/kg at 8 hourly intervals |
| Chloral hydrate | Per rectum | 30 mg/kg initially, then 20 mg/kg 2 hourly for 6 hours, then 20 mg/kg 6 hourly. |

*Drugs to reduce brain swelling:*

(1) Mannitol intravenously 0.5–1.5 g/kg over 10–30 minutes, repeated 8 hourly (total dose of 6 g/kg per 24 hours).
(2) Dexamethasone intravenously 2–4 mg initially followed by 1–2 mg 6-hourly, or 0.5 mg/kg per 24 hours.

pentobarbitone is discussed by Simon (1985). *General anaesthesia with halothane* combined with neuromuscular blockade is described by Delgado-Escueta *et al.* (1982). A continuous infusion of *lidocaine* (lignocaine) has been used successfully in adults and children, including neonates, in a dosage of 3.5 mg/kg per hour and is reported as effective and safe (Pascual *et al.*, 1988). *Chlormethiazole*, a sedative–hypnotic drug derived from the thiazole part of the vitamin B1 molecule, has been shown to have an anticonvulsant effect and is used to treat convulsions associated with alcoholism. It has been used to treat status epilepticus but should not be combined with diazepam, since synergism and marked sedation with a risk of respiratory depression may occur. It is given as an 0.8% solution, starting with 5 mg/kg per hour, increasing to 10 mg, then 20 mg to a maximum of 25 mg/kg per hour (Lingam *et al.*, 1980). The dose is titrated for maximum control of seizures and EEG monitoring is helpful.

*Paraldehyde* has a long and honourable history in the treatment of convulsive status epilepticus and can probably control status in the majority of patients. Difficulties with administration are the main problem. It is probably the best of all agents for intramuscular use initially (1 ml per year of age up to a maximum of 5 ml), but is slow to take effect. Although an extremely safe drug in most respects, it nevertheless has an unpleasant odour and, because it is excreted through the lungs, it should be avoided in children with chronic pulmonary disease. It can be used intravenously, with caution, as a bolus dose of 1 ml of sterile paraldehyde injection B.P. diluted in 25 ml of saline but may cause phlebitis. Rectally, diluted in twice its volume of olive or arachis oil, it is slow and unpredictable in its action but is useful for maintenance therapy when seizures are recurring intermittently. Dosage is similar to the intramuscular dosage and should not exceed 5 ml in a young child. The dose may be repeated after 1 hour. Tolerance to the drug, unlike diazepam, is not a problem.

Two other drugs which have been used to treat refractory status are sodium valproate and chloral hydrate. *Sodium valproate* has been used rectally with success (Snead and Miles, 1985) but is slow to take effect. Sodium valproate syrup (200 mg per 5 ml) is used, diluted 1:1 with tap water and administered in a loading dose of 10–20 mg/kg. Maintenance dosage per rectum is 10–15 mg/kg every 8 hours, preferably combined with blood level monitoring. A recent report by Lampl *et al.* (1990) has claimed successful control of convulsive status in adults using *chloral hydrate* rectally. The dosage schedule consisted of 30 mg/kg of chloral hydrate rectally, followed by 20 mg/kg every 2 hours for 6 hours, followed by 20 mg/kg every 4 hours for a total of 48 hours. No serious side-effects were reported.

## Mortality and morbidity

Status epilepticus is a serious and potentially fatal complication of the epilepsies. Prior to the advent of modern intensive care technology, Aicardi and Chevrie (1970) found a mortality of 11% in a series of 239 children less than 15 years old. Death during status is associated with respiratory or cardiac arrest or may sometimes be due to overtreatment with sedative drugs, particularly barbiturates. In a recent mainly prospective study of convulsive status treated in a modern intensive care unit, in which the condition was defined as lasting longer than 30 minutes, 7 (3.6%) of 193 children died within 3 months of the episode of status and all of these had either an acute CNS insult or progressive encephalopathy (Maytal *et al.*, 1989). No deaths occurred among the 137 children with idiopathic or febrile status. Status was relatively brief in most cases and it was considered that the mortality rate reflected the severity of the underlying disorder causing the status rather than the severity of the status. Mortality and the incidence of sequelae are usually related to the cause of the status, the outcome in symptomatic cases where there is an acute CNS insult or a progressive or non-progressive encephalopathy being significantly worse than in idiopathic or febrile status. Age and duration of status are also significant unfavourable factors, children under 3 years doing particularly badly (Chevrie and Aicardi, 1978). This relationship appears to reflect the fact that acute symptomatic status epilepticus, due to conditions such as acute bacterial meningitis, is far more common in the younger age groups. Duration of status is often greater in these cases also. However, the incidence of neurological sequelae in aggressively treated status epilepticus in children today, in the absence of an acute neurological insult or chronic or progressive encephalopathy, is low (Maytal et al., 1989). Following febrile status in otherwise normal children, Maytal and Shinnar (1990) did not find a significantly increased risk for subsequent febrile (brief or prolonged) or afebrile seizures. However, as already emphasized, follow-up needs to be lengthy before possible temporal lobe damage can be completely ruled out.

## Non-convulsive status epilepticus

### Clinical features

The earlier concept of status epilepticus was restricted to convulsive status. Non-convulsive status epilepticus is difficult to define and the literature is confusing. The reader is recommended to read the excellent review by Stores (1986). He defines non-convulsive status as an electroclinical syndrome in which the most fundamental feature is a change in the patient's behaviour. This change may be difficult to recognize in many patients, especially in young retarded children who may have persistent abnormalities of behaviour anyway. As a result, the onset and duration of this type of status may be difficult to judge. Clinically, there is usually a variable degree of clouding of mental processes, ranging from drowsiness to stupor and encompassing subtle changes such as slowness, moodiness, disinterest in play, and confusion. During the episodes, the children are slow to react to stimuli, are unable to concentrate, become disorientated and develop dysphasia or lose speech. The fluctuating nature of the symptoms is very characteristic. Intermittent ataxia may be a feature or sometimes a 'pseudoataxia', a term used by Brett (1966) to describe a situation where the intrusion of subtle repeated myoclonic jerks may simulate ataxia.

### Incidence and diagnosis

Most cases of non-convulsive status epilepticus occur in children under 10 years of age and diagnosis is dependent on clinical suspicion and careful EEG examination, including a sleep record, if possible. Combined video/EEG monitoring is a very useful aid, if available. The majority of children presenting with this type of status will have a history of previous epilepsy but, in some, non-convulsive status may be the presenting feature of the epileptic illness and, in these especially, the insidious nature and subtlety of the symptoms may result in delay in making a precise diagnosis (Manning and Rosenbloom, 1987). Misdiagnosis is also frequent, the symptoms being ascribed to antiepileptic drug intoxication, prolonged postictal state, acute encephalopathy, neurodegenerative disorder or primary psychiatric cause, including depression, hysteria or psychosis (Stores, 1986). A useful clinical clue to diagnosis is the unexpected return of the child to his usual self, a reversal of the so-called 'pseudodementia' of non-convulsive status, suggestive that there is an epileptic cause.

## Varieties of non-convulsive status epilepticus

Generalized non-convulsive status epilepticus is now often called *absence status* (Gastaut, 1983) but this term is unsatisfactory, in the author's view, to describe cases with only mild blunting of consciousness. In many respects, Brett's (1966) imprecise term 'minor epileptic status' is preferable since it does cover the diverse manifestations of this condition. The term 'petit mal status' is misleading, since it implies a close relationship with childhood absence epilepsy (petit mal) and, in the author's experience, such an association with that primary generalized epilepsy is exceptionally rare. Ohlahara *et al.* (1979) have described such cases. In cases where the EEG shows prolonged electrical 3 Hz spike-wave status with only occasional clinical absences, one should suspect the existence of another syndrome and, in one such personal case, the patient was later shown to have electrical status epilepticus during sleep (the ESES syndrome), a condition first described by Patry, Lyagoubi and Tassinari (1971) and discussed in detail in Chapter 17.

The absences, when they occur in non-convulsive status, are quite atypical compared with the simple absences of petit mal. They are often prolonged and may be associated with other clinical manifestations such as myoclonic jerks, atonic features, and ataxia. There are, in addition, often behavioural changes. The EEG usually shows continuous, bilaterally synchronous, symmetrical epileptic activity. Spike-wave activity is usually at a slow rate (2–2.5 Hz) and is often irregular and arrhythmic. Bursts of frontal slow activity and of fast activity are also present. Rarely, there may be evidence of focal abnormalities.

In the author's experience, most cases of non-convulsive status epilepticus in young children occur in association with one of the secondary generalized epilepsies, particularly the early severe secondary myoclonic epilepsies. Children with the *Lennox–Gastaut syndrome* are very likely to develop this complication. The association with serious secondary generalized epilepsy probably explains why the long-term outlook for intellectual function in these children is so poor (Brett, 1966; Manning and Rosenbloom, 1987). As Aicardi (1986) has suggested, both the electrical status and the behavioural deterioration may be secondary to some severe ongoing cerebral process.

However, this poor prognosis is not invariable for children who have experienced non-convulsive status. Doose (1983) has described the occurrence of non-convulsive status in non-retarded children with primary or idiopathic *myoclonic–astatic epilepsy* who have a genetically determined susceptibility to epilepsy. In these, remission of seizures and normal psychomotor development later are not uncommon (see Chapter 5).

The *treatment* of non-convulsive status may be very difficult. Intravenous diazepam is the usual initial therapy but this type of status can be resistant to benzodiazepines, especially when the patient has already been taking one of these drugs orally. Occasionally, a paradoxical response may occur with the induction of convulsive seizures (Livingston and Brown, 1987). Other drugs which should be considered are sodium valproate and ethosuximide. Browne (1983) has recommended a trial of intravenous acetazolamide (250 mg for children weighing less than 35 kg and 500 mg for those over that weight) for resistant cases of what he terms absence status. ACTH or corticosteroids are also effective on occasions (Robinson, 1985).

*Complex partial status epilepticus* is another variety of non-convulsive status which has been described mainly in adults but has also been documented in children (Stores, 1986). The condition usually consists of frequently repeated episodes of typical or atypical complex partial seizures without full recovery of consciousness interictally. This causes a fluctuating mental state with least responsiveness during the ictal episodes and varying degrees of confusion in between. Rarely, complex partial status may exist as a continuous clouding of consciousness and it may then be difficult to differentiate from other types of absence status. Stereotyped automatisms may be a feature. Prolonged memory disturbances and cognitive defects may follow the ictal event. The EEG is essential for establishing a correct diagnosis. The presence of a frontal or temporal focus of spikes unilaterally makes the diagnosis easier but, unfortunately, frequent secondary generalization of discharges makes identification of a focus and correct interpretation of the record difficult.

Aggressive treatment is recommended along the lines suggested for generalized tonic–clonic status, in order to reduce the incidence of post-ictal memory and cognitive sequelae. Intravenous diazepam and phenytoin are the most useful parenteral drugs (Holmes, 1987).

## Conclusion

As has been reiterated several times, status epilepticus, especially generalized tonic–clonic status, is a major paediatric emergency which can result in permanent brain damage or death. It is important to recognize when this dangerous situation exists or is imminent, and to know how to institute appropriate therapy. It is best for a clinician to choose one particular line of treatment which can be executed comfortably and expeditiously in his or her clinical situation and to become familiar with it. An inadequate response to treatment may result from the initial administration of the chosen drug at too low a dosage, or by some route other than intravenous; failure to repeat the dose when the first dose is ineffective; failure to identify a treatable underlying cause; and failure to institute appropriate maintenance therapy. At all times, it is necessary to tread the difficult path between undertreatment and overtreatment in order to secure a successful outcome.

## References

AICARDI, J. (1986) *Epilepsy in Children* Raven Press, New York pp. 240–259
AICARDI, J, and CHEVRIE, J. J. (1970) Convulsive status epilepticus in infants and children. A study of 239 cases. *Epilepsia*, 11, 187–197
ASCONAPE, J. and PENRY, J. K. (1984) Some clinical and EEG aspects of benign juvenile myoclonic epilepsy. *Epilepsia*, 25, 108–114
BITTENCOURT, P. R. M. and RICHENS, A. (1981) Anticonvulsant-induced status epilepticus in Lennox–Gastaut syndrome. *Epilepsia*, 22, 129–134
BRETT, E. M. (1966) Minor epileptic status. *Journal of the Neurological Sciences*, 3, 52–75

BROWNE, T. R. (1983) Status epilepticus. *In Epilepsy, Diagnosis and Management* (eds T. R. Browne and R. G. Feldman), Little, Browne and Co., Boston, pp. 341–354

BROWN, J. K. and HABEL, A. H. (1975) Toxic encephalopathy and acute brain swelling in children. *Developmental Medicine and Child Neurology*, **17**, 659–679

BROWN, J. K. and HUSSAIN (1991 a and b) Status epilepticus. I(a) Pathogenesis II(b) Treatment. *Developmental Medicine and Child Neurology*, **33**, (I-a) 3–17; (II-b) 97–109

CHEVRIE, J. J. and AICARDI, J. (1978) Convulsive disorders in the first year of life: neurologic and mental outcome and mortality. *Epilepsia*, **19**, 67–74

CORSELLIS, J. A. N. and BRUTON, C. J. (1983) Neuropathology of status epilepticus in humans. In *Advances in Neurology*, Vol. **34**, Status Epilepticus (eds. A. V. Delgado-Escueta, C. G. Wasterlain, D. M. Treiman and R. J. Porter), Raven Press, New York, pp. 129–139

CRAWFORD, T. O., MITCHELL, W. G. and SNODGRASS, S. R. (1987) Lorazepam in childhood status epilepticus and serial seizures. *Neurology*, **37**, 190–195

DELGADO-ESCUETA, A. V., WASTERLAIN, C., TREIMAN, D. M. and PORTER, R. J. (1982) Current concepts in neurology. Management of status epilepticus. *New England Journal of Medicine*, **306**, 1337–1340

DOOSE, H. (1983) Non-convulsive status epilepticus in childhood: clinical aspects and classification. In *Advances in Neurology*, Vol. **34**, Status Epilepticus (eds A. V. Delgado-Escueta, C. G. Wasterlain, D. M. Treiman and R. J. Porter), Raven Press, New York, p. 83

DULAC, O., AICARDI, J., REY, E. and OLIVE, G. (1978) Blood levels of diazepam after single rectal administration to infants and children. *Journal of Pediatrics*, **93**, 1039–1041

FALCONER, M. A., SERAFETINIDES, E. A. and CORSELLIS, J. A. N. (1964) Etiology and pathogenesis of temporal lobe epilepsy. *Archives of Neurology*, **10**, 233–248

GASTAUT, H. (1983) Classification of status epilepticus. In *Advances in Neurology*, Vol. 43. Status Epilepticus (eds. A. V. Delgado-Escueta, C. G. Wasterlain, D. M. Treiman and R. J. Porter), Raven Press, New York, p. 15

GASTAUT, H., POIRIER, F., PAYER, H., *et al.* (1960) HHE syndrome. Hemiconvulsions, hemiplegia, epilepsy. *Epilepsia*, **1**, 418–447

GASTAUT, H., ROGER, J., OUAHCHI, S., *et al.* (1963) An electroclinical study of generalized epileptic seizures of tonic expression. *Epilepsia*, **4**, 15–44

GOUTIÈRES, F. and AICARDI, J. (1985) Atypical presentation of pyridoxine-dependent seizures. A treatable cause of intractable epilepsy in infants. *Annals of Neurology*, **17**, 117–120

GRAND, W. (1975) The significance of post-traumatic status epilepticus in childhood. *Journal of Neurology, Neurosurgery and Psychiatry*, **37**, 178–180

GUERRINI, R., DRAVET, C., RAYBAUD, C. *et al.* (1992) Epilepsy and focal gyral anomalies detected by MRI: electroclinicomorphological correlations and follow-up. *Developmental Medicine and Child Neurology*, **34**, 706–718

HANSON, P. A. and CHODOS, R. (1978) Hemiparetic seizures. *Neurology*, **28**, 920–923

HOLMES, G. L. (1987) Status epilepticus. In *Diagnosis and Management of Seizures in Children*. W. B. Saunders Company, Philadelphia, London, pp. 262–276

LAMPL, Y., ESHEL, Y., GILAD, R. and SAROVA-PINCHAS, I. (1990) Chloral hydrate in intractable status epilepticus. *Annals of Emergency Medicine*, **19**, 674–676

LINDSAY, J., GLASER, G., RICHARDS, P. and OUNSTED, C. (1984) Developmental aspects of focal epilepsy treated by neurosurgery. *Developmental Medicine and Child Neurology*, **26**, 574–587

LINGAM, S., BERWHISTLE, H., ELLISTON, H. M. and WILSON, J. (1980) Problems with intravenous chlormethiazole (Heminevrin) in status epilepticus. *British Medical Journal*, **280**, 155–156

LIVINGSTON, J. H. and BROWN, J. K. (1987) Non-convulsive status epilepticus resistant to benzodiazepines. *Archives of Disease in Childhood*, **62**, 41–44

LIVINGSTON, J. H. and BROWN, J. K. (1988) Diagnosis and management of non-convulsive status epilepticus. *Paediatric Review and Communications*, **2**, 283–315

MANNING, D. J. and ROSENBLOOM, L. (1987) Non-convulsive status epilepticus. *Archives of Disease in Childhood*, **62**, 37–40

MAYTAL, J. and SHINNAR, S. (1990) Febrile status epilepticus. *Pediatrics*, **86**, 611–616

MAYTAL, J., SHINNAR, S., MOSHÉ, S. L. and ALVAREZ, L. A. (1989) Low morbidity and mortality of status epilepticus in children. *Pediatrics*, **83**, 323–331

MELDRUM, B. S. and BRIERLEY, J. B. (1973) Prolonged epileptic seizure in primates: ischaemic cell change and its relations to ictal physiological event. *Archives of Neurology*, **28**, 10–17

NELSON, K. B. and ELLENBERG, J. H. (1978) Prognosis in children with febrile seizures. *Pediatrics*, **61**, 720–727

OHTAHARA, S., OKA, E., YAMATOGI, Y. *et al.* (1979) Non-convulsive status epilepticus in childhood. *Folia Psychiatr. Neurol. Jpn*, **33**, 345–351

PASCUAL, J., SEDANO, M. J., POLO, J. M. and BERCIANO, J. (1988) Intravenous lidocaine for status epilepticus. *Epilepsia*, **29**, 584–589

PATRY, G., LYAGOUBI, S. and TASSINARI, C. A. (1971) Subclinical 'electrical status epilepticus' induced by sleep in children. *Archives of Neurology*, **24**, 242–252

ROBINSON, R. O. (1985) Seizures and steroids. *Archives of Disease in Childhood*, **60**, 94–95

SIMON, R. P. (1985) Management of status epilepticus. In *Recent Advances in Epilepsy*, No. 2 (eds T. A. Pedley and B. S. Meldrum) Churchill Livingstone, Edinburgh, London, pp. 137–160.

SNEAD, O. C. and MILES, M. V. (1985) Treatment of status epilepticus in children with rectal sodium valproate. *Journal of Pediatrics*, **106**, 323–325

STORES, G. (1986) Non-convulsive status epilepticus in children. In *Recent Advances in Epilepsy*, No. 3 (eds T. A. Pedley and B. S. Meldrum) Churchill Livingstone, Edinburgh, London, pp. 295–310

WEINER, H. L., URION, D. K. and LEVITT, L. P. (1982) *Pediatric Neurology for the House Officer*, 3rd Edition Williams and Wilkins, Baltimore, London, pp. 49–51

# Chapter 12

# Reflex epilepsy

Seizures triggered by a sensory stimulation are sometimes called 'reflex epileptic seizures', since the nerve structure responsible for the seizure is situated between the sensory afferent pathway and the efferent tract responsible for the epileptic phenomena, thus acting as a reflex centre. This concept of reflex epilepsy was very fashionable in the nineteenth century when it was considered that a major cause of epilepsy, particularly in children, was chronic sensory irritation produced by such varied causes as intestinal worms, phimosis, refractive errors and teething. Part of this belief lingers on in the lay mind, and perhaps the association between chronic constipation and epilepsy in the folklore of epilepsy is a part of it.

## Criteria

When strict criteria are used for defining 'reflex' epilepsy it is found to be relatively rare. Gastaut and Tassinari (1966) made the point that true 'reflex' epilepsy should be clearly distinguished from the part played by non-sensory epileptogenic factors which seem to act by affecting certain biological constants and modifying the threshold of cerebral excitability. These factors include hyperventilation; hyperthermia; the ingestion of alcohol; metabolic disorders of various kinds, including hypocalcaemia and hypoglycaemia; extreme physical or emotional stress, particularly when accompanied by sleep deprivation; and perhaps hormonal changes occurring at menstruation or during puberty.

### Photosensitivity and television-induced epilepsy

By far the most frequent of true reflex epileptic seizures are those produced by visual stimuli (i.e. visually evoked reflex epilepsy), although even those are relatively rare in relation to the overall frequency of epileptic attacks. Photosensitivity can be investigated in the EEG laboratory by applying a very bright rhythmically repeating white flash (intermittent photic stimulation) to the whole of the visual fields of both eyes, open and shut, for short periods. Single visual-evoked responses can then be recorded over the occipital areas at slow rates of flicker and continuous rhythmic waveforms occur at faster rates of flicker. These responses do not irradiate anteriorly and cease with the final flash of the stimulating sequence. It is essential to remember that these responses are a normal finding. The most common abnormality following photic stimulation is that induced in the photosensitive epilepsies. This consists of a burst of bilaterally symmetrical generalized multiple spikes (poly-spikes) or spike and wave complexes (*Figure 12.1*). These generalized discharges usually appear after very brief stimulation and may sometimes outlast the period of stimulation. This type of response is termed the photoconvulsive response. It may be seen in up to 1% of normal children (Driver and MacGillivray, 1976) and in a few normal adults. In any individual exhibiting the photoconvulsive response the period of stimulation should be brief in case a seizure is induced.

Some individuals are exquisitely photosensitive and may have a seizure provoked by intermittent light stimulation under natural conditions, for example the play of light through trees or on water or on snow or reflected from a brilliant object. There is a less sensitive group in which clinical seizures can be induced by flickering from a light source of high intensity with relatively darker surroundings. This is the situation which obtains in *television-induced epilepsy* which is by far the commonest type of photosensitive epilepsy today. Gastaut and Tassinari (1966) summarized the characteristic features of television-induced seizures as those occurring essentially but not exclusively in children, being almost always of the primary generalized major tonic–clonic type, being sometimes preceded by generalized myoclonic jerks and almost always showing spike and wave complexes or polyspike and wave discharges during intermittent photic stimulation in the EEG laboratory. An absence, lasting 5–15 seconds, may also be induced by intermittent photic stimulation. Children with photosensitivity are mainly at risk when viewing television while being seated close to a normally functioning set. Neither faulty functioning of the television set producing a flicker effect (as with a faulty line hold) nor the usual play of images on the screen seems to play any significant part in causing seizures, except perhaps in a few very sensitive individuals. The proximity of the screen is of paramount importance in triggering an attack which may occur when the subject approaches the set to adjust it. Some photosensitive children seem compulsively drawn to the screen and may occasionally seem to enjoy the sensation produced, although usually they fear it. Nearness to the screen means that a larger area of the retina is stimulated by flicker, and viewing in subdued ambient lighting may also increase the contrast effect produced by the brightly lit screen. Sensitive subjects are equally at risk from black-and-white television and colour television. There is no convincing evidence that any particular component of the colour spectrum is more epileptogenic than others. Using a portable TV set with a small screen may reduce the risk (Editorial, 1978).

Bower (1963) and Troupin (1966) drew attention to the fact that epilepsy induced by television viewing was less commonly encountered in the USA than in Europe. This has been shown to be due to higher frequency of the AC mains supply in the USA which alternates at 60 Hz compared with 50 Hz in Europe. The normally functioning television set produces flicker at the mains frequency and at half that rate, and the slower flicker rates in Europe (50 Hz and 25 Hz) are more likely to produce a photoconvulsive response in photosensitive patients. In the EEG laboratory the great majority of patients with photosensitivity will show photoconvulsive responses (polyspikes, polyspikes and waves or spike-wave complexes at 3 Hz) at flicker frequencies of 15–20 flashes per second. Similar discharges occur on eye closure in the resting EEG in about 20% of sensitive patients, and this finding usually indicates that photoconvulsive responses will follow during photic stimulation.

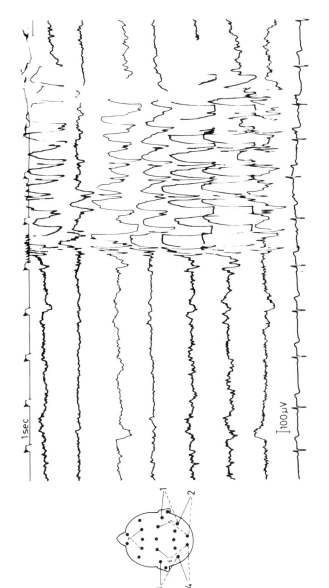

*Figure 12.1* Girl aged 12 years and awake with eyes open. EEG shows paroxysmal spike–wave complexes occurring in response to intermittent photic stimulation at 20 flashes per second

## Photosensitive epilepsy: age of onset and prognosis

Photosensitive epilepsy usually begins in the decade 6–15 years, never earlier and rarely later. It commences most frequently between the ages of 12 and 13 years, which suggests a possible link with early puberty. There is a higher incidence of the condition in females. Studies of the long-term prognosis of photosensitivity (Jeavons and Harding, 1975) suggest that photosensitivity continues for at least 10 years and usually into the third decade of life. Jeavons, Bishop and Harding (1986), after a prolonged follow-up study, concluded that photosensitivity disappeared earlier in patients treated with sodium valproate (mean age of 22.9 ± 2.5 years) than in untreated subjects (24.5 ± 4.9 years). They pointed out that it was uncommon in their series to find evidence of photosensitivity in the EEGs of the parents of photosensitive children, even when one or other parent described symptoms associated with flicker at an earlier age. The general experience is that it is unusual to encounter clinical photosensitive epilepsy in adults.

## Photosensitivity: genetics

Doose *et al.* (1969) surveyed the hereditary aspects of the EEG abnormalities induced by photic stimulation. They found that 26.2% of the siblings of patients with photosensitive epilepsy showed a photoconvulsive EEG response, compared with 6.7% in healthy controls. They concluded that the photoconvulsive response could be a symptom of a very widespread genetically determined susceptibility to convulsions of the primary generalized type originating from the brain-stem, and that the actual morbidity for epilepsy was low. A symptomatic photosensitivity is very rarely associated with organic brain lesions such as brain tumours or after encephalitis, and is a characteristic finding in neuronal ceroid lipofuscinosis (Batten–Vogt syndrome) where discharges occur in the EEG in response to very low rates of intermittent photic stimulation (Pampiglione and Harden, 1977). Paroxysmal abnormalities in  the EEG in response to photic stimulation may be seen very early in the course of severe myoclonic epilepsy in infancy (Dravet, *et al.*, 1992) and are regarded as an ominous finding.

## Prevention and Treatment

The photosensitive patient should always watch television from a distance of not less than 3 metres and the room should be well lit. He or she should be dissuaded from approaching the set in order to adjust it or to change the channel; however, if this is absolutely necessary one eye should be covered with the palm of the hand as this will usually help to block the photoconvulsive response (Jeavons and Harding, 1970). Polarized sunglasses are helpful outdoors in preventing attacks in bright sunlight. The patient whose seizures are entirely photosensitive may not need antiepileptic therapy, although there are many exceptions, particularly where there are epileptic discharges in the resting EEG in addition to those produced by flicker or when clinical seizures are frequent, and when the environmental risks are increased (see later). The patient who has epilepsy other than that produced by flicker (a point difficult to establish with certainty in the very sensitive patient) and who also has definite photosensitive epilepsy will need regular long-term anticonvulsant medication. Although all the commonly used antiepileptic drugs have been tried for this purpose, there is evidence (Jeavons, Clark and Maheshwari, 1977) that sodium valproate is particularly effective in this regard. Many parents ask whether the images on a cinema screen constitute a risk for a photosensitive patient, but in fact the flickering is at too high a frequency to induce an attack. The flicker effect used in discothèques, on the other hand, may provoke seizures in sensitive individuals, and in 1971, the Greater London Council forbade the use of flicker rates faster than 8 flashes per second; a slow frequency reduces the risk but does not abolish it altogether. Even watching the movement of an escalator may be provocative in some individuals.

Gastaut (1952) was probably the first person to describe *self-induced photosensitive epilepsy* when he wrote: 'One of our young patients provoked his absences voluntarily by placing rhythmically his hand, fingers open, in front of his eyes when he looked at the sun. A little girl took a mischievous pleasure in provoking her absences by moving her head very quickly from right to left behind a window trimmed with stained glass panes brilliantly illuminated by the sun.' The mechanism in this rare form of epilepsy (perhaps commoner, as Gastaut remarks, beneath 'the luminous sky of Provence') consists of the rhythmical interruption of natural or artificial light and is similar to the effects produced by watching sunlight flickering through trees while being driven in a car or by watching the rotation of the blades of a helicopter against a bright sky. Sherwood (1962) collectively reviewed cases of self-induced epilepsy.

In recent times, the increase in video games using television sets has led to reports of what has been called 'space-invader epilepsy' (Rushton, 1981; De Marco and Ghersini, 1985). This is, of course, another instance of photosensitive epilepsy. The increasing use of visual display units with home computers and of computers in schools also presents a risk to the photosensitive individual because such equipment requires close viewing. Jeavons, Bishop and Harding (1986) commented that because of these various new risks, it had become necessary to treat more photosensitive subjects with sodium valproate than heretofore – in order to enable them to lead as normal a life as their peers (including visiting discotheques). They also cautioned them against withdrawing medication prematurely from the adolescent or young adult lest they lose a driving licence or, as the author has witnessed on more than one occasion, a job. Another argument for the increasing use of drug therapy in these patients is the observation by Jeavons and his colleagues that photosensitivity seems to disappear earlier in the treated compared with the untreated.

Jeavons (1977) has differentiated patients with what he terms '*photomyoclonic epilepsy*' from the general body of the patients with photosensitive epilepsy. These are patients, usually adolescents, who show spontaneous spike and wave discharges in their EEGs and also have similar discharges during intermittent photic stimulation. He has described two subgroups comprising, first, those patients who have myoclonic jerks of head and arms, occurring spontaneously and during photic stimulation and, secondly, those patients who demonstrate rapid jerking movements of the eyelids immediately after eye closure (associated with bilateral spike and wave activity) and who have brief absences associated with spike-wave discharges at 3 Hz which occur both spontaneously and during photic stimulation. He entitled the latter 'eyelid myoclonia with absences'. The recommended treatment is with sodium valproate.

Before leaving the subject of visually evoked reflex epilepsy, the condition of *pattern-evoked epilepsy* needs to be mentioned. In this unusual entity seizure discharges are produced in the EEG by looking at certain patterns, either lined or squared. Episodes of staring triggered by vertical lines such as striped or corduroy trousers and absences precipitated by other vertical lines such as air vents, tiles or bedspreads have been reported (Chatrian *et al.*, 1970). Pattern-evoked responses probably play a part in reading epilepsy, mentioned below.

## Non-visual precipitating factors

The most common modality of sensory precipitation in reflex epilepsy is visual, but there are rarer sensory precipitants including sound, touch, proprioception and also possibly visceral, olfactory and vestibular stimuli. Seizures may be triggered by a particular mental activity, such as hearing or performing music, reading, writing, specific visual or auditory imagery or mathematical calculation. The term 'startle epilepsy' is sometimes applied to brief clonic or tonic–clonic seizures provoked by auditory stimuli or by touch. Acoustimotor seizures may occur in infants with diffuse brain disease or abnormality, classically in those with $GM_2$ gangliosidosis (Tay–Sachs disease). Similar brief attacks are also seen in older children and are provoked by a violent and unexpected noise, almost always in children with epilepsy due to diffuse organic brain disease. The author has seen them especially in mentally handicapped children who had previously suffered from infantile spasms or who had one of the secondary generalized epilepsies of the myoclonic type. These seizures are particularly resistant to drug therapy, but treatment with carbazepine may be beneficial (Sáenz-Lope, Herranz and Masdeu, 1984).

A different type of '*startle epilepsy*' may be elicited by touching the patient or by sudden movements which elicit a proprioceptive response. However, such stimuli may prove ineffective unless combined with an element of surprise. This type of startle response may occur following a sudden tap or blow on the head and must be distinguished from reflex anoxic syncope, a much commoner cause of such an event. Rarely, immersion of the lower parts of the body in water, as when bathing a child, may lead to a reflex epileptic seizure occurring (Shaw *et al.*, 1988; also see Appendix 2). Reflex anoxic syncope may also follow sudden immersion in cold water (see Chapter 22). Another type of attack provoked by movement is that usually entitled 'paroxysmal choreoathetosis' (Perez-Borja, Tassinari and Swanson, 1967). These attacks, which can occur either in children or in adults, are facilitated by anxiety, tension, a fright, and especially by a sudden movement, but not during exercise. The patient stiffens, stares, adducts the lower limbs, and dystonic or writhing movements of trunk and limbs occur accompanied by grimacing. Many authorities have considerable reservations about the genuinely epileptic nature of this curious condition. It is important to remember, however, that persistent choreoathetoid involuntary movements can also occur in epileptic patients with chronic phenytoin toxicity (McLellan and Swash, 1974). Another non-epileptic condition bearing the name *startle disease* or *hyperekplexia* has been described (Andermann and Andermann, 1984). It is inherited as an autosomal dominant trait. Excessive startle, sudden falling following a startle stimulus, nocturnal jerking of the legs and, in infancy, generalized stiffness are the main features.

The wider one casts the net of reflex epilepsy, the more one realizes that the strict distinction between genuine sensory and non-sensory precipitating factors cannot be maintained. For example, *reading epilepsy* (Critchley, 1962) is accompanied by patterned visual and proprioceptive stimuli which could act as triggers, and some patients with reading epilepsy are also photosensitive. Others, however, are affected only by interesting, difficult or emotionally charged reading material. In some, reading is only one of several activities associated with language which induce seizures. In the form of evoked seizures in which the stimuli are complex, such as a particular type of music or a particular type of reading material, part of the response may, in that particular patient, be secondary to emotional factors causing a conditioned response in a Pavlovian sense. In the rare patient whose seizures are precipitated by eating or gustatory sensations, a conditioned reflex is almost certainly responsible. Telemetric and ambulatory monitoring techniques have been particularly useful in these and other types of rare epilepsy (Binnie, Rowan and van Wieringen, 1982). Of interest is the fact that in some of these evoked or reflex epilepsies the patient may be deconditioned to the particular stimulus involved (Forster *et al.*, 1969). A somewhat analogous situation exists in the case of certain partial motor or sensory seizures precipitated by sensory stimuli in which the patient can abort the attack by counterstimulation, for example by vigorously rubbing the hand and arm if the attack has started there.

In conclusion, it must be emphasized that reflex epilepsies, apart from photosensitive epilepsy, are very rare, But, just as their dramatic nature has always intrigued the lay observer, their underlying mechanisms have also greatly interested the leading minds in the world of epileptology in efforts to understand the basic pathophysiology of epilepsy. Interested readers are referred to the Symposium on Reflex Mechanisms in the Genesis of Epilepsy, published in *Epilepsia* in 1962. The monograph entitled *Photosensitivity and Epilepsy* by Newmark and Penry (1979) is another valuable review.

## References

ANDERMANN, F. and ANDERMANN, E. (1984) Startle disease or hyperekplexia. *Annals of Neurology*, 16: 367–368

BINNIE, C. D., ROWAN, A. J. and VAN WIERINGEN. A. (1982) Eating epilepsy: report of 4 cases with review of the literature. *Electroencephalography and Clinical Neurology*, 53, 47P

BOWER, B. D. (1963) Television flicker and fits. *Clinical Pediatrics*, 2, 134–138

CHATRIAN, G. E., LETTICH, E., MILLER, L. H. and GREEN, J. R. (1970). Pattern sensitive epilepsy: Part I. *Epilepsia*, 11. 125–149

CRITCHLEY, M. (1962) Reading epilepsy. *Epilepsia*, 3, 402–406

DE MARCO, P. and GHERSINI, L. (1985). Videogames and epilepsy. *Developmental Medicine and Child Neurology*, 27, 519–521

DOOSE, H., GERKEN, H., HIEN-VOLGEL, K. F. and VOLZKE, E. (1969) Genetics of photosensitive epilepsy. *Neuropädiatrie*, 1, 56–73

DRAVET, C., BUREAU, M., GUERRINI, I. et al. (1992). *Epileptic Syndromes in Infancy, Childhood and Adolescence* 2nd edn (eds J. Roger, C. Dravet, *et al.*), John Libbey, London, Paris, pp. 75–88

DRIVER, M. V. and MACGILLIVRAY, B. B. (1976) Electroencephalography. In *A Textbook of Epilepsy*, 1st edn (eds J. Laidlaw and A. Richens), Churchill Livingstone, Edinburgh, London, New York, pp. 109–144

EDITORIAL (1978) Television-induced epilepsy and its prevention. *British Medical Journal*, 2, 1301–1302

FORSTER, F. M., HANASTIA, P., CLEELAND, C. S. and LUDWIG, A. (1969) A case of voice induced epilepsy treated by conditioning. *Neurology*, 19, 325–331

GASTAUT, H. (1952) Effects de la S.L.I. sur l'activité nerveuse centrale et sur ses composantes somatiques, végétatives et psychiques. In *Compte Rendus du Bième Congrès Technique National de Sécurité et d'Hygiène du Travail*, Foulon, Paris, pp. 1–10

GASTAUT, H. and TASSINARI. C. A. (1966) Triggering mechanisms in epilepsy. The electroclinical point of view. *Epilepsia*, 7, 85–138

JEAVONS, P. M. (1977) Nosological problems of myoclonic epilepsies in childhood and adolescence. *Developmental Medicine and Child Neurology*, **19**, 3–8

JEAVONS, P. M. and HARDING, G. F. A. (1970) Television epilepsy. (letter) *Lancet*, **2**, 926

JEAVONS, P. M. and HARDING, G. F. A. (1975) *Photosensitive Epilepsy*, Clinics in Developmental Medicine, No. 56, Spastics International/Heinemann Medical, London

JEAVONS, P. M., CLARK, J. E. and MAHESHWARI, M. C. (1977) Treatment of generalised epilepsies of childhood and adolescence with sodium valproate (Epilim). *Developmental Medicine and Child Neurology*, **19**, 9–25

JEAVONS, P. M., BISHOP, A. and HARDING, G. F. A. (1986) The prognosis of photosensitivity. *Epilepsia*, **27**, 569–575

MCLELLAN, D. L. and SWASH, M. (1974) Choreo-athetosis and encephalopathy induced by phenytoin. *British Medical Journal*, **2**, 204–205

NEWMARK, M. E. and PENRY, J. K. (1979) *Photosensitivity and Epilepsy: a Review*. Raven Press, New York

PAMPIGLIONE, G. and HARDEN, A. (1977) So-called neuronal ceroid lipofuscinosis. Neurophysiological studies in 60 children. *Journal of Neurology, Neurosurgery and Psychiatry*, **40**, 323–330

PEREZ-BORJA, C., TASSINARI, A. C. and SWANSON, A. G. (1967) Paroxysmal choreoathetosis and seizures induced by movement (reflex epilepsy). *Epilepsia*, **8**, 260–270

RUSHTON, D. N. (1981) 'Space Invader' epilepsy. (letter) *Lancet*, **1**, 501

SAENZ-LOPE, E., HERRANZ, F. J. and MASDEU, J. C. (1984) Startle epilepsy, a clinical study. *Annals of Neurology*, **16**, 78–81

SHAW, N. J., LIVINGSTON, J. H., MININS, R. A., and CLARKE, M. (1988) Epilepsy precipitated by bathing. *Developmental Medicine and Child Neurology*, **30**, 108–114

SHERWOOD, S. L. (1962) Self induced epilepsy, a collection of self induced epilepsy cases. *Archives of Neurology*, **6**, 49–65

SYMPOSIUM ON REFLEX MECHANISMS IN THE GENESIS OF EPILEPSY (1962) *Epilepsia*, **3**, 209–468

TROUPIN, A. S. (1966) Photic activation and experimental data concerning coloured stimuli. *Neurology*, **16**, 269

# Chapter 13

# Epilepsy in the adolescent

Epilepsy is the most common neurological disorder in adolescence. In one American clinic specifically for adolescent patients, epilepsy accounted for 63% of the neurological problems seen and for 9.9% of the total patients seen (Castle and Fishman, 1973). Cooper (1965), in his large study of children with epilepsy, found a total prevalence rate of 8.2/1000 at the age of 15 years (4.7 new and 3.4 old cases). In Kurland's (1959–60) study the average annual incidence rate for seizures between the ages of 10 and 14 years and between the ages of 15 and 19 years was, respectively, 24.7/100 000 and 18.6/100 000 population, with higher incidence rates for males occurring with all types of seizures. In a survey of adolescent services in the USA and Canada, Garell (1965) found that convulsive disorders ranked among the five most frequently encountered conditions in most clinics. The frequency with which epilepsy occurs in adolescence and the interaction between the condition and the special problems of adolescence make it necessary to consider the problem and its management in this age group separately. The problem may conveniently be divided into epilepsy beginning before adolescence and epilepsy arising *de novo* during adolescence. The clinical aspects were very well reviewed by Gascon (1974) using this subdivision.

## Prepuberty epilepsy

Epilepsy beginning in childhood may improve or deteriorate with the onset of puberty. In considerably more than 50% of children with childhood absence epilepsy (petit mal) arrest of the condition or very marked improvement will have taken place. In others, however, primary generalized epilepsy of the grand mal type will complicate their seizure problem. The prognosis of petit mal is discussed in more detail elsewhere (page 85). Benign partial epilepsy of childhood, also described elsewhere (page 103), tends to arrest in early or mid-adolescence. Primary generalized epilepsy with generalized tonic–clonic seizures (grand mal) beginning in later childhood, may worsen coincidentally with the growth spurt at puberty and then improve or remit when the growth spurt ceases (Niijima and Wallace, 1989). A similar upsurge in tonic–clonic seizures or the onset of such seizures may occur in girls in relation to the menarche when there may be a close temporal relationship between seizures and the menses (Rosciszewska, 1987). Epilepsy occurring only around the time of menstruation (catamenial epilepsy) is, however, quite rare. Any patient with chronic epilepsy who suffers marked deterioration in his symptoms or whose seizure patterns change in adolescence should be suspected of having a slow growing brain tumour (Lee *et al.*, 1989) and should have the appropriate neuroradiological investigations instituted. However, it should be remembered that established temporal lobe epilepsy may be increasingly complicated by behavioural disorders in adolescence, and these should be distinguished from genuine seizure patterns.

## Epilepsy starting at puberty

When epilepsy arises *de novo* in this age group, it is important to inquire into any previous history of possible seizures which may have been missed or forgotten, for example, the brief staring attacks of petit mal or febrile convulsions in early childhood. True primary generalized epilepsy of the petit mal type rarely presents in early adolescence and extremely rarely after the age of 15 years (Livingston, 1972). When absences present in adolescence, it is important to remember that they may, in fact, be of the temporal lobe type rather than the true petit mal type. Prolonged and/or atypical attacks should suggest this and careful EEG examination, including a sleep record and perhaps telemetry if available, should be performed (see Chapter 23). Juvenile absence epilepsy is a distinct syndrome from childhood absence epilepsy. It is a primary generalized epilepsy with an age-related onset, usually at puberty. The absences do not differ from those of childhood, but occur much less frequently, even sporadically. There may be associated grand mal seizures on awakening and perhaps some myoclonic jerking. The EEG shows characteristic 3 Hz spike and wave activity. The response to sodium valporate is good (Wolf, 1992).

*Primary brain tumours*, arising in the cortex, are much more likely to present in adolescence than they are in early childhood when subtentorial tumours predominate (see Chapter 16). Partial epilepsy may occasionally be the presenting symptom of such a tumour, and certainly it looms largely in parents' minds when their son or daughter develops epilepsy in adolescence. Nevertheless, brain tumours are a rare cause of epilepsy presenting during adolescence. A syndrome of *benign partial epilepsy in the adolescent* has been described (Loiseau and Orgogozo, 1978). The onset is between 10 and 20 years with a peak at 13–14 years. Males predominate and a family history of epilepsy is rare. The condition presents in otherwise normal adolescents with either a single simple or complex partial seizure or with a cluster of attacks occurring over 24 hours. An isolated seizure occurs in 80% of cases and a brief cluster of attacks in the remainder. The EEG is normal. There are no recurrences and the aetiology is unknown.

*Photosensitive epilepsy* may present for the first time in adolescence and the mechanism triggering the first attack may be the flashing stroboscopic lights used in the subterranean darkness of a discothèque!

*Primary generalized epilepsy of the grand mal type* may also present for the first time in adolescence, and the initial attack may be precipitated by lack of adequate sleep, excessive fatigue, overindulgence in alcohol or drug abuse or withdrawal. Characteristically, the seizures occur on awakening and may begin with clonic movements followed by a brief tonic–clonic seizure and loss of consciousness. This particular epileptic syndrome is now usually entitled *epilepsy with grand mal seizures on awakening*. There may be associated photosensitivity. The response to sodium valproate is usually good and a permanent remission is the rule in the majority of cases (Delgado-Escueta, Treiman and Walsh, 1983). This condition and juvenile absence epilepsy are closely related to the following important and underdiagnosed epileptic syndrome.

## Juvenile myoclonic epilepsy

This epilepsy was first described by Herpin (1867), who observed the myoclonic jerks in his own son. Since 1957, in a series of publications, Janz has drawn attention to this epileptic syndrome and aroused worldwide interest in it. It is now often called juvenile myoclonic epilepsy of Janz or the Janz syndrome. Janz has used the term impulsive petit mal in some of his publications (Janz and Christian, 1957; Janz, 1985, 1989). He considers that, in an unselected patient population comprising children, adolescents and adults in equal measure, this epilepsy will account for about 7–9% of cases. The sex incidence is equal. This is a genetically determined primary generalized epilepsy and the gene locus has been identified on chromosome 6 (Delgado-Escueta et al., 1989). The prevalence of close relatives with afebrile epileptic seizures is 5–6%.

This epilepsy typically begins in early adolescence, with a peak age of onset between 13 and 15 years of age. However, diagnosis may be delayed considerably because of failure by parents (and doctors) to recognize the myoclonic jerks as seizures (Dreifuss, 1989). It is important to note that the disorder may begin either earlier or later than usual, indeed at any time of life (Gram et al., 1988). One of the author's cases occurred in a medical student in his early twenties, and was unrecognized in a medical family.

The epilepsy typically commences with early morning jerks of the head, neck and upper limbs. They may occur singly, or in clusters of a few jerks of varying intensity at irregular intervals. They may be so violent that the patient may throw down objects being held – the so-called 'flying cornflakes syndrome'. Unlike absences, consciousness is unimpaired during the jerks, a distinguishing feature from myoclonic absences (see Chapter 7). All patients with the syndrome have myoclonic jerks and, after a variable interval, generalized seizures develop also in over 80% of cases (Janz, 1989). These consist most commonly of generalized tonic-clonic seizures occurring most frequently on awakening. A minority of patients also experience absences. Precipitating factors leading to seizures are of the greatest importance in this syndrome. These include sudden awakening from sleep, sleep deprivation, stress and the consumption of alcohol. Janz (1989) comments that alcohol appears to act indirectly by leading to sleep deprivation, persuading the patient to conceal his or her natural fatigue and stay up late.

The interictal EEG pattern consists of polyspike-wave discharges combined with a relatively normal background activity. A burst of spikes occurs simultaneously with the myoclonic jerks. Photosensitivity is common, occurring in 40% of the author's series (O'Donohoe, 1990). As befits a true primary generalized epilepsy of genetic origin, the patients are usually of average or superior intelligence, neurological abnormalities are absent and brain scan examinations are normal.

The prognosis for juvenile myoclonic epilepsy is favourable for control of seizures, provided the appropriate diagnosis is made early and antiepileptic drug treatment instituted at once. Ideally, treatment should be started before major seizures develop and this implies recognition of the syndrome when myoclonic jerks are the sole manifestation.

Modification of the patient's life style is of supreme importance if treatment is to be successful. Alcohol should be eschewed, except in great moderation, adequate sleep is essential and sudden awakening of the patient should be avoided. The condition presents a particular problem for young doctors who have or who develop the condition, since medicine often necessitates an irregular life with loss of sleep, sudden awakening from sleep and chronic fatigue as everyday problems.

Sodium valproate is the drug of choice for treatment and successful control of seizures has been reported in over 80% of cases (Penry, Dean and Riela, 1989). However, relapses are common and are usually precipitated by fatigue, noncompliance, stress, sleep deprivation, and alcohol consumption. Adequate dosage of the drug is essential and at least 15–20 mg/kg per day should be given. Primidone has been suggested as the best alternative antiepileptic drug if sodium valproate is ineffective or unsuitable for the patient (Dreifuss, 1989).

Unfortunately, there is now an increasing awareness that this epilepsy does not resolve with time and that treatment and modification of lifestyle may need to be lifelong. Relapses have been reported in at least 75% of cases when treatment is discontinued or omitted (Dreifuss, 1989). It is fair to say that no other epilepsy or epileptic syndrome illustrates so clearly the need for precise diagnosis and proper counselling of the patient and relatives as does the Janz syndrome of juvenile myoclonic epilepsy.

## Differential diagnosis

Careful history taking and physical examination are as important in adolescence as in any other age group. The differential diagnosis is, however, rather different from that in childhood. Syncope is more common in early adolescence and 'dizzy spells', occurring perhaps under emotional stress, also need to be distinguished from minor epileptic attacks. Malingering and hysterical attacks may also have to be considered, and loss of consciousness provoked by hyperventilation is still seen occasionally in hysterical girls. One should beware of any attack which can be produced 'on request' or before an audience, where the seizure patterns change from attack to attack, where bodily injury never occurs in the seizure, and where recovery is unexpectedly rapid and the usual postictal symptoms of sleep, stupor, confusion and headache do not follow an apparent major tonic–clonic convulsion. The hysterical patient may betray herself by being able to give an account of events which coincided with her actual attack or she may clearly be imitating the genuine seizure patterns of another patient in the same hospital ward. Hysteria and other non-epileptic attacks are discussed in detail by Trimble (1981) and by Betts (1990), and the reader is also referred to Chapter 24. The possibility of a degenerative disease such as subacute sclerosing parencephalitis (SSPE), presenting with myoclonic jerks, should be borne in mind in the differential diagnosis of juvenile myoclonic epilepsy.

## Investigations

The investigation of epilepsy in adolescence should be limited to the basic tests, including EEG examination, unless there is some specific indication for proceeding to a more detailed study of the patient. EEG examination may show the presence of focal spikes or typical or atypical spike-wave patterns. Interseizure EEG records, both in waking and in sleeping, may be quite normal in primary generalized epilepsy (grand mal) of the idiopathic type in which genetic factors are aetiologically predominant. Partial or focal motor convulsions alone are not an indication for extensive neuroradiological investigations unless there are some associated abnormal neurological findings. Careful clinical assessment of the individual patient should remain the essential guide to whether detailed investigation is necessary or not. CT scanning may be advisable when a partial epilepsy is of recent onset, when there are associated neurological abnormalities on examination, or where there is evidence of progression or deterioration in the clinical state. It must be remembered that elaborate or painful investigations are particularly alarming for the adolescent, and this includes the performance of a lumbar puncture. Examination of CSF for measles antibodies is, of course, essential in suspected SSPE.

## Therapy

The general problems of anticonvulsant therapy in adolescence are similar to those which obtain in childhood generally, but there are special difficulties peculiar to this age group. *The commonest reason for failure to obtain control or for loss of control of seizures in adolescents is the patient's intentional or unintentional failure to take his medication regularly.* The patient should be seen frequently in the early stages of therapy and carefully instructed about the nature of his illness and the need to take his drugs conscientiously.

The use of the word 'drug' in this age group is probably a mistake anyway and the word 'medication' may be preferable. The adolescent is particularly concerned about his appearance, his need to conform with his peers, his sense of personal identity and the need to break away from dependence on his parents; the stress of an unpredictable condition such as epilepsy and the need to take regular treatment may place intolerable burdens on him. He will be aware of the social implications of having epilepsy and of the public prejudice about the condition and he may attempt to refute the diagnosis by omitting his drugs. Sudden withdrawal of medication is, of course, a potent cause of status epilepticus at any age. Monitoring of serum levels may be necessary at regular intervals in order to test the patient's compliance with medical advice about treatment (*see* Chapter 25).

The patient will need constant support and encouragement, and family counselling and planning regarding vocational aspirations should start at this time. It should be appreciated that the earlier one recognizes disabling emotional reactions to epilepsy, the easier it will be to alleviate them and to ensure that the patient will maintain a stable personality. The help of a psychiatrist skilled in the management of adolescent problems may be invaluable. The expense of therapy in some countries should also be remembered.

It should not be assumed that those adolescents with less serious and often well controlled epilepsy are free of emotional difficulties related to epilepsy. Hodgman *et al.* (1979), studying the emotional complications of adolescent grand mal epilepsy, found poor self-image, pessimism about future expectations, and a consciousness of the social stigma of epilepsy even though seizure control was good and neurological impairment was absent. Ross and Tookey (1988), reporting earlier studies of secondary schoolchildren with epilepsy in Bristol, found that divorce and death of one parent, particular fathers, were more common than expected, reflecting the burden thrown by the handicapped child on to the family. In a more encouraging recent survey of adolescents with epilepsy, Clement and Wallace (1990) did not find a similar occurrence of marital breakdown and related problems.

The patient should be encouraged to wear a Medic-Alert bracelet indicating the nature of his complaint, especially if his attacks are frequent and major in type, but many adolescents will refuse to do this. In those patients whose epilepsy began before adolescence and who have had some years of remission on treatment, the question of withdrawing treatment will arise. As discussed elsewhere (p. 287), there is controversy about whether withdrawing treatment during puberty leads to relapse, but evidence suggests that this may not be so (Holowach, Thurston and O'Leary, 1972).

## Drugs of choice

If possible, the drugs chosen for treatment should be those which do not interfere with concentration and with academic, social and physical activities. For this reason barbiturates should probably be avoided. Ingesting alcohol with an anticonvulsant such as phenobarbitone will result in a summation of sedative effects, and adolescents with epilepsy should be discouraged from taking alcohol which may in itself provoke a seizure in a susceptible individual. Furthermore, it should be remembered that in depressed adolescents barbiturates are among the most lethal of the common anticonvulsants used in attempted suicide. Carbamazepine is, in the author's experience, an excellent anticonvulsant for general use in adolescence. The problems of using phenytoin at any age are discussed elsewhere but, in the adolescent, thickening of facial tissues, gum hyperplasia and hirsutism may be intolerable side-effects, especially in girls (see Chapter 26). There is no convincing evidence that anticonvulsants, including phenytoin, exacerbate or cause adolescent acne (Greenwood, Fenwick and Cunliffe, 1983). Sodium valproate is now extensively used in different epilepsies in this age group and is notably free of depressant side effects. However, in those cases where it causes excessive weight gain and/or hair loss, the patient may react by withdrawal and with depression and the drug may have to be stopped (Egger and Brett, 1981).

## Withdrawal of therapy

In the author's experience the adolescent with epilepsy lives for the day when treatment is terminated. Withdrawal of therapy should depend on the following considerations:

1   That he/she has been seizure free for a period of 2–4 years, preferably the latter.
2   That his/her epilepsy was of a type which responded promptly to treatment in the first instance.
3   That intelligence is unimpaired and that no underlying neurological disease or serious psychological disorder exists.
4   That care is exercised in withdrawing drugs slowly, especially in girls at puberty.
5   That EEG abnormalities have not persisted or worsened during therapy.

It should also be remembered, when withdrawing therapy in late adolescence, that even a single seizure may prohibit the patient from obtaining a driving licence or it may cause the loss of one already obtained, thereby perhaps causing the loss of a job also. Therefore, drugs should be withdrawn very slowly (taking 6–8 months for the process), each drug should be withdrawn independently if two are being used concurrently and, if a relapse occurs, medication should be restarted immediately at the dosage levels which previously controlled the epilepsy. It must be emphasized again, however, that insofar as withdrawal of drug therapy is concerned, the patient with juvenile myoclonic epilepsy should be regarded as probably needing treatment indefinitely.

## General advice

The patient and his parents will be concerned about participation in sports and other physical activities. There is evidence that physical exercise actually raises the seizure threshold (Götze, Munter and Teichmann, 1967) and it is not necessary to place unusual restrictions on the patient which will, in any case, only increase his sense of being different from his peers and draw their attention to the difference. Swimming alone should, however, be prohibited and he should be encouraged to take showers rather than baths. (*See also* Appendix 2.)

In late adolescence the patient and his parents will be concerned about vocational training, university education, the prospects of marriage and the genetic risks of epilepsy. The wish to obtain a driving licence will also arise and legal regulations about this vary from country to country, and in the USA from state to state.

To sum up, the adolescent patient with epilepsy needs good and regular medical care, an explanation about his illness and constant encouragement. He requires as good an education or vocational training as possible, support and advice to ensure that normal personality development occurs and, perhaps the most important of all, enlightened attitudes about epilepsy from parents, peers, teachers and prospective employers.

## References

BETTS, T. (1990) Pseudoseizures: seizures that are not epilepsy. *Lancet*, **336**, 231–234

CASTLE, G. F. and FISHMAN, L. S. (1973) Seizures in adolescent medicine. *Pediatric Clinics of North America*, **20**, 819–835

COOPER, J. E. (1965) Epilepsy in a longitudinal study of 5000 children. *British Medical Journal*, 1, 1020–1022.

CLEMENT, M. J. and WALLACE, S. J. (1990) A survey of adolescents with epilepsy. *Developmental Medicine and Child Neurology*, **32**, 849–857

DELGADO-ESCUETA, A. V. TREIMAN, D. M. and WALSH, G. O. (1983) The treatable epilepsies I. *New England Journal of Medicine*, **308**, 1508–1514

DELGADO-ESCUETA, A. V. GREENBERG, D. A., TREIMAN, L. et al. (1989) Mapping the gene for juvenile myoclonic epilepsy. *Epilepsia*, **30**, Supplement 4, S8–S18

DREIFUSS, F. E. (1989) Juvenile myoclonic epilepsy. Characteristics of a primary generalized epilepsy. *Epilepsia*, **30**, Supplement 4, S1–S7

DREIFUSS, F. E. (1989) Panel discussion on juvenile myoclonic epilepsy. *Epilepsia*, **30**, Supplement 4, S24–S27

EGGER, J. and BRETT, E. M. (1981) Effects of sodium valproate in 100 children with special reference to weight. *British Medical Journal*, **283**, 577–580

GARELL, D. C. (1965) A survey of adolescent medicine in the U.S. and Canada. *American Journal of Diseases of Children*, **109**, 314–317

GASCON, G. G. (1974) Epilepsy in the adolescent. *Postgraduate Medicine*, **55**, 111–117

GÖTZE, W., MUNTER, ST., K. M. and TEICHMANN, J. (1967) Effects of exercise on seizure threshold: investigated by electroencephalographic telemetry. *Diseases of the Nervous System*, **28**, 664–667

GRAM, L., ALVING, J., SAGILD, J. C. and DAM, M. (1988) Juvenile myoclonic epilepsy in unexpected age groups. *Epilepsy Research*, **2**, 137–140

GREENWOOD, R., FENWICK, P. B. C. and CUNLIFFE, W. J. (1983) Acne and anticonvulsants. *British Medical Journal*, **287**, 1669–1670

HERPIN, T. H. (1987) *Des Accès Incomplets d'Epilepsie*. Balliere, Paris

HODGMAN, C. H., MCANARNEY, E. R., MYERS, G. J. (1979) Emotional complications of adolescent grand mal epilepsy. *Journal of Pediatrics*, **95**, 309–312

HOLOWACH, J., THURSTON, D. L. AND O'LEARY, J. L. (1972) Prognosis in childhood epilepsy. *New England Journal of Medicine*, **286**, 169–174

JANZ, D. (1985) Epilepsy with impulsive petit mal (juvenile myoclonic epilepsy). *Acta Neurologica Scandinavica*, **72**, 449–459

JANZ, D. (1989) Juvenile myoclonic epilepsy: epilepsy with impulsive petit mal. *Cleveland Clinic Journal of Medicine*, **56**, Supplement, Part 1, S23–S33

JANZ, D. AND CHRISTIAN, W. (1957) Inpulsiv-Petit Mal. *Dtsch Z. Nervenheilk*, **176**, 346–386

KURLAND, L. T. (1959–1960) The incidence and prevalence of convulsive disorders in a small urban community. *Epilepsia*, **1**, 143–161

LEE, T. K. Y., NAKUSA, Y., JEFFREE, M. A. et al. (1989) Indolent glioma: a cause of epilepsy. *Archives of Disease in Childhood*, **64**, 1666–1671

LIVINGSTON, S. (1972) *Comprehensive Management of Epilepsy in Infancy, Childhood and Adolescence*. Charles C. Thomas, Springfield, Illinois; p. 58

LOISEAU, P. AND ORGOGOZO, J. M. (1978) An unrecognized syndrome of benign focal epileptic seizures in teenagers. *Lancet*, **2**, 1070–1071

NIIJIMA, S.-I. AND WALLACE, S. J. (1989) Effects of puberty on seizure frequency. *Developmental Medicine and Child Neurology*, **31**, 174–180

O'DONOHOE, N. V. (1990) Juvenile myoclonic epilepsy (Janz syndrome). *Irish Journal of Medical Science*, **159**, 192

PENRY, J. K., DEAN, J. C. and RIELA, A. R. (1989) Juvenile myoclonic epilepsy. Long-term response to therapy. *Epilepsia*, **30**, Supplement 4, S19–S23

ROSCISZEWSKA, D. (1987) Epilepsy and menstruation. In *Epilepsy* (ed. A. Hopkins), Chapman and Hall, London, pp. 373–376.

ROSS, E. M. and TOOKEY, P. (1988) Educational needs and epilepsy in childhood. In *Epilepsy, Behaviour and Cognitive Function* (eds M. R. Trimble, E. H. Reynolds), John Wiley and Sons, Chichester, pp. 87–96

WOLF, P. (1992) Juvenile absence epilepsy. In: *Epileptic Syndromes in Infancy, Childhood and Adolescence*, 2nd edn (eds J. Roger, M. Bureau, et al.), John Libbey, London, Paris, pp. 307–312.

Chapter 14

# Post-traumatic epilepsy

The remarkable improvements in modern obstetrics have made brain injury at birth a rarity. The avoidance of breech delivery has been particularly important in this respect. However, the battering of babies (euphemistically called non-accidental injury) has reached epidemic proportions in many Western societies, and injuries to the head and face are all too common. Battering is probably the commonest single cause of subdural haematoma in infancy today. Furthermore, as Caveness (1976) has written: 'accidental death and disability in our time has achieved a magnitude comparable to the plagues of the Middle Ages'. The frequency of post-traumatic epilepsy is increasing, in children as well as adults, because of the larger number and greater severity of head injuries, particularly those caused by traffic accidents (Jackson, 1978). Lesions occur as a result of contusions and lacerations, not only at the actual site of injury but also in distant and opposite regions of the brain. Quite apart from cortical damage, lesions are frequent in the brain-stem in many cases of severe head injury. Anoxic damage to the brain and the consequences of cerebral oedema and haemorrhage are additional features. In those who survive, several epileptic foci may develop in different parts of the brain and atrophic changes may also be present. About 15% of those suffering cranial trauma will have severe brain injury. Less than 50% of these will survive their injury and those who do survive are at substantial risk for later epilepsy, ranging from 10 to 15% (Hauser, 1990).

Children, particularly boys, are at risk of sustaining head injuries as a result of their adventurous play. Potentially dangerous toys, such as skateboards, may add to the risk unless protective headgear is worn. The value of such headgear for cyclists is also widely acknowledged. Jennett (1973) estimated that 100 000 patients are admitted to British hospitals with head injuries every year and approximately one-quarter of these are under 16 years of age.

## Seizures occurring soon after injury

Seizures in the first week after injury are much commoner than those occurring in any of the succeeding weeks. Epilepsy in the first week (early epilepsy) differs significantly from that which occurs later. Approximately one-third of early fits occur within an hour of injury, about a third during the rest of the first day and the remainder during the first week.

155

Traumatic epilepsy of this type is most common in young children. The incidence of early seizures is almost twice as great in the under-fives as in the over-fives (Annegers *et al.*, 1980). Any seizures in the first week after injury should be taken seriously (particularly in young children) because of the immediate risk of status epilepticus developing, even after relatively mild injuries (Shoek, Minderhoud and Wilmink, 1984). The special significance of early epilepsy after a head injury is that it carries four times the risk of the patient developing late epilepsy. Of people who have a seizure in the first week after injury, 75% never experience another. However, 25% do have a subsequent seizure, and this represents a very significantly increased risk when compared with patients who do not suffer an early convulsion and where the risk of later epilepsy is only 3%. Jennett (1987) found the risk to be exactly the same, even when the injury was trivial, i.e. where no fracture, no unconsciousness or post-traumatic amnesia and no intracranial haematoma occurred. Even a single seizure in the first hour signifies a considerable risk, and may influence the decision about whether or not to use prophylactic antiepileptic medication.

Three conditions contribute to a higher risk of late epilepsy, namely a seizure occurring in the first week, a depressed fracture and an acute intracranial haematoma. Post-traumatic amnesia lasting for more than 24 hours, the presence or absence of both dural tears and focal signs are all of predictive value in estimating the risk of late epilepsy. By using all this information it is possible for the neurosurgeon to identify high-risk patients and to consider recommending prophylactic antiepileptic medication (Jennett, 1975, 1987). In Jennett's opinion, evidence is available to enable the neurosurgeon to assess the risk of late epilepsy in any individual case of head injury and to offer the patient advice about prophylaxis. As already stated, the risk of late epilepsy never disappears completely, but of those who are going to develop it nearly three-quarters will do so by the end of the second year after the accident. Several authors, including Jennett and van de Sande (1975), found EEG studies unhelpful in predicting the possibility of late epilepsy. However, EEG abnormalities are commoner in those who develop late epilepsy and this only reflects the greater degree of brain damage in these patients. Also, there are patients who develop EEG abnormalities but who never have a seizure and some who develop post-traumatic epilepsy and have normal EEGs.

Although antiepileptic drugs are commonly used to prevent the development of post-traumatic seizures, their use remains controversial. Phenytoin has been the drug most frequently employed and a recent controlled study (Temkin *et al.*, 1990) suggests that, although an appropriate dose of this drug reduces the incidence of seizures in patients at high risk after severe head injury, it does not seem to be as effective in preventing the development of later epilepsy. What is required is an antiepileptic drug which will interfere with the processes, whatever they are, which lead to the development of later epilepsy, and studies are continuing in a search for such a drug (Hauser, 1990).

A specific form of post-traumatic epilepsy in children relates to seizures in response to the insertion of ventricular shunts for the treatment of hydrocephalus (Ines and Markand, 1977). The seizures are usually simple partial in type and their onset may be delayed for years. They should be distinguished from convulsive or other attacks consequent on shunt malfunction. Diffuse brain disease or atrophy associated with hydrocephalus may be responsible for secondary generalized seizures.

## Prophylaxis after injury

As already indicated, the question of pharmacological prophylaxis of post-traumatic epilepsy has aroused considerable interest among those dealing with injured adults. This problem arises because of the clinical phenomenon of the latent period, which may be measured in years, between the brain trauma and the appearance of late epilepsy. It has been suggested that a period of 'ripening' of the epileptogenic lesion is required before clinical epilepsy develops. It may be that anticonvulsant drugs can suppress this process long enough for it to disappear, perhaps because damaged neurons die. It is known, from the evidence of experimental neurophysiological research, that the interictal cortical spike may propagate via association tracts to the homologous region of the opposite hemisphere evoking a secondary spike. In chronic preparations in animals such a region of secondary spiking may become independently active, forming a 'mirror' focus, which may persist even after the primary focus becomes inactive or is ablated. Mirror foci are not limited to the cortex, but may also develop in the limbic and other subcortical systems where they are synaptically related to a primary subcortical focus (Proctor, Prince and Morrell, 1966). It seems clear, therefore, that bombardment by neurons of the primary focus alters neurons of the mirror area so that they become independently epileptic.

The related phenomenon called 'kindling', the knowledge of which is based on animal studies (Moshé and Ludvig, 1988), is also important in this context and has been discussed in detail in Chapter 2. Kindling has been defined as the facilitation of seizure pathways by repeated seizures until, ultimately, spontaneous seizures develop. It has been proposed that the kindling process could explain the latent period that exists between the occurrence of a causative insult such as head trauma and the actual onset of epilepsy (Goddard, 1983) and it has been argued that prophylactic antiepileptic medication may prevent the process and may also interfere with the development of mirror foci.

## Medicolegal aspects

Paediatricians are sometimes faced with the medicolegal problem of trying to decide whether a child is genuinely experiencing post-traumatic epilepsy or not. Usually, the first question to consider is whether the child is having genuine epilepsy or not, and the case history and the EEG examination are helpful here. Secondly, he should consider whether the type of epilepsy which is occurring is one which is likely to follow trauma. Clearly, a condition such as primary generalized epilepsy of the petit mal type is not a post-traumatic sequela. Thirdly, he should examine the circumstances of the original injury and decide whether it was of sufficient severity to cause brain injury and subsequent epilepsy. A pitfall here has already been mentioned, namely that even trivial head injuries may be followed by late epilepsy, especially in those who have seizures in the first week after the accident. In any event, head injuries and later epilepsy are closely associated in the lay mind and it may be very difficult to convince a court that a cause and effect situation does not exist in any particular case.

# References

ANNEGERS, J. F., GRABOW, J. D., GROOVER, R. V. *et al.* (1980) Seizures after head trauma: a population study. *Neurology*, **30,** 683–689

CAVENESS, W. F. (1976) Epilepsy: a product of trauma in our time. *Epilepsia*, **17,** 207–215

GODDARD, G. V. (1983) The kindling model of epilepsy. *Trends in Neuroscience*, **7,** 275–279

HAUSER, W. A. (1990) Prevention of post-traumatic epilepsy. *New England Journal of Medicine,* **323,** 540–541

INES, D. F. and MARKLAND, O. M. (1977) Epileptic seizures and abnormal electroencephalographic findings in hydrocephalus and their relation to shunting procedures. *Electroencephalography and Clinical Neurophysiology*, **42,** 761–768

JACKSON, R. H. (1978) Hazards to children in traffic. *Archives of Disease in Childhood*, **53,** 807–813

JENNETT, B. (1973) Trauma as a cause of epilepsy in childhood. *Developmental Medicine and Child Neurology*, **15,** 56–62

JENNETT, B. (1975) *Epilepsy after Non-missile Head Injuries,* 2nd edn, Heinemann Medical, London

JENNETT, B. (1987) Epilepsy after head injury and intracranial surgery. In *Epilepsy* (ed. A. Hopkins), Chapman and Hall, London, pp. 401–412

JENNETT B. and VAN DE SANDE, J. (1975) EEG prediction of post-traumatic epilepsy. *Epilepsia*, **16,** 251–256

MOSHÉ, S. L. and LUDVIG, N. (1988) Kindling. In *Recent Advances in Epilepsy,* NO. 4 (eds T. A. Pedley and B. S. Meldrum), Churchill Livingstone, Edinburgh, London, pp. 21–44

PROCTOR, F., PRINCE, D. and MORRELL, F. (1966) Primary and secondary spike foci following depth lesions. *Archives of Neurology*, **15,** 151–162

SHOEK, J. W., MINDERHOUD, J. M. and WILMINK, J. T. (1984) Delayed deterioration following mild head injury in children. *Brain*, **107,** 15–36

TEMKIN, N. R., DIKMEN, S. S., WILENSKY, A. J. *et al.* (1990) A randomized, double-blind study of phenytoin for the prevention of post-traumatic seizures. *New England Journal of Medicine*, Vol. 323.

# Chapter 15

# Mental handicap and epilepsy

## Overall frequency of epilepsy

Epilepsy is one of the most frequently associated handicaps occurring in mentally retarded children, and it is of considerable significance in their management. It is difficult to get a true estimate of the prevalence of epilepsy in the mentally handicapped, but it is certain that the proportion rises steadily as the degree of retardation increases. Tizard and Grad (1961), in a survey of severely retarded children at home and in institutional care, found that 18% suffered from seizures and that the seizures were more frequent among those who were institutionalized. Corbett (1974) reported an epidemiological study of retarded children in Camberwell, London, in which parents were questioned in detail; over 80% of the children had EEGs and all were neurologically assessed. He found that, of 155 children with an IQ under 50 or with one of the syndromes associated with severe retardation, 32% had a history of epilepsy at some time during life, while 19% had had at least one seizure during the previous year. In the children with an IQ of less than 50, a quarter under the age of 5 years had had a fit in the previous year in comparison with an incidence of 18% between the ages of 5 and 10 years and 5% between the ages of 10 and 15 years. Seizures in the mentally handicapped are therefore a particular problem of early childhood. The frequency of epilepsy in the mildly mentally handicapped is less certain and is probably in the order of 3–6% depending on whether uncomplicated epilepsy or epilepsy associated with other neurological handicaps is considered (Rutter, Graham and Yule, 1970). In the mildly mentally handicapped social and environmental factors are probably as important as organic factors in the aetiology of their condition, and therefore it is not surprising that epilepsy is less frequent in this group. Corbett in 1985 and 1990 has again reviewed the topic of epilepsy associated with mental retardation, and the interested reader should also consult the proceedings of an important symposium edited by Wood (1985).

## Variation with different syndromes

The occurence of epilepsy varies considerably in the different syndromes associated with mental handicap. It is relatively uncommon in Down's syndrome. A recent retrospective study of this condition found an overall frequency of seizures of 6.4% (Stafstrom *et al.*, 1991). The authors emphasize that it should not be assumed that epilepsy in Down's syndrome is a direct consequence of abnormal brain development. They found an identifiable aetiology in 62% of their cases and this was usually related to the common medical complications of the condition. In early-onset epilepsy, hypoxic–ischaemic damage resulting from perinatal problems, hypoxia or cerebral artery occlusion from congenital heart disease, and CNS and other infections were important factors. During later childhood and adolescence, head injury and the consequences of congenital heart disease were the main aetiologies. Where no cause for the epilepsy was identified, seizures could begin at any time from infancy onwards. Infantile spasms may occur in association with Down's syndrome, but it is worth nothing that febrile convulsions are rare (Tatsuno *et al.*, 1984). Epilepsy may commence or reappear in the fourth decade in association with the early onset of Alzheimer's dementia in these patients (Evenhuis, 1990).

In tuberose sclerosis, on the other hand, epilepsy is very common, particularly infantile spasms (Riikonen and Simell, 1990). Chronic intractable epilepsy may follow this early onset. It is important to remember that tuberose sclerosis may be the cause of epilepsy presenting at any age. There is a close relationship in this inherited disorder between the time of onset of seizures and the degree of mental handicap. In those with seizures commencing prior to 1 year of age, less than 10% will later prove to have normal intelligence (Gomez, 1988). In Rett's syndrome, in which progressive deceleration of psychomotor development and loss of acquired cognitive and motor skills occur in females after an initial 6–18 months of apparently normal development, various types of seizures have been reported in up to 80% of cases (Rett Syndrome Work Group, 1988). Epilepsy is usually a late development in the severely mentally handicapped ataxic children with Angelman's 'happy puppet' syndrome but the diagnosis may be suspected from the characteristic EEG pattern of diffuse rhythmic high voltage slow activity present in infancy (Boyd, Harden and Patton, 1988).

Seizures are also a frequent problem in children with cerebral palsy. It has been estimated that approximately 20% of cases of childhood epilepsy are the result of brain lesions which also cause cerebral palsy (Aicardi, 1990). However, the various types of cerebral palsy are not equally associated with epilepsy. The incidence is highest in patients with quadriplegia and hemiplegia and lowest in those with dystonic cerebral palsy and spastic diplegia. The more severe and generalized the cerebral palsy and the more profound the mental retardation, the greater will be the incidence of epilepsy. However, even in the presence of a morphological organic brain lesion causing cerebral palsy, the influence of a familial predisposition to epilepsy may be important in determining whether or not the individual patient develops seizures (Aksu, 1990). Children with cerebral palsy who develop epilepsy, when compared with neurologically normal children who do so, will usually have an earlier age of onset of seizures and are likely to prove more resistant to antiepileptic drug therapy (Hosking, Miles and Winstanley, 1990). The occurrence of epileptic seizures in patients with structural brain damage or abnormality is always a serious event, since epilepsy in such cases tends to be severe and disruptive for children who already have other disabilities. However, approximately half of all children with epilepsy and either cerebral palsy or mental retardation will eventually respond to antiepileptic drug therapy (Brorson and Wranne, 1987) and, in other cases, surgical treatment is offering new possibilities for amelioration of the epilepsy (Aicardi, 1990, also see Chapter 27).

## Behavioural disturbances and epilepsy

The associations between epilepsy and behavioural disturbances in children of normal intellect, and between structural brain lesions, epilepsy and behavioural disorders will be discussed in Chapter 20. Severely retarded children with epilepsy may also have troublesome behaviour problems, and it is most important to bear in mind that these may be a consequence of overenthusiastic antiepileptic medication. Seizures in these children are often refractory to therapy and parents and doctors, especially doctors working with institutionalized children, may be tempted to use excessive doses of drugs or to indulge in gross polypharmacy in attempts to control the attacks. As a result, the patient may become overactive, aggressive, destructive and even uncontrollable, or alternatively he or she may become apathetic and somnolent. Progressive mental deterioration may be suspected as a result. The seizures may even increase in frequency, leading to yet more medication. The epilepsy may be blamed for the deterioration in the intellectual level or a condition of minor status epilepticus may be suspected. The EEG is useful in diagnostic differentiation here but it may be difficult to arrange one urgently for children in institutions for the mentally handicapped. Estimating serum levels of antiepileptic drugs is mandatory in this situation and this service should be available for the severely mentally handicapped with epilepsy. It should also be noted that chronic toxic effects of drugs such as folate deficiency, vitamin D deficiency and the various effects of phenytoin overdosage are commoner in institutionalized mentally handicapped children with epilepsy than they are in normal children with epilepsy living at home (*see* Chapter 26).

The importance of correctly diagnosing and managing epilepsy in mentally handicapped and brain-injured children cannot be overemphasised. Treatment of epilepsy is an integral part of the comprehensive care of these children and should be under the direction of doctors who are familiar with the problems presented by seizures in childhood and skilled in their management.

## EEG findings

Corbett, Harris and Robinson (1975) summarized their EEG findings of the Camberwell study of 155 children with moderate and severe mental handicap aged from 2 to 15 years at the time of the survey. They categorized their results as follows. Some records failed to show any abnormality while others showed mild abnormalities only. Clearly abnormal records, including those with unequivocal epileptic abnormalities, occurred twice as frequently in children who had a history of epilepsy. They commented on the difficulties experienced in obtaining satisfactory records in these patients. The recording should preferably be done by a technician experienced in dealing with children, and stick-on electrodes are essential if unacceptable movement artefacts are to be avoided.

## Drug treatment

The drug treatment of epilepsy in the mentally handicapped should be subject to the same precautions that are applied to normal children with epilepsy. However, it must again be emphasized that children with moderate or severe handicap and those with neurological deficits, such as spastic cerebral palsy, tend to develop troublesome side-effects, particularly abnormal overactivity and irritability, when treated with phenobarbitone and primidone. In an excellent review of the problems posed by the use of the older antiepileptic drugs in mentally handicapped individuals, Schain (1979) considered that special attention should be directed to choosing drugs for long-term administration which do not interfere with the maximum possible rehabilitation of these patients. Drugs which are free of undesirable mental or cosmetic side-effects are best, and he favoured carbamazepine and sodium valproate among those in current use.

## Does epilepsy lead to mental deterioration?

The parents of any child with epilepsy frequently ask if their child will become mentally subnormal as a consequence of his complaint. Epilepsy and mental abnormality are closely associated in the lay mind, partly because the moderately and severely retarded often have epilepsy as a symptom of their basic brain disease, and partly because the myth of the 'epileptic personality' dies hard and the fear of mental deterioration in the child haunts the parents. The latter problem is discussed fully in Chapter 20. However, parents should be assured that although a very small number of children with epilepsy undoubtedly show deterioration of intellect and personality (e.g. some children with infantile spasms and the myoclonic epilepsies and cases of degenerative disease presenting with epilepsy) the vast majority are of normal and often superior intelligence and remain so in spite of their complaint. A prospective study (Bourgeois *et al.*, 1983) tested the stability of the IQ in children with epilepsy and found that the score did not alter appreciably with time. Early onset of epilepsy, frequent seizures which were difficult to control and chronic drug toxicity were, however, correlated with a decline in the IQ score in a minority of cases.

### References

AICARDI, J. (1990) Epilepsy in brain-injured children. *Developmental Medicine and Child Neurology*, **32**, 191–202

ASKU, F. (1990) Nature and prognosis of seizures in patients with cerebral palsy. *Developmental Medicine and Child Neurology*, **32**, 661–668

BOURGEOIS, B. F. D., PRENSKY, A. L., PALKES, H. S. *et al.* (1983) Intelligence in epilepsy: a prospective study in children. *Annals of Neurology*, **14**, 438–444

BOYD, S. G., HARDEN A. and PATTON, M. A. (1988) The EEG in early diagnosis of Angelman's (happy puppet) syndrome. *European Journal of Pediatrics*, **147**, 508–513

BRORSON, L. O., WRANNE, L. (1987) Long-term prognosis in childhood epilepsy: survival and seizure prognosis. *Epilepsia*, **28**, 324–330

CORBETT, J. A. (1974) Epilepsy in children with severe mental handicap. *Proceedings of Symposia 16* (ed. F. P. Woodford), Institute for Research into Mental and Multiple Handicap, London, pp. 27–41

CORBETT, J. A. (1985) Epilepsy as part of a handicapping condition. In *Paediatric Perspectives on Epilepsy* (eds E. Ross and E. Reynolds), John Wiley, London, pp. 79–89

CORBETT, J. A. (1990) Epilepsy and mental retardation. In *Comprehensive Epileptology* (eds M. Dam and L. Gram), Raven Press, New York, pp. 271–280

CORBETT, J. A., HARRIS, R. and ROBINSON, R. G. (1975). Epilepsy. In *Mental Retardation and Developmental Disabilities* (ed. J. Wortis), Brunner Mazel, New York, Vol VII, pp. 81–111

EVANHUIS, H. M. (1990). The natural history of dementia in Down's syndrome. *Archives of Neurology*, **47**, 263–267

GOMEZ, M. R. (1988) *Tuberous Sclerosis*, 2nd Edition, Raven Press, New York

HOSKING, G., MILES, R. and WINSTANLEY, P. (1990) Seizures in patients with cerebral palsy. *Developmental Medicine and Child Neurology*, **32**, 1026–1027

RETT SYNDROME DIAGNOSTIC CRITERIA WORK GROUP (1988) Diagnostic Criteria for Rett syndrome. *Annals of Neurology*, **23**, 425–428

RIIKONEN, R. and SIMELL, O. (1990) Tuberous sclerosis and infantile spasms. *Developmental Medicine and Child Neurology*, **32**, 203–209

RUTTER, M., GRAHAM, P. and YULE, W. (1970) A Neuropsychiatric Study in Childhood. *Clinics in Developmental Medicine*, Nos. 35/36, Spastics International/Heinemann Medical, London

SCHAIN, R. J. (1979). Problems with the use of anticonvulsant drugs in mentally retarded individuals. *Brain and Development*, **2**, 77–82

STAFSTROM, C. E., PATXOT, O. F., GILMORE, H. E. and WISNIEWSKI, K. E. (1991) Seizures in children with Down's syndrome: etiology, characteristics and outcome. *Developmental Medicine and Child Neurology*, **33**, 191–200

TATSUNO, M., HAYASHI, M., IWAMOTO, H. *et al*. (1984) Epilepsies in childhood Down's syndrome. *Brain and Development*, **6**, 37–44

TIZARD, J. AND GRAD, J. C. (1961) The mentally handicapped and their families. *Maudsley Monograph*, No. 7, Oxford University Press, London

WOOD, C. (ed. 1985) *Epilepsy and Mental Handicap*. Royal Society of Medicine Round Table Series, No. 2. Royal Society of Medicine Services and Labaz Sanofi, UK, Ltd, London

# Chapter 16

# Epilepsy and brain tumours

Brain tumours have a notorious reputation as a cause of late-onset epilepsy in adults, even though they are responsible for only about 10% of such cases. As the most frequent solid tumours occurring in childhood, brain tumours constitute an important part of paediatric oncology. Brain tumours and epilepsy are inextricably linked in the lay mind and many parents are deeply concerned about this possibility, particularly when their child has his first seizure or when the attacks are refractory to treatment. *In fact, brain tumours are a very rare cause of childhood epilepsy.* Nevertheless, as Rasmussen (1983) has emphasized, the possibility of an indolent glioma causing a chronic partial or focal epilepsy should be remembered at all ages in childhood, especially if intracranial calcification is present. A CT examination is then mandatory, and surgical excision may be curative.

In a review of tumours in infancy and childhood (edited by Jones and Campbell, 1976), 30 consecutive children with intracranial tumours, the majority treated at the Royal Children's Hospital, Melbourne, were analysed. Tumours occurring in the posterior cranial fossa were the most common and accounted for 51% of their series. Others have put the incidence of subtentorial tumours in childhood as high as two-thirds of all cases (Wilson, 1975). Subtentorial tumours commonly present with signs and symptoms of cerebellar involvement, with evidence of raised intracranial pressure and occasionally with cranial nerve palsies. Seizures are almost unknown in such a situation, although the intermittent decerebrate posturing of a child with a cerebral tumour compressing the midbrain may be mistaken for an epileptic seizure on occasions. The second most common group of cerebral tumours in children consists of those found in the region of the third ventricle and includes craniopharyngiomata, tumours of the optic nerves and chiasma, and tumours of the walls and floor of the ventricle. These are usually non-epileptogenic, although thalamic tumours may sometimes be associated with seizures (Hirose, Lombroso and Eisenberg, 1975). Superficial tumours of the cerebral cortex accounted for 10% of the Melbourne series (Jones and Campbell, 1976) and these were usually highly malignant. Non-malignant tumours such as meningiomata were exceedingly rare, difficult to eradicate and not necessarily associated with seizures, probably because the brain had ample time to adapt to their presence. In contrast, the rare cortical oligodendroglioma presents with seizures in the majority of cases (Backus and Millichap, 1962).

Malignant cortical tumours in the Melbourne series (Jones and Campbell, 1976) were evenly distributed over the first three quinquennia of childhood and early adolescence. The commonest locations were in the parietal and frontal lobes, and much less frequently they were in the temporal and occipital lobes. Epilepsy occurred in 26% of those with cortical tumours and was usually focal or partial. Generalized seizures can occur, however, and frontal lobe tumours have a sinister reputation for presenting with status epilepticus in both children and adults (Rowan and Scott, 1970). The other symptoms and signs of cortical tumours in children are headache, vomiting, papilloedema and the occasional development of a hemiparesis (O'Donohoe, 1982). Despite the rarity of this association between brain tumours and epilepsy, fundoscopy should be the rule in all children presenting with their first seizure.

Lee *et al.* (1989) from Oxford have published an important paper concerning the need to suspect the possible existence of a slow-growing glioma in children with long-standing partial epilepsy which is proving difficult to control. The mean age of onset in their series was $3\frac{1}{2}$ years, but the average age of diagnosis was nearly 5 years later. In some of their patients, it was inferred that the tumours may have been present from birth. The delay in diagnosis was ascribed to misinterpretation of CT scans in which there had been a failure to recognize characteristic indentation of the inner table of the skull by the localized space-occupying lesion. They emphasized that surgery was capable of removing the tumour and curing the epilepsy. Unfortunately, surgery achieves complete removal in only a minority of other malignant tumours, especially in the very young (Dropcho *et al.*, 1987). Other methods of treatment, including chemotherapy, are being actively investigated. The review by Cohen and Duffner (1984) provides an exhaustive review of intracranial tumours in childhood in all their aspects.

Intracranial parenchymal arteriovenous fistulae may also lead to the occurrence of severe epilepsy, behaving as a space-occupying lesion in this respect (Kelly, Mellinger and Sundt, 1978). Small lesions tend to be deep and are often silent until rupture, when they bleed massively. Large lesions are characterized by seizures and progressive motor deficit. CT scanning with contrast enhancement is the most useful diagnostic test. In a personal case of the author's, surgical removal of the lesion produced dramatic improvement in the patient's epilepsy.

## References

BACKUS, R. E. and MILLICHAP, J. G. (1962) The seizure as a manifestation of intracranial tumor in childhood. *Pediatrics*, **29**, 978–984

COHEN, M. E. and DUFFNER, P. K. (1984) *Brain Tumors in Children. Principles of Diagnosis and Treatment.* The International Review of Child Neurology, Raven Press, New York

DROPCHO, E. J., WISOFF, J. H., WALKER, R. W. and ALLEN, J. C. (1987) Supratentorial malignant gliomas in childhood. A review of fifty cases. *Annals of Neurology*, **22**, 355–364

HIROSE, G., LOMBROSO, C. T. and EISENBERG, H. (1975) Thalamic tumors in childhood. *Archives of Neurology*, **32**, 740–744

JONES, P. G. and CAMPBELL, P. E. (1976) *Tumours of Infancy and Childhood*, Blackwell Scientific, Oxford, London, Edinburgh, Melbourne, pp. 231–287

KELLY, J. J., MELINGER, J. F. and SUNDT, T. M. (1978) Intracranial arteriovenous malformations in childhood. *Annals of Neurology*, **3**, 338–343

LEE, T. K. Y., NAKASU, Y., JEFFREE, M. A. *et al.* (1989) Indolent glioma: a cause of epilepsy. *Archives of Disease in Childhood*, **64**, 1666–1671

O'DONOHOE, N. V. (1982) Headache and tumours in children. *British Medical Journal*, **285**, 4–5

RASMUSSEN, T. (1983) Cortical resection in children with focal epilepsy. In *Advances in Epileptology: The XIVth Epilepsy International Symposium* (eds M. Parsonage, R. H. E. Grant, A. G. Craig and A. A. Ward), Raven Press, New York pp. 249–254

ROWAN, A. J. and SCOTT, D. F. (1970) Major status epilepticus. A series of 42 patients. *Acta Neurologica Scandinavica*, **46**, 573–584

WILSON, C. B. (1975) Diagnosis and surgical treatment of childhood brain tumors. *Cancer*, **35**, 950–956

# Chapter 17

# Epilepsy and sleep

Consideration is given to various non-epileptic paroxysmal nocturnal events in the text on the differential diagnosis of epilepsy (pages 221–222). These include night-mares, night terrors and nocturnal enuresis. In the author's opinion, neither these nor other phenomena such as sleep-walking should be designated as 'epileptiform' or as 'epileptic equivalents'. However, the close relationship between true epileptic attacks and sleep has been well known since earliest times and the rapidly increasing knowledge of the physiology of sleep-in recent years has led to a corresponding interest in the association between sleep and epilepsy.

Since the earliest use of the EEG in clinical research, there has been a close interest in the altered electrophysiological state occurring in sleep and in the relationship between sleep and epilepsy. Janz (1974) reviewed the information concerning epilepsy and the sleeping–waking cycle available at that time and Kellaway and Frost (1983) have also published an extensive review.

It is recognized that sleep may be divided into four stages, called 1 to 4 or, sometimes A to D (Loomis, Harvey and Hobart, 1937; Dement and Kleitman, 1957). The first stage (stage A) is really not sleep at all but represents drowsiness with eyes closed. The alpha rhythm (8–13 Hz) persists in the EEG but, as drowsiness passes into sleep, it gives way to a flatter wave pattern characterized by slower more irregular theta waves (4–7 Hz) and by low-voltage fast or beta activity (8–13 Hz). This is the second stage of sleep or stage B. In the third stage (stage C), the pattern of the second stage gives way to more irregular and slower waves of higher voltage (frequency 1–6 Hz). From time to time spindles of faster waves occur in the anterior areas and are known as sleep spindles. In this stage an appropriate external stimulus, such as a sudden loud noise, will give rise to a characteristic wave pattern known as a 'K' complex. This consists of a small sharp wave succeeded by one or more larger slow waves which are then followed by fast waves. Finally, in stage 4 (stage D) slow irregular high-voltage delta waves (1–3 Hz) replace all other forms of activity and the individual is deeply asleep. Some have distinguished two separate stages (D and E) in deep sleep, depending on whether stimulation elicits 'K' complexes or not. In the understanding of the sleep process, the concept of continuous activity of the cortex as shown by the EEG is essential. Except in the deepest stage of sleep, when stimuli may provoke no reaction, 'cerebral vigilance' remains. This is something quite distinct from normal consciousness. Consciousness depends on a steady activation flow from the reticular formation in the brain-stem

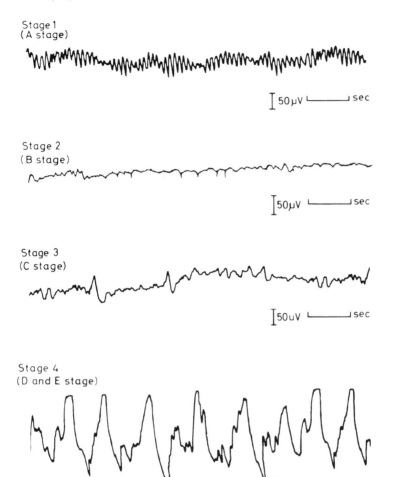

*Figure 17.1* The EEG stages of sleep (1 to 4 or A to D and E). (*Courtesy of Roche Products Ltd., London*)

to the cortex. When this activation flow diminishes or ceases, as it does in sleep, contact with reality, or consciousness as we know it, is lost but cerebral vigilance, although lowered, remains with us until the deepest stages of sleep are reached. Even in the deepest stage of sleep, however, a stimulus with special relevance to the sleeping person may produce arousal, as, for example, when a sleeping mother awakens to her baby's faint cry from another room.

The mechanism *of arousal* is centred in the reticular formation of the midbrain and hindbrain, and without the activation (which the reticular formation gives to the cortex) consciousness would not be possible. In sleep these two parts of the brain behave differently. During the deepest stage of cortical sleep the hindbrain is relatively active, and when cortical sleep lightens the hindbrain sleep deepens producing a situation called 'paradoxical sleep'. During paradoxical sleep, the cortical EEG is characterized by a near-wakefulness pattern, and rapid bilateral synchronous eye movements occur. The latter have resulted in paradoxical sleep being called *rapid eye movement or REM sleep*. Cortical vigilance is high in REM sleep and one might also expect consciousness to be present, but the latter is not the case because of the relative inactivity of the reticular formation. The subject is, in fact, difficult to awaken from this type of sleep. During REM sleep there is a suppression of muscle tone and accelerated irregular respiration and heart rates, whereas in non-REM sleep (stages 1–4) muscle tone is present because of the activity of the reticular formation, and heart and respiration rates are slow and regular. Dreaming is generally believed to take place during REM sleep. The pattern of a normal night's sleep is to pass initially into stage 4 sleep and, during the rest of the night, to rise and fall through progressively lighter stages until finally awakening. Superimposed on this pattern are periods of REM sleep which occupy 15–25% of the total sleep time of adults. In the newborn, however, REM sleep occupies 45–50% of total sleep time, but with increasing age the proportion of quiet non-REM sleep soon increases and adult sleep patterns are reached in later childhood.

## Non-epileptic disorders which may be confused with epilepsy

Disorders other than epilepsy which are associated with sleep and which may be confused with epileptic events were reviewed by Anders and Weinstein (1972) and by Stores (1991). Nocturnal enuresis, sleep walking, sleep talking and night terrors are associated with emergence from stage 3 and/or 4 non-REM sleep and are defined as disorders of arousal. The disorders of arousal appear to be associated especially with the presence of normal neurological immaturity in young children. Narcolepsy, on the other hand, is associated with the abnormal occurrence of REM sleep and is regarded as a disorder of sleep. Enuresis is one of several possible manifestations of obstructive sleep apnoea in children, which tend to be more varied than in adults where loud snoring is the predominant sign. Other nocturnal symptoms in this condition that might be misinterpreted are difficulty in breathing, restless sleep and intense sweating (Editorial, 1989). Rarely, episodes of automatic behaviour during the sleeping hours, sometimes with hallucinations and followed by amnesia, may be mistaken for complex partial seizures or even for non-convulsive status epilepticus. EEG monitoring during the episodes will make the distinction in difficult cases (Stores, 1986, 1991).

## Stages of sleep and waking related to seizures

Gibbs and Gibbs (1952), in their classic atlas of the EEG, were among the first investigators to emphasize the fact that seizure discharges were much more frequent in sleep than in the waking state and that such discharges were particularly frequent in symptomatic epilepsy. They showed that a sleep EEG was much more likely to demonstrate a temporal lobe epileptic focus than was a waking record. This is not invariable, however, and Matthes (1961) stressed that sleep may not activate the epileptic focus but may actually cause a decrease in temporal lobe activity in a proportion of children. In using sleep as an initiator of epileptic activity in children, it is important not to be misled by the occurrence of sharp waves and rhythmic spike waves over the vertex during drowsiness and light sleep, findings which many consider normal phenomena.

When the times at which seizures occur in the context of the sleeping–waking cycle are recorded, it will be found that they tend to occur as follows:

1   Within the first or second hour after going to sleep, i.e. during deep sleep.
2   One to 2 hours before the usual time of awakening, i.e. during lighter sleep.
3   Within the period of a few minutes to 2 hours after awakening (early morning seizures).

Epilepsy occurring exclusively during sleep is uncommon at all ages (Gibberd and Bateson, 1974).

When the chronological approach is applied to the various types of childhood epilepsy, both generalized and partial, it will be found that these epilepsies often have fairly clear relationships to the sleeping–waking cycle. Infantile spasms are frequent during drowsiness and just after awakening and may be repeated. Although the EEG pattern of hypsarrhythmia is generally present in both the sleeping and waking states, it may be apparent only during sleep, particularly non-REM sleep, in certain cases. A sleep record should therefore be performed in all patients who have a clinical history suggestive of the condition, but who show a normal or non-hypsarrhythmic record at the onset of the illness (Hrachovy and Frost, 1989).

The sudden bodily jerks of the whole or part of the body upon falling asleep are a very familiar experience and are often accompanied by sudden and violent sensations, particularly by a feeling of falling. The individual usually awakens in an alarmed state. *Sleep jerks* occur at the stage of disappearance of the alpha rhythm and the appearance of low-voltage slow waves in the EEG. They are certainly not an epileptic phenomenon and, indeed, there is no evidence for the existence of any type of epilepsy having as its sole symptom the occurrence of epileptic myoclonias on falling asleep or during sleep (Lugaresi *et al.*, 1970).

In the *primary and secondary generalized myoclonic epilepsies* of late infancy and early childhood, including those preceded by infantile spasms, nocturnal seizures are common and, as Janz (1974) has said: 'when the parents take their ailing child into bed with them, the child's myoclonic jerking throughout the night may give them not a moment's rest'. Short generalized tonic flexion spasms may occur in the severe varieties of myoclonic epilepsy, such as the Lennox–Gastaut syndrome (Gastaut *et al.* 1966), particularly during the deeper stages of sleep. Drop seizures of the akinetic type often occur following arising, both after awakening from nocturnal and from afternoon sleep. Myoclonic absences are also frequent at these times. In the EEG diagnosis of these epilepsies it is important to remember that the slow spike-wave pattern may be activated by sleep.

The *less serious varieties* of childhood epilepsy also have a close relationship to the sleeping–waking cycle. Lennox-Buchthal (1973), in her monograph on febrile convulsions, emphasized that the attacks occurred during sleep in half the cases studied and that they were related to sleep (on going to sleep or on awakening) in another quarter. Any family doctor or paediatric hospital resident will be only too well aware of this association.

*Primary generalized epilepsy of the petit mal type*, on the other hand, occurs most frequently after children have awakened, and attacks are particularly common after arising in the early morning, although they may occur at any time of the day. The attacks do not, as a rule, occur during sleep, although the EEG discharges may be recorded in sleep. Lack of sleep for any reason may result in an increased number of absences the next day. Where petit mal and grand mal are combined, the major attacks tend to occur in the waking state, often after awakening (Janz, 1974).

Awakening clonic–tonic–clonic seizures may be triggered by sleep deprivation, by excessive fatigue and by alcohol intake, especially during adolescence. The awakening grand mal of puberty, as it has been called, is probably one of the phenotypes of Janz's syndrome of juvenile myoclonic epilepsy (Delgado-Escueta, Treiman and Walsh, 1983). It has a good prognosis, over 80% of cases remitting with sodium valproate therapy, although relapse is common after withdrawal of treatment.

In *juvenile myoclonic epilepsy* itself, bilateral myoclonic jerks, especially of shoulders and arms, are frequent after awakening and major seizures may also occur after awakening. In some photosensitive individuals, the spike and wave activity which occurs after eye closure and which may be accompanied by eyelid flicker and brief absences, is not usually a problem in the dark when the person retires to bed, according to Jeavons (1977). However Tassinari *et al.* (1977) reported myoclonic jerks which were related to eye closure and occurred at bedtime in five children, four of whom showed photosensitivity. These jerks were noted before actual sleep ensued and so could be distinguished from the normal sleep jerks. In doubtful cases the EEG helps to make the distinction. Children and adolescents with marked photosensitivity may also suffer from myoclonic jerks after awakening in the morning, particularly when sunlight shines into bedrooms as curtains are drawn or when natural or artificial light is reflected from bathroom tiles or mirrors. One of the author's patients, with discharges occurring after eye closure, experienced absences when he dipped his head towards a washbasin to wash his face.

*Primary generalized epilepsy of the grand mal type* is relatively uncommon during sleep in childhood. When attacks do occur they tend to exhibit two peaks, either soon after falling asleep or during early morning sleep. Secondarily generalized tonic–clonic seizures in patients with partial epilepsy are much commoner than primary generalized epilepsy of the grand mal type but they are difficult to distinguish from generalized tonic–clonic attacks without focal onset because sleep conceals their initial motor phenomena, such as versive movements or unilateral clonic movements which may be easily observed during wakefulness. By far the commonest epilepsy of this type manifesting itself in sleep is that known as benign partial epilepsy of childhood with centro-temporal spikes, which is fully described in Chapter 9. In one large series (Beaussart, 1972), 51% of the cases had their attacks exclusively during sleep. Ambrosetto and Gobbi (1975) were able to record an EEG during nocturnal sleep in a 10-year-old boy and noted that the spike discharges were activated both in REM sleep and in slow-wave sleep. The actual attack occurred as the boy appeared to be awakening and while he was still in a drowsy state. The seizures may be misinterpreted as primary generalized seizures rather than partial attacks with secondary generalization. The EEG discharges are activated by sleep in benign partial epilepsy of childhood with centro-temporal spikes, making it likely that the attacks actually start during sleep and wake the patient before secondary generalization occurs and consciousness is lost. In about one-third of patients, the spike discharges are only present during sleep (Loiseau and Duché, 1989). It is important to remember, however, that there is no direct quantitative relationship between the overall amount of focal spike activity and the number of clinical seizures experienced in this type of epilepsy (Kellaway and Frost, 1983).

*Partial seizures with complex symptomatology* are uncommon during drug-induced or natural sleep, despite the fact that sleep is usually a potent activator of focal EEG discharges in this type of epilepsy. Partial deprivation of sleep prior to EEG examination is often used to encourage the patient to fall asleep naturally during the recording. Temporal lobe attacks, when occurring in sleep, tend to do so after the patient has fallen asleep rather than in the second half of the night, and they may also occur during an afternoon nap.

Exclusively nocturnal temporal lobe seizures are extremely rare (Tassinari *et al.*, 1977) and similar attacks are nearly always experienced in the daytime also. The practical importance of this observation is that one should be cautious about diagnosing complex nocturnal behavioural manifestations as being epileptic in nature unless similar diurnal episodes are observed. Diagnostic accuracy may depend on monitoring of the EEG and of other physiological events during sleep. Portable cassette systems for home monitoring of children's sleep are now available (Stores and Bergel, 1989). Complex partial seizures of frontal lobe origin may also present problems in diagnosis, since they may be associated with bizarre clinical manifestations at night and be misdiagnosed as nightmares (Stores, Zaiwalla and Bergel, 1991). Precise diagnosis is essential and may require an actual ictal EEG recording.

Tassinari *et al.* (1977) have described a very rare type of *epileptic encephalopathy* occurring during slow-wave sleep and associated with subclinical status epilepticus. EEG sleep recordings are essential for diagnosis. Continuous high-voltage diffuse slow spike-wave discharges appear as soon as the patient falls asleep and persist throughout non-REM sleep. This makes it impossible to distinguish the stages of sleep. The electrical status disappears in REM sleep phases. The syndrome begins in childhood between the ages of 4 and 10 years. Infrequent nocturnal seizures, diurnal absences, behavioural disorders and deterioration in intellectual capacity, language function and social performance may occur. The behavioural disorders may be prepsychotic in type and associated with a relative lack of interest in the environment and in normal activities. There are also disturbances of memory and of temporo-spatial orientation. Antiepileptic drugs are largely ineffective in abolishing the electrical status although they may control the clinical seizures to an extent. The duration of the syndrome is variable but there is a prospect of remission during adolescence. Tassinari *et al.* (1992) reviewed their experience with this rare syndrome in great detail and have suggested that the substitution of the continuous spike-wave discharges for the normal physiological sleep pattern of non-REM sleep over many years could be responsible for the appearance of complex and severe neurological impairment, mainly involving language function, and with associated mental and psychiatric disturbances. They postulate analogies with the Landau–Kleffner syndrome of acquired aphasia in childhood (see Chapter 21). Donat and Wright (1989) have published a comprehensive review of current knowledge concerning the relationships between sleep, the epileptic syndromes and the EEG in infancy and childhood.

## Effects of drug treatment

How may these considerations regarding epilepsy and sleep affect general management and treatment? Since overfatigue and insufficient sleep may affect seizure frequency in some childhood epilepsies, it follows that an ordered life with a regular bedtime and hour for rising should be beneficial. There has long been much interest in the effects of drugs on sleep patterns. Barbiturates and related drugs increase the amount of deep sleep. In deep sleep, as already described, the hindbrain and its reticular formation are active and this may facilitate the genesis and propagation of discharges in primary and secondary generalized epilepsies, including those originating in the temporal lobes. Phenobarbitone has long been considered by many as unsuitable for the treatment of epilepsy during sleep (Janz, 1974). In paradoxical or REM sleep, although cortical vigilance is high, there is relative inactivity of the reticular formation and a consequent reduction in epileptogenesis may take place (Montplaisir *et al.*, 1980). Drugs with a reduced hypnotic effect, such as phenytoin and carbamazepine, and drugs which increase the amount of REM sleep, such as the benzodiazepines, may be more effective in sleep epilepsies than those drugs with a marked hypnotic effect.

Finally, it must be admitted that there is a great deal that is unknown concerning the relationship between sleep and epilepsy. Factors involved must include endocrine and metabolic phenomena because some hormones show circadian rhythms and there are changes in body temperature, in water and electrolyte balances, and in neurotransmitter mechanisms during sleep. The circadian sleep-wake cycle and the REM/non-REM sleep cycle are endogenous rhythms which appear to be autonomous.

Experimental evidence indicates that there are two major circadian pacemakers in humans and that these control the rhythms of various physiological subsystems. One controls the rhythm of REM sleep, plasma cortisol concentration, core body temperature, and urinary potassium secretion. The other controls the cycle of slow-wave sleep, serum growth hormone secretion, skin temperature, and urinary calcium excretion. Under normal conditions, these two pacemakers are interactive and internally synchronized. It seems certain that the epileptic process in the brain is subject to biorhythmic modulation. Research suggests that this modulatory action mainly affects the elaboration of the epileptic process rather than primary epileptogenesis (Kellaway and Frost, 1983; Kellaway, 1985).

The mechanism whereby slow-wave sleep enhances the elaboration and spread of epileptiform activity in the brain may be explained on the basis of the synchronizing effect of slow-wave sleep which facilitates recruitment of increased numbers of neurons into time-locked firing patterns. REM sleep usually has the opposite effect, but may sometimes be associated with augmentation of discharges also. The worldwide research interest in the physiology of sleep will surely throw further light on these processes in the future.

# References

AMBROSETTO, G. and GOBBI, G. (1975) Benign epilepsy of childhood with Rolandic spikes, or a lesion?: EEG during a seizure. *Epilepsia*, **16**, 793–796

ANDERS, T. F. and WEINSTEIN, P. (1972) Sleep and its disorders in infants and children: a review. *Pediatrics*, **50**, 312–324

BEAUSSART, M. (1972) Benign epilepsy of childhood, with Rolandic (centrotemporal) paroxysmal foci: a clinical entity. Study of 221 cases. *Epilepsia*, **13**, 795–811

DELGADO-ESCUETA, A. V., TREIMAN, D. M. and WALSH, G. O. (1983) The treatable epilepsies. 1. *New England Journal of Medicine*, **308**, 1508–1514

DEMENT, W. and KLEITMMAN, N. (1957) Cyclic variations in EEG during sleep and their relation to eye movements, body motility and dreaming. *Electroencephalography and Clinical Neurophysiology*, **9**, 673–690

DONAT, J F. and WRIGHT, F. S. (1989) Sleep, epilepsy and the EEG in infancy and childhood. *Journal of Child Neurology*, **4**, 84–94

GASTAUT, H., TASSINARI, C. A., REGIS, H. *et al.* (1966) Childhood, epileptic encephalopathy with diffuse slow spike waves (otherwise known as 'petit mal variant or Lennox syndrome'). *Epilepsia*, **7**, 139–179

GIBBERD, F. B. and BATESON, M. C. (1974) Sleep epilepsy: its pattern and prognosis. *British Medical Journal*, **2**, 403–405

GIBBS. F. A. and GIBBS, E. L. (1952) *Atlas of Electroencephalography*, Vol. 2: *Epilepsy*, Addison-Wesley, Cambridge, MA

HRACHOVY, R. A. and FROST, J. D. (1989) Infantile spasms. *Cleveland Clinic Journal of Medicine*, **56**, Supplement Part I, S10–S17

JANZ, D. (1974) Epilepsy and the sleeping-walking cycle. In *Handbook of Clinical Neurology*, Vol. 15: *The Epilepsies* (eds P. J. Vinkeri and G. W. Bruyn), North Holland, Amsterdam, pp. 457–490

JEAVONS, P. M. (1977) Nosological problems of myoclonic epilepsies in childhood and adolescence. *Developmental Medicine and Child Neurology*, **19**, 3–8

KELLAWAY, P. (1985) Sleep and epilepsy. *Epilepsia*, Supplement I, S15–S30

KELLAWAY, P. and FROST, J. D. (1983) Biorhythmic modulation of epileptic events. In *Recent Advances in Epilepsy*. No. 1 (eds T. A. Pedley and B. S. Meldrum), Churchill Livingstone, Edinburgh and London, pp. 139–154

EDITORIAL (1989) Airway obstruction during sleep in children. *Lancet* ii, 1018–1019 (vol. **334**)

LENNOX-BUCHTHAL, M. A. (1973) Febrile convulsions: a reappraisal. *Electroencephalography and Clinical Neurophysiology*, Suppl. **32**, pp. 38–40

LOISEAU, P. and DUCHE, B. (1989) Benign childhood epilepsy with centrotemporal spikes. *Cleveland Clinic Journal of Medicine*. Supplement Part I, S17–S22

LOOMIS. A. L., HARVEY, E. N. and HOBART, G. A. (1937) Cerebral states during sleep as studied by human brain potentials. *Journal of Experimental Psychology*, **21**, 127–144

LUGARESI, E., COCCAGNA. G., MANTOVANI, M. *et al.* (1970) The evolution of different types of myoclonus during sleep: a polygraphic study. *European Neurology*, **4**, 321–331

MATTHES, A. (1961) Die psychomotorische Epilepsie in Kindesalter. 11. *Zeitschrift fur Kiriderheilkunde*, **85**, 472–492

MONTPLAISIR, J., SAINT-HILAIRE, J. M., LAVERDIÈRE, M. *et al.* (1980) Contribution of all-night polygraphic recording to the localization of primary epileptic foci. In *Advances in Epileptology: The XIth Epilepsy International Symposium* (eds R. Canger, F. Angeleri and J. K. Penry), Raven Press, New York, pp 135–138

STORES, G. (1986) Non-convulsive status epilepticus in children. In *Recent Advances in Epilepsy* 1 (eds T. A. Pedley and B. S. Meldrum), Churchill Livingstone, Edinburgh, London, pp. 295–310

STORES, G. (1991) Confusions concerning sleep disorders and the epilepsies in children and adolescents. *British Journal of Psychiatry*, **158**, 1–7

STORES, G. and BERGEL, N. (1989) Clinical utility of cassette EEG in childhood seizures disorders. In *Ambulatory EEG Monitoring* (ed. J. S. Ebersole), Raven Press, New York, pp. 129–139

STORES, G., ZAIWALLA, Z. and BERGEL, N. (1991) Frontal Lobe complex partial seizures in children: a form of epilepsy at particular risk of misdiagnosis. *Developmental Medicine and Child Neurology*, **33**, 998–1009

TASSINARI, C. A., TERZANO, G., CAPOCCHI, G. *et al.* (1977) Epileptic seizures during sleep in children. In *Epilepsy, The Eight International Symposium* (ed. J. K. Penry), Raven Press, New York, pp. 345–354

TASSINARI, C. A., BUREAU, M., DRAVET, C., DALLA BERNARDINA, B. and ROGER J. (1992) Epilepsy with continuous spikes and waves during slow sleep — otherwise described as ESES (epilepsy with electrical status epilepticus during slow sleep).In: *Epileptic Syndromes in Infancy, Childhood and Adolescence*, 2nd edn (eds J. Roger, M. Bureau, C. Dravet *et al.*), John Libbey, London, Paris, pp. 245–256

# Chapter 18

# Unusual manifestations of childhood epilepsy

References to the less usual varieties of childhood epilepsy are made elsewhere in this book. These include the syndrome of acquired aphasia associated with a convulsive disorder, the unusual types of nocturnal epilepsy and psychotic behaviour and also so-called abdominal epilepsy. Neurologists have always been fascinated by the desire to classify and categorize the many clinical fragments of an epileptic attack. A peculiar or unusual clinical manifestation may be either a facet of a complex seizure or may represent the patient's only presenting symptom. The latter situation may be present when uncontrollable pathological laughter occurs as an epileptic phenomenon, a condition termed gelastic epilepsy (*gelos* = mirth). There is usually a subjective experience of merriment, and complex co-ordinate movements with grinning, giggling or joyful weeping may occur. Gascon and Lombroso (1971) wrote of this unusual complaint in children and adolescents, and they adopted strict criteria for its diagnosis. These are as follows:

1   Stereotyped recurrence of the attack.
2   The absence of external precipitating factors.
3   Concomitance of other manifestations generally accepted as epileptic, eg. tonic and clonic movements, disturbance of consciousness and/or automatisms.
4   Interictal and/or ictal discharges being present in the EEG.

In four of their ten patients they observed bursts of uncontrollable laughter occurring simultaneously with discharges in the EEG. They were careful to distinguish between the ictal laughter and the postictal laughter which may occur after seizures of various types. Half of their patients had interictal discharges of the generalized spike-wave type while the rest had discharges located over one or other temporal lobe.

It has been suggested that there is a motor centre for laughter in or near the hypothalamus. Laughing attacks may occur with hypothalamic lesions sometimes causing precocious puberty (Williams, Schutt and Savage, 1978). The usual hypothalamic lesion is a hamartoma. Symptoms may begin very early, even in infancy, and characteristically consist of frequent brief repetitive outbursts of laughter, usually mechanical and mirthless in type. Normal early psychomotor development is succeeded by cognitive deterioration and behavioural problems later. Magnetic resonance imaging is the most effective method of demonstrating these lesions (Berkovic *et al.*, 1988). The prognosis for seizure control by drugs is poor and surgical removal of the lesions is extremely difficult.

Involuntary laughter may also be associated with lesions involving frontal or temporal lobes and with many other different types of pathology (Leading article, 1977). Gascon and Lombrusco (1971) thought that gelastic epilepsy should be considered as being due to pathological discharges traversing complex neuronal circuits subserving laughter, and arising at quite different levels in different cases. Most authors agree that possible subcortical sites for emotional epilepsy are the limbic system and the hypothalamus. Parts of the limbic system, notably the hippocampus and the amygdala, lie within the temporal lobe and are frequently involved in the pathogenesis of epilepsy. Quite apart from gelastic epilepsy, crying epilepsy (quiritarian or dacro-cystic) and running epilepsy (cursive) have been described with temporal lobe lesions, including tumours. Turning of the head may occur with these types of temporal lobe epilepsy, and epigastric auras may precede the attack, indicating juxtaposition in the temporal lobe of brain centres for visceral and affective functions. In 'epilepsia cursiva' or 'running seizures' the patient becomes confused, out of contact with his surroundings and thus starts running (Walsh, 1974). In certain cases the patient may be exteriorizing inner feelings of fear or terror as attempts at flight. A generalized seizure may follow if there is diffuse spread of the epileptic discharge. Alternatively, the patient may become combative and violent. Usually, however, any acts of aggression which may occur in temporal lobe attacks are brief and nonpurposeful and are responses to attempted restraint during an automatism (Special Report, 1981). Exercise in itself may sometimes induce seizures (Ogunyemi, Gomez and Klass, 1988)

## Changes in mood, attitude and social behaviour

Williams (1966) wrote about the dilemma of recognizing what is truly ictal or epileptic in nature and of avoiding the ambiguity of phrases such as *epileptic equivalent states and epileptiform attacks* in relation to temporal lobe epilepsy. Patients with this type of epilepsy usually have a structural abnormality or disordered function of the temporal lobe or lobes, i.e. those parts of the brain which are responsible for the integration of all sensation into total experience. Since such experience is primarily responsible for behaviour, it is not surprising that this type of epilepsy is associated with psychological disorders reflected in disturbance of mood or attitude or evident in disturbed social behaviour. Williams (1966, 1981) recommended that the clinician keep clearly before him the distinction between what happens in the attack and what results from the postictal confusional state, and that he should divorce these events from the total behaviour of the patient. He noted that many people with aggressive psychopathic behaviour also have disturbance in the temporal lobe areas reflected in the EEG or in morbid anatomical studies, even though they may never suffer from epilepsy. The importance of these observations resides in the fact that frequently a diagnosis of temporal lobe epilepsy is made in individuals, including children, who demonstrate disturbed behaviour and who may have an EEG abnormality over a temporal lobe, without any clinical evidence that they suffer from the paroxsymal disorder of epilepsy. Another common error is to categorize as 'temporal lobe epilepsy' any epilepsy with an EEG spike focus over one or other lobe. This is unfortunate, since one of the commonest epileptic syndromes in late childhood is that known as benign partial epilepsy with centrotemporal spikes, in which such an EEG abnormality is usually present but where the clinical history is totally different from that of secondary partial epilepsy causing temporal lobe seizures.

**Table 18.1 Complex partial seizures categorized according to their initial symptoms**

*With disturbance of thought*
Dreamy states with clouding of consciousness
Illusional or hallucinatory experiences resembling a dream
Feelings of familiarity in strange surroundings (déjà vu)
Visual illusions in which objects appear smaller (micropsia) or larger (macropsia)
Auditory illusions in which sounds become fainter (microacusia) or louder (macroacusia)
Illusions of depersonalization and unreality, e.g. the illusion of observing oneself from outside the body
Sudden compulsive thoughts, often of an unpleasant or bizarre nature

*With disturbance of language*
Episodes of dysphasia where seizure discharge involves the dominant hemisphere
Speech automatisms with utterance of identifiable words

*With complex motor behaviour*
Motor automatisms with confusion, incoherent mumbling, repetitive actions and inappropriate behaviour
Prolonged 'fugue states' – largely confined to adults

*With antisocial behaviour*
Moodiness, irritability and anger may occur periodically as epileptic manifestations

*With affective disturbance*
Feelings of fear which may be intense
Sensations of pleasure or wellbeing
Gelastic epilepsy

*With olfactory disturbances*
Hallucinations of smell which may be intense and unpleasant (uncinate fits)
Licking and smacking of lips may occur

*With visual symptoms*
Simple visual hallucinations – lights, stars
Complex visual hallucinations of familiar scenes

*With vertiginous symptoms*
Sensations of spinning, usually on a vertical axis
Sensations of falling

*Abdominal and alimentary sensations*
Epigastric sensations which are difficult to describe
A desire to defaecate

*With cardiovascular symptoms*
Precordial discomfort
Fluttering sensations in the left chest
Tachycardia

# Bizarre manifestations

It is difficult to list all the unusual, bizarre and often baffling clinical manifestations of epilepsy. In this section, one has merely tried to indicate some of the more dramatic possibilities and a more comprehensive list is provided in *Table 18.1*. It is most important to realize that complex partial seizures in children as in adults, may have their origin in the frontal lobes in some cases, although they most commonly originate in the temporal lobes (Stores, Zaiwalla and Bergel, 1991). The interested reader who desires more information on the subject is also requested to consult William Lennox's classic book (1960) with its numerous case histories, particularly the chapter on psychomotor epilepsy.

## References

BERKOVIC, S. F., ANDERMANN, F., MELANSON, D. *et al.* (1988) Hypothalamic hamartomas and ictal laughter. Evolution of a characteristic epileptic syndrome and diagnostic value of magnetic resonance imaging. *Annals of Neurology*, **23**, 429–439

GASCON, G. G. and LOMBROSO, C. T. (1971) Epileptic (gelastic) laughter. *Epilepsia*, **12**, 63–76

LEADING ARTICLE (1977) Less usual forms of epilepsy. *British Medical Journal*, **275**, 127–128

LENNOX, W. G. (1960) *Epilepsy and Related Disorders*, Vol. 1, J. and A. Churchill, London, Little, Brown, Boston, pp. 227–321

OGUNYEMI, A. O., GOMEZ, M. R. and KLASS, D. W. (1988) Seizures induced by exercise. *Neurology*, **38**, 633–634

STORES, G., ZAIWALLA, Z. and BERGEL, N. (1991) Frontal lobe complex partial seizures in children: a form of epilepsy at particular risk of misdiagnosis. *Developmental Medicine and Child Neurology*, **33**, 998–1009

SPECIAL REPORT (1981) The nature of aggression during epileptic seizures. *New England Journal of Medicine*, **305**, 711–716

WALSH, G. O. (1974) Unusual presentations of epilepsies. *Pediatrics*, **53**, 548–551

WILLIAMS, D. (1966) Temporal lobe epilepsy. *British Medical Journal*, **1**, 1439–1442

WILLIAMS, D. (1981) The emotions and epilepsy. In *Epilepsy and Psychiatry* (eds E. H. Reynolds and M. R. Trimble), Churchill Livingstone, Edinburgh and London, pp. 49–59

WILLIAMS, M., SCHUTT, W. and SAVAGE, D. (1978) Epileptic laughter with precocious puberty. *Archives of Disease in Childhood*, **53**, 965–966

# Chapter 19

# Intractable epilepsy in childhood

## Introduction

Intractable epilepsy may be defined as epilepsy with seizures which have remained uncontrolled for years despite accurate diagnosis and investigation and following appropriate therapy. Accurate diagnosis of epilepsy is an essential first step. Most doctors who deal with epilepsy at a consultant level will have shared the experience of Jeavons (1983), who reported that 25% of children referred to an epilepsy clinic with a diagnosis of epilepsy had non-epileptic events, particularly syncopal attacks and psychiatric disorders.

Pseudoseizures present an especially difficult problem in differential diagnosis, especially in adolescence (Finlayson and Lucas, 1979). The undiagnosis of epilepsy may be particularly difficult once a misdiagnosis has been made. The misdiagnosis of the precise type of seizure which is occurring is another frequent error. For example, mistaking complex partial seizures for childhood absence epilepsy, and vice versa, leads to incorrect therapy and faulty prognostic advice.

## Some causes of intractability

The patient may not be fortunate enough to see a doctor with an interest in epilepsy. Sadly, epilepsy is still not a fashionable complaint, even among neurologists! The doctor may select the wrong drug for the particular type of epilepsy or give the right drug in the wrong amounts, i.e., too little or too much. He may show lack of patience with the problem or resign from it prematurely.

Furthermore, the patient (or the parents) may arbitrarily change the antiepileptic drug or change from doctor to doctor without showing patience with the problem or even optimism about it. Many parents will only accept full seizure control and are plunged into despair by even an occasional attack. This attitude also produces feelings of anxiety and pessimism in the patient. It is difficult to convince some parents that their child is better off living an essentially normal life between occasional non-incapacitating seizures than being seizure-free and in a perpetual state of drug-induced drowsiness and confusion. Gordon (1988) has emphasized for many years the importance of avoiding overdosage with antiepileptic drugs, since this may actually cause an increase in the frequency of seizures. During adolescence, a disorderly or disorganized way of life as, for example, lack of adequate sleep, excess of alcohol, overwork and exhaustion, and emotional difficulties may lead to poor seizure control. The prime importance of inadequate sleep as a triggering factor for seizures in juvenile myoclonic epilepsy has been emphasized elsewhere in this book. Compliance with drug therapy is essential and 'just keep taking the tablets' is far from being a joke where epilepsy is concerned. It has been estimated (E. R. Grass, 1974, personal communication) that simply persuading patients to take their medication regularly and in the right doses will improve epilepsy control by 15–20% over all. The importance of regular medication cannot be overstressed, since haphazard treatment or the sudden withdrawal of treatment (as may happen with the misguided practice of stopping treatment before an EEG) can lead to the occurrence of status epilepticus.

## Metabolic disease and tumours

Treatment may fail because there is serious associated brain disease. Metabolic brain diseases, especially those involving cortical grey matter, may cause intractable seizures. Neuronal ceroid lipofuscinosis (Batten's disease) can mimic the Lennox–Gastaut syndrome (Harden and Pampiglione, 1982). Biotinidase deficiency, treatable with biotin orally, may present with drug-resistant seizures and psychomotor retardation in infancy (Wolf et al., 1983) and molybdenum co-factor deficiency may also be overlooked as a cause of refractory seizures during infancy (Aukett, Bennett and Hosking, 1988). Pyridoxine dependency may present in an atypical fashion and should be considered as a possible cause of intractable epilepsy in infants and young children (Goutières and Aicardi, 1985). Indolent cerebral gliomata should always be remembered as a cause of intractable seizures (Lee et al., 1989). It is essential, as Aicardi (1988) advises, that any patient with intractable epilepsy should be periodically reassessed with an open mind, since the true diagnosis may remain hidden for years. Modern neuroimaging techniques have made exact aetiological diagnosis easier in recent years.

## Structural brain disease

Structural brain disease in any highly epileptogenic area is likely to lead to difficulties with seizure control and this is seen, for example, with mesial temporal sclerosis causing complex partial seizures. Diffuse brain disease, such as exists in some moderately and many severely mentally handicapped children, is frequently a cause of intractable epilepsy and these children are quite often the victims of well-intentioned polypharmacy which compounds their many problems. The lack of facilities for the investigation and treatment of epilepsy in such children often leads to poor results being obtained and this has produced a demand for the establishment of special clinics and centres to deal with the problem. Recent studies suggest that 10% of children with mental retardation alone (IQ less than 70) or with cerebral palsy alone will also have epilepsy. The more severe the mental retardation, the greater is the likelihood of co-existent epilepsy. When mental retardation and cerebral palsy are combined, there is a 50% chance of epilepsy also being present (Hauser and Nelson, 1989).

# Epileptic syndromes and intractability

In approaching the problem of intractable epilepsy in infancy, childhood and adolescence, one should, if possible, utilize a syndrome-oriented rather than a seizure-oriented approach since, in many of these cases, a variety of seizure types and even episodes of status epilepticus will be encountered. Although seizures may draw attention to the existence of a syndrome, the syndrome itself is composed of the 'running together' (the meaning of 'syndrome') of other components including family history, age of onset, abnormal neuropsychiatric features or their absence, interictal and ictal EEG, natural history leading to remission or chronicity and response to medication (Dreifuss, 1990). The delineation of epileptic syndromes permits a reasonably reliable estimate of the natural history and prognosis to be made (O'Donohoe, 1992). The resistance to treatment of infantile spasms and the Lennox–Gastaut syndrome is well known. Early myoclonic encephalopathy, including Ohtahara's syndrome, has its onset before 3 months of age, and the overall prognosis is very poor. Severe myoclonic epilepsy in infancy, originally described by Dravet (1978), also has an exceptionally poor outlook.

Epilepsy with continuous spike-wave discharges during slow-wave sleep, also called the ESES syndrome (epilepsy with electrical status epilepticus during slow-wave sleep), first described by Patry, Lyagoubi and Tassinari (1971), is another very drug-resistant condition. Epilepsy with myoclonic absences, although apparently idiopathic or primary in aetiology, can prove very resistant to drug therapy (Tassinari, Bureau and Thomas, 1992). The syndrome of gelastic epilepsy associated with a hamartoma of the floor of the fourth ventricle (Breningstall, 1985) is another condition which is almost invariably drug-resistant.

Pellock (1989), reviewing chronic epilepsy in children, makes the important point that some epileptic syndromes, regarded as relatively benign and responding well to antiepileptic drugs, may qualify as potentially chronic forms of epilepsy because of their tendency to relapse when treatment is inadequate or has been stopped. Juvenile myoclonic epilepsy is the outstanding example of this. Patients with this disorder require relatively high dosage of medication, usually sodium valproate, and relapse may be expected in 75–100% of cases, even after many years of freedom from seizures, if the dosage is reduced or the drug discontinued (Janz, 1989). Treatment usually needs to be life-long if relapse is to be avoided. A somewhat similar situation obtains in the case of childhood absence epilepsy. Generalized tonic–clonic seizures may develop during adolescence, years after apparent remission of this epileptic syndrome. The occurrence of generalized tonic–clonic seizures during the evolution of the absences indicates the likelihood of later persistent seizures (Loiseau et al., 1983).

# Factors predictive of chronic epilepsy

It should be emphasized that there are limitations to the concept of epileptic syndromes and some of the most difficult cases of intractable epilepsy cannot be so categorized. Aicardi (1988) mentions several factors which may be predictive of chronic epilepsy. Early age of onset, especially in infancy, has been identified with a poorer prognosis in terms of intellectual function and the development of other neurological abnormalities. However, studies showing an association between early seizure onset and poor prognosis have drawn their populations from highly selected sources, chiefly teaching hospitals and special clinics. In such studies, conditions such as infantile spasms are likely to be over-represented. Ellenberg *et al.* (1984) were unable to confirm such an association in their huge prospective study of children followed to age 7 years. The connection between intractability and organic brain damage has already been mentioned. Certain seizure types (tonic, atonic, flexor or extensor spasms) are likely to resist treatment and the child with multiple seizure types, very frequent seizures, clusters of seizures, and recurrent episodes of status epilepticus will often prove very difficult to control. Long duration of epilepsy, with or without treatment, and failure of previous treatments are unfavourable prognostic indicators. An abnormal EEG, especially when the background activity is constantly disturbed and when paroxysmal abnormalities are frequent, is a useful prognostic aid but it must be considered within the context of the overall clinical picture.

## Incidence

The actual frequency of intractable epilepsy is difficult to estimate. The overall remission rate ascertained by longitudinal studies following the diagnosis of epilepsy in patients of all ages has been reported as about 70% (Annegers, Hauser and Elveback, 1979). However, higher remission rates have been reported in children, except when serious handicapping conditions with signs of neurodeficit and frequent and diverse seizures are present. Bronson and Wranne (1987), in a 12-year follow-up study of children aged 0–19 years, showed that for those who were mentally and neurologically normal and had a low seizure frequency, prognosis was excellent, only 11% having active epilepsy after 12 years.

## Treatment

The preferred method of treatment of chronic epilepsy in childhood is by the use of a single drug. Polytherapy in this situation, as in others, is often associated with pharmacokinetic interactions which may result in a higher incidence of side-effects and poorer control of seizures. In any patient on multiple drugs for chronic intractable epilepsy, an attempt should be made to return again to the use of single drugs in full therapeutic dosage. This will frequently lead to an improvement in seizure control (Shorvon and Reynolds, 1977) and in general performance (Trimble and Cull, 1988). However, it must be said that reduction in polytherapy is more likely to be successful when there is only one seizure type (Albright and Bruni, 1985).

Maximum clinically tolerated doses of a single drug should be given before it is discarded. This has been shown to be particularly important with a drug such as sodium valproate (Ohtsuka *et al*, 1992). Substitution by a second drug given alone is the next step, and the dosage should again be pushed to the upper limit of clinical toleration.

If monotherapy fails, consideration must be given to using two drugs together. In general, the literature on the use of two-drug combinations is not encouraging and they may even result in an increase in seizure frequency, probably as a result of a decline in individual serum concentrations due to drug interactions. It is doubtful if antiepileptic drugs act synergistically, although there is some evidence that barbiturates and phenytoin may do so and it is possible that ethosuximide and sodium valproate do so when they succeed in controlling childhood absence epilepsy which is refractory to either drug used alone (Rowan *et al.*, 1983).

A form of polytherapy which has gained some legitimacy is what is usually called adjunctive or 'add on' therapy. Clobazam has been the main drug used in this respect and initial improvement in seizure control has been reported in about 60% of patients following the addition of this drug to other antiepileptic agents (Callaghan and Goggin, 1988). However, as so often happens with the benzodiazepine drugs, less than half of those showing a dramatic initial response will maintain that response for longer than a year and often only do so for much shorter periods. For this reason, repeated courses of clobazam rather than continuous therapy may be more effective. Benzodiazepines often appear to work best in conjunction with sodium valproate. Another add-on drug which is sometimes surprisingly effective, especially when used in combination with carbamazepine for the control of the refractory partial seizures, is acetazolamide (Oles *et al.*, 1989) and it should also be given a trial in patients with resistant absence attacks.

The newer antiepileptic drugs have also shown promise as adjunctive therapy in some of the resistant chronic epilepsies of infancy and early childhood. Vigabatrin has been helpful in the treatment of infantile spasms, halving the number of attacks in patients in one large series (Chiron *et al.*, 1991). Improvement has also been reported in some cases of Lennox–Gastaut syndrome and the drug has been particularly effective in resistant partial epilepsies of various types (Dulac *et al.*, 1991). Lamotrigine, again employed as adjunctive therapy, has also been reported to produce significant improvement in a wide variety of chronic seizure disorders in children, the response of atypical absences being particularly impressive (Gibbs *et al* 1992).

In cases of drug-resistant chronic epilepsy in childhood, the intermittent use of *steroids* and corticotrophin (ACTH) as adjunctive therapy may be beneficial (Robinson, 1985). Consideration should also be given to a trial of *the medium-chain triglyceride [MCT] diet*, because it may be remarkably successful in controlling seizures, particularly when frequent and disabling tonic–clonic, myoclonic and drop attacks are occurring (Sills *et al*, 1986). The diet is discussed in detail in Appendix 1.

## Surgical treatment

Epilepsy surgery is increasingly advocated for children whose seizures are refractory to medical therapy. A number of surgical procedures is available, including temporal lobectomy, hemispherectomy and corpus callosotomy. These procedures are discussed in the chapter on the surgical treatment of epilepsy. Modern neuroimaging has made it possible to identify lesions such as hemimegalencephaly, the removal of which may alleviate chronic seizures (King *et al.*, 1985).

An increasing number of other related focal neuronal migration disorders associated with chronic partial seizures in childhood are being identified, especially by MRI, and are proving amenable to surgical removal (Palmini *et al.*, 1991). On the other hand, Huttenlocher and Hapke (1990) caution against the over-enthusiastic early use of surgery, especially mutilating procedures such as callosotomy and hemispherectomy, in chronic cases, pointing out that the natural history of intractable seizures in children in their large and lengthy study was one of slow linear improvement for at least 18 years after onset.

## Psychosocial management

It should be remembered that there are many aspects to intractable childhood epilepsy other than eventual seizure control and the possible effects of seizures on intellectual function. Farrell (1989), emphasizing the psychosocial management of these children, points to their lower self-esteem, their limited social skills, the higher incidence of psychiatric disturbance, the overprotectiveness of parents, and the general public prejudice about epilepsy and its victims. The small but definite mortality from uncontrolled seizures should not be overlooked. Not only the children but also their families suffer long-term stress as a result of chronic epilepsy (Hoare and Kerley, 1991) and the parents need constant support and encouragement in handling the many problems that arise. In the author's view, this is best achieved in a special out-patient clinic for children with epilepsy where the family is likely to receive continuing help and advice from skilled and familiar medical, nursing and social services personnel.

## References

AICARDI, J. (1988) Clinical approach to the management of intractable epilepsy. *Developmental Medicine and Child Neurology*, **30**, 429–440

ALBRIGHT, P. and BRUNI, J. (1985) Reduction of polypharmacy in epileptic patients. *Archives of Neurology*, **42**, 797–799

ANNEGERS, J. F., HAUSER, W. A. and ELVEBACK, L. R. (1979) Remission of seizures and relapse in patients with epilepsy. *Epilepsia*, **20**, 729–737

AUKETT, A., BENNETT, M. J. and HOSKING, G. P. (1988) Molybdenum co-factor deficiency: an easily missed inborn error of metabolism. *Developmental Medicine and Child Neurology*, **30**, 531–535

BRENINGSTALL, G. N. (1985) Gelastic seizures, precocious puberty, and hypothalamic hamartoma. *Neurology*, **35**, 1180–1183

BRONSON, L. O. and WRANNE, L. (1987) Long-term prognosis in childhood epilepsy: survival and seizure prognosis. *Epilepsia*, **28**, 324–330

CALLAGHAN, N. and GOGGIN, T. (1988) Adjunctive therapy in resistant epilepsy. *Epilepsia*, **29**, Supplement 1, S29–S35

CHIRON, C., DULAC, O., BEAUMONT, D. *et al.* (1991) Therapeutic trial of vigabatrin in refractory infantile spasms. *Journal of Child Neurology*, **6**, Supplement 2, S52–S59

DRAVET, C. (1978) Les épilepsies graves de l'enfant. *Vie Medicale*, **8**, 543–548

DREIFUSS, F. E. (1990) The epilepsies: clinical implications of the International Classification. In: Epileptic Syndromes: genetic, diagnostic and therapeutic aspects. *Epilepsia*, **31**, Supplement 3, S3–S10

DULAC, O., CHIRON, C., LUNA, D. *et al.* (1991) Vigabatrin in childhood epilepsy. *Journal of Child Neurology*, **6**, Supplement 2, S30–S37

ELLENBERG, J. H., HIRTZ, D. G. and NELSON, K. B. (1984) Age of onset of seizures in young children. *Annals of Neurology*, **15**, 127–134

FARRELL, K. (1989) Management of chronic epilepsy in children. In *Chronic Epilepsy: Its Prognosis and Management* (ed. M. R. Trimble), John Wiley and Sons, Chichester, New York, pp. 151–164

FINLAYSON, R. E. and LUCAS, A. R. (1979) Pseudoepileptic seizures in children and adolescents. *Mayo Clinic Proceedings*, **54**, 83–87

GIBBS, J., APPLETON, R. E., ROSENBLOOM, L. and YUEN, W. C. (1992) Lamotrigine for intractable childhood epilepsy: a preliminary communication. *Developmental Medicine and Child Neurology*, **34**, 369–71

GORDON, N. (1988) Intractable epilepsy. *Developmental Medicine and Child Neurology*, **30**, 830

GOUTIÈRES, F. and AICARDI, J. (1985) Atypical presentations of pyridoxine-dependent seizures: a treatable cause of intractable epilepsy in infants. *Annals of Neurology*, **17**, 117–120

HARDEN, A. and PAMPIGLIONE, G. (1982) Neurophysiological studies (EEG, ERG, VEP, SEP) in 88 children with so-called neuronal ceroid lipofuscinosis. In *Ceroid-Lipofuscinosis [Batten's Disease]* (eds D. Armstrong, N. Koppang and J. A. Rider), Elsevier, Amsterdam, pp. 61–70

HAUSER, W. A. and NELSON, K. (1989) Epidemiology of epilepsy in children. *Cleveland Clinic Journal of Medicine*, **56**, Supplement Part 2, S185–194

HOARE, P. and KERLEY, S. (1991) Psychosocial adjustment of children with chronic epilepsy and their families. *Developmental Medicine and Child Neurology*, **33**, 201–215

HUTTENLOCHER, P. R. and HAPKE, R. J. (1990) A follow-up study of intractable seizures in childhood. *Annals of Neurology*, **28**, 699–705

JANZ, D. (1989) Juvenile myoclonic epilepsy: epilepsy with impulsive petit mal. *Cleveland Journal of Medicine*, **56**, Supplement Part 1, S23–S33

JEAVONS, P. M. (1983) Non-epileptic attacks in childhood. In *Research Progress in Epilepsy* (ed. F. C. Rose), Pitman, London, pp. 224–230

KING, M., STEPHENSON, J. B. P., ZIERVOGEL, M. *et al.* (1985). Hemimegalencephaly – a case for hemispherectomy? *Neuropediatrics*, **16**, 46–55

LEE, T. K. Y., NAKASU, Y., JEFFREE, M. A. *et al.* (1989) Indolent glioma: a cause of epilepsy. *Archives of Disease in Childhood*, **64**, 1666–1671

LOISEAU, P., PESTRE, M., DARTIGUES, J. F. *et al.* (1983) Long-term prognosis in two forms of childhood epilepsy: typical absence seizures and epilepsy with rolandic (centrotemporal) EEG foci. *Annals of Neurology*, **13**, 642–648

O'DONOHOE, N. V. (1992) Delineation of epileptic syndromes. *Current Paediatrics*, **2**, 68–72

OHTSUKA, Y., AMANO, R., MIZUKAWA, M. *et al.* (1992) Treatment of intractable childhood epilepsy with high-dose valproate. *Epilepsia*, **33**, 158–164

OLES, K. S., PENRY, J. K., COLE, D. L. W. and HOWARD, G. (1989) Use of acetazolamide as an adjunct to carbamazepine in refractory partial seizures. *Epilepsia*, **30**, 71–78

PALMINI, A., ANDERMANN, F., OLIVIER, A. *et al.* (1991) Focal neuronal migration disorders and intractable partial epilepsy: results of surgical treatment. *Annals of Neurology*, **30**, 750–757

PATRY, G., LYAGOUBI, S. and TASSINARI, C. A. (1971) Subclinical 'electrical status epilepticus' induced by sleep in children. *Archives of Neurology*, **24**, 242–252

PELLOCK, J. M. (1989) Syndromes of chronic epilepsy in children. In *Chronic Epilepsy: Its Prognosis and Management* (ed. M. R. Trimble), John Wiley and Sons, Chichester, New York, pp. 73–85

ROBINSON, R. O. (1985) Seizures and steroids. *Archives of Disease in Childhood*, **60**, 94–95

ROWAN, A.J., MEIJER, J. W. A., DE BEER-PAWLIKOWSKI, N. (1983) Valproate-ethosuximide combination therapy for refractory absence seizures. *Archives of Neurology*, **40**, 797–802

SHORVON, S. D. and REYNOLDS, E. H. (1977) Unnecessary polypharmacy for epilepsy. *British Medical Journal*, **1**, 1635–1637

SILLS, M. A., FORSYTHE, W. I., HAIDWKEWYCH, D. *et al.* (1986) The Medium Chain Triglyceride diet and intractable epilepsy. *Archives of Disease in Childhood*, **61**, 1168–1172

TASSINARI, C. A., BUREAU, M. and THOMAS, P. (1992) Epilepsy with myoclonic absences. In *Epileptic Syndromes in Infancy, Childhood and Adolescence.* (eds J. Roger, M. Bureau, C. Dravet *et al.*), 2nd Edition, John Libbey, London, Paris, Rome, pp. 151–160

TRIMBLE, M. R. and CULL, C. (1988) Children of school age: the influence of antiepileptic drugs on behaviour and intellect. *Epilepsia*, **29**, Supplement 3, S15–S19

WOLF, B., GRIER, R. E., ALLEN, R. S. *et al.* (1983) Phenotypic variation in biotinidase deficiency. *Journal of Pediatrics*, **103**, 233–237

# Chapter 20

# Emotional and psychiatric aspects of epilepsy

> The good physician is concerned not only with turbulent brain waves but with disturbed emotions and with social injustice, for the epileptic is not just a nerve–muscle preparation; he is a person, in health an integrated combination of the physical, the mental, the social and the spiritual. Disruption of any part can cause or aggravate illness (Lennox and Markham, 1953)

Many writers have suggested that the main handicap associated with epilepsy is of the psychological kind. Observations of the mental peculiarities of epileptic persons extend across recorded medical history (Temkin, 1971). While some individuals with epilepsy may have behavioural disorders as a concomitant of underlying brain disorders, it is of first importance to realize that they may also have psychological morbidity as a result of their failure to adapt to their milieu and as a consequence of the failure of society to encompass them and their disabilities. The impact of chronic epilepsy on a child's emotional and personality development will vary at different ages and it should be clearly understood that there is no single or characteristic mental state or behaviour pattern consequent on chronic epilepsy. The factors which tend to increase psychiatric morbidity are as follows:

1  Early age of onset and chronicity.
2  Adverse environmental circumstances, including a disturbed family background.
3  The occurrence of certain specific varieties of epilepsy such as temporal lobe epilepsy.
4  The presence of structural or organic brain disorders.

It is highly improbable that any single form of personality disturbance could emerge in persons with different degrees and types of cerebral damage or with no evidence of damage, with different genetic endowments and environmental circumstances, and who are differently affected by epilepsy. Nevertheless, there persists in the lay mind, and even in the medical mind, a mistaken concept of what has been called 'the epileptic personality'. This was described by Aretaeus of Cappodocia (Temkin, 1971) as follows: 'They became languid, spiritless, stupid, inhuman, unsociable, and not disposed to hold intercourse, nor to be sociable, at any period of life; sleepless, subject to many horrid dreams, without appetite, and with bad digestion; pale, of a leaden color; slow to learn from torpidity of the understanding and of the senses'. Since this first description there have been many other equally pejorative accounts of the sufferer from epilepsy, right up to the present century.

Happily, however, this century has seen the abandonment of such an unscientific and prejudiced view of the person with epilepsy. It has been replaced both by concern for the predicament in which the patient finds himself and by increased understanding of the disadvantages which his condition and society have placed on him.

Accounts of the emotional and psychiatric disorders associated with epilepsy in general and with childhood epilepsy in particular are complex and often confusing. In an attempt to give an orderly account it is proposed to discuss the problem under the following headings:

1   Environmental influences including the attitudes of society.
2   The influences of age and development.
3   The role played by specific varieties of epilepsy.
4   The factor of structural or organic brain abnormality.
5   The influence of drugs.
6   The relationship to serious psychiatric disorders, particularly psychosis.

## Environmental influences including the attitudes of society

The psychological effects of seizures on the patient's family will be discussed in Chapter 24 and have been well described by Lindsay (1972). She has pointed out that when parents first see their child having a seizure their immediate reaction is often 'I thought he was dead'. This shock to the parents can then set up long-lasting reverberations in their relationships not only with the child himself, but also between themselves and with those who care for him and teach him. Even though the child recovers in a few minutes, the parents are often left with an abiding fear that at any time and without warning they could lose their child. Prompt attention to the child and careful explanation to the parents at the time of the first seizure may be very important in preventing later abnormal relationships.

If, following the first seizure, the child is left with a chronic physical handicap, such as a hemiplegia, or if the epilepsy becomes recurrent and chronic then a change in parental attitudes is inevitable. They tend to adopt attitudes of either rejection or overprotection, more commonly the latter. The child is overindulged and carefully protected from stress. The extent of the handicap is denied and the child is treated as if he were still a baby. This is, of course, more likely to happen when the epilepsy begins in early childhood and if the attacks are severe and/or frequent and if they are associated with mental or physical handicap. The early age of onset, chronicity and associated structural or organic brain abnormality have constantly been shown to increase psychiatric morbidity in the individual with epilepsy.

Rejection is a less common response by parents, but some react in this way because, as Lindsay (1972) has pointed out, the child has a disorder which makes him untrustworthy in the sense that cataclysmic breakdowns in his behaviour may happen without warning. His whole existence as a person may then be denied. The cataclysmic nature of the seizure and its effect on observers will be discussed again later, but its critical importance in developing attitudes to the affected individual cannot be overemphasized. The fear of the child's death may concern the parents, and this is not unreasonable.

Sillanpää (1973), in his lengthy review from Finland of the medicosocial prognosis of children with epilepsy, found that deaths were unexpectedly high, with a loss of

1% per year from status epilepticus, chest infections and other complications. Among 245 children studied, 5 drowned, emphasizing the need for some restrictions even with the benefits of modern therapy (*see* Appendix 2). Sillanpää (1973) also found a higher incidence of marital breakdown and divorce among the parents and guardians of the epileptic children studied when compared with the normal population. He stressed that chronic tension within the family and the effects of uncertainty and the restrictions imposed on the child might actually make the epilepsy worse, thereby creating a vicious circle. Lindsay (1972) has stressed the contagious nature of the breakdowns which can have their origins in the patient's epilepsy, and it is in such a situation that there may be a need to place the child in a calm and orderly environment and institute psychotherapy for the child and the family. Hoare (1984), in a study from Oxford, demonstrated an increased rate of psychiatric disturbance among the siblings and mothers of children with chronic epileptic disorders.

## Social aspects

One should enquire into why seizures constitute socially unacceptable behaviour and why, in consequence, there is so much prejudice in the public mind concerning epilepsy. Why it is necessary constantly to prove that it is possible to suffer epilepsy and still be of sound mind? To some extent it is connected with the fact that epilepsy is not a trivial matter. Many people with multiple handicaps suffer from epilepsy as a secondary effect of the initial brain disease or damage which caused their handicaps. There are also some sufferers from epilepsy who, even though of normal intelligence and free from other handicaps, may nevertheless have their whole lives marred by epilepsy. On the other hand, there are many whose seizure disorder is trouble free. As Ann Hackney (1976) has written: 'Any single encounter with epilepsy will tell only part of the tale and may lead to unfair generalizations. The condition is too complex, with its wide variety of causes, manifestations and effects. Unfortunately, there are still stereotyped images of epileptic personalities and mentalities which may be true, in part, of some, but are inadequate and unjust to most.' The very complexity and diversity of epilepsy, therefore, is the first reason for public misunderstanding and prejudice.

What is the nature of this innate *prejudice against epilepsy*? There is evidence of its pervasiveness in different kinds of cultures, both pretechnological and technological, and even among otherwise rational individuals, including physicians. Bagley (1972), in his very perceptive analysis of the problem, felt that the basis of the prejudice was: 'fear, of the sudden loss of physical and emotional control'. He found evidence of social prejudice at all levels – in the field of employment, education and even in medical care – and also found that people with epilepsy were regarded with more hostility than the mentally ill or people with cerebral palsy. He found significant correlations between a scale measuring racial prejudice and one measuring attitudes to the handicapped, the latter being dominated by hostile attitudes towards epilepsy. In addition, he remarked that there were affinities between the two insofar as racial prejudice also involved a fear of the unknown and the unpredictable. Bagley (1972) felt that people with epilepsy are seen in hostile terms which are as great as or greater than those in which ethnic minorities are viewed. 'The man with epilepsy is feared and hated because he does what we are afraid we will do ourselves. He loses control – basic control of his motor movements. He reverts to the "primitive", so that the punishment of him (by social rejection and ostracism) appears to be justified.' Bagley (1972) went on to say that widespread social rejection of people with epilepsy may well be largely responsible for the increased prevalence of behaviour disorders among them.

Taylor (1969), discussing prejudice against epilepsy, wrote that the social structure survives through its experience of the value of control, order and reason, and that the two things which most threaten our control over the environment are madness and death. To an observer without medical knowledge an epileptic fit appears as 'a brief excursion through madness into death'. Society has developed mechanisms for coping with these two eventualities, but the psychological difficulty in accepting epilepsy is that having severed human relationships briefly in a similar fashion to madness or death the seizure is then followed by recovery. Every recurring seizure subsequently reinforces the view of witnesses that the epileptic cannot be relied upon to participate fully in society because he is liable, at any time, to go out of control. Therefore, unless he can be cured he must be set apart: he must be reformed or else rejected. Furthermore, every seizure with its humiliations reinforces for the epileptic the failure of society to help him, and this accentuates his feeling of being different. Taylor (1969) also pointed out that, because epilepsy has its greatest incidence in early childhood, the young child with chronic epilepsy has no experience of normality. His experience of epilepsy is his experience of life. If the epileptic tendency passes away he is left unable to take up normality again, as he might do after a transient illness, because he has to build it for the first time. He is then in danger of the epilepsy becoming a way of life and of relying on the fact of his being different as a protection from the demands of good social behaviour.

In further analyses of the problem of prejudice and epilepsy, Taylor (1973a, 1987) considered the stigmas of epilepsy. (A stigma may be defined as a blemish or a token of disgrace or a mark of infamy.) The clearest stigma of epilepsy is the seizure itself with its overt implications of total loss of control. There are other more subtle stigmas too, including the need to take medication regularly, the restrictions on activity, the days off school or work, the periods of hospitalization in some cases and the mysterious injuries that may occur. Consider, for example, the stigma of having to wear a protective helmet. Taylor (1973a) concluded that the only way to combat prejudice is by diminishing ignorance through education, and that we should teach people to tolerate uncertainty and to try to control ancient prejudices by an effort of will.

Livingston (1972) emphasizes that a teacher should explain to a class in which there is a child with epilepsy that it is not contagious, must not convey prejudice and must give a simple explanation to the other children about the nature of the seizures. To do this satisfactorily, however, the teacher should be well informed about the child's problems and about the nature of the epilepsy. A teacher who knows what to expect can be prepared to deal with a seizure in the classroom, both in the terms of helping the child and in terms of helping the child's classmates to understand what has happened (Vining, 1989a). It is notable how well other children will accept epilepsy if the general attitude is sensible. It is essential, however, that the same discipline should apply to the child with epilepsy as to the rest of the class. The child will rapidly learn to dominate the class situation if he knows that he will not be punished like the other children. Unfortunately, some doctors still make the excuse that the child cannot help his behaviour because he is an epileptic. This particular attitude is very likely to lead to a personality disturbance and to the development of behavioural disorders in the child.

## The influences of age and development

Normal personality development takes place by intimate interaction of the individual with the environment. The environment will have a generally consistent component, either 'good' or 'bad', in the case of a normal child. Where the child has a chronic illness, such as epilepsy, a new variable component is introduced depending on the ways in which the illness of the individual is perceived by various people around him at different times. Taylor (1971a) adapted a scheme or model of normal personality development devised by Erikson (1966, 1977) in order to illustrate the effects of chronic epilepsy on personality development during the various stages of the child's development.

## Infancy

During infancy it is normal for the parents to love their child and for the child to feel loved. Seizures during the neonatal period and during infancy frequently have an ominous prognosis. Death, neurological disability, intellectual impairment and later chronic epilepsy are common. For a mother, an infantile convulsion means that her child is manifestly abnormal. The child may be deprived of mothering through special nursing requirements, through separation or through rejection. The very existence of the child is threatened by the possibility of death and, as we have seen, the parallels between an epileptic seizure and sudden unexpected death are very close. The violence of infantile spasms and the appearance of the child in an attack often give the impression of great and inexplicable pain and anguish for the child. The parents feel cut off from their normal response of giving comfort to the child in his predicament. Furthermore, this very serious disorder is likely to be followed by gross mental defect or by what Ounsted (1970) has called 'a phenocopy of infantile autism' or by both. In these circumstances the mother's trust and the infant's autonomy are threatened. She is afraid to leave her child alone and imposes limitations on his movements. For a child of unimpaired intelligence who is struggling to establish independence this may lead to conflict and humiliation. As Taylor (1971a) said, psychological difficulties are grafted on to a disordered neurological substrate and they impose their own limitations on growth and development. The child's developing sense of separation from the mother and his sense of personal identity may be affected adversely.

## Later infancy and early childhood

In later infancy and early childhood the development of the myoclonic epilepsies may have equally disturbing effects on the mother–child relationship. Catastrophic falls to the ground, so characteristic of these epilepsies, may make the erect posture unreliable and dangerous. This leads to great parental anxiety with increased restrictions on a child who is in the exploratory phase of learning and is actively using walking and climbing for that purpose. Febrile convulsions, commonest between 6 months and 4 years of age, frequently lead the parents to believe that their child has died (Clare, Smith and Wallace, 1978). Green and Solnit (1964) described what they called the 'vulnerable child' syndrome in which the parents, having so powerfully experienced the belief that their child was dead or going to die, regard their child quite differently in the event of his recovery. They may feel that the child is on loan and that he might be snatched away at any time. In recurrent epilepsy this proximity to death may regularly occur, constantly reinforcing the parents' beliefs concerning the eventual loss of their child. Thus, although parents often display considerable devotion and withdraw from social pleasures in order to protect the child, the basis of trust is seriously disrupted. The children themselves experience years of treatment with drugs for a condition which they cannot remember experiencing and which is not freely discussed with them. However, their parents' anxiety is communicated to them, in fact so much so that, as Livingston (1972) has pointed out, some children may express a fear of dying during or as a result of a seizure. Children with epilepsy are significantly more anxious, inattentive, overactive and socially isolated than normal children, and boys appear to suffer more in this respect than girls (Stores, 1977). Maladjustment may show itself as feelings of insecurity, inadequacy, various degrees of nervous tension, anxiety and irritability. The child may become withdrawn and defeatist in his attitude or, on the other hand, hostile, aggressive and antisocial in his behaviour. Enuresis, encopresis, temper tantrums, nail-biting and so on may all occur.

Taylor (1971a), again using Erikson's model, pointed out that the development of petit mal absences may often coincide with what Erikson called the 'phase of initiative'. Children with petit mal have been found to be more neurotic and less antisocial than children with other forms of epilepsy. The inception of petit mal is usually preceded by some years of normal development so that trust and autonomy will already have been established. Petit mal absences then make frequent breaks in consciousness, disrupting the child's awareness of what is happening around him. Children with petit mal tend to become compliant and non-assertive, uniformly quiet and well behaved. They tend to fade into the background and these personality traits may persist into adult life. In one long-term follow-up of children with petit mal absences, one-third had a social maladjustment in adult life (Loiseau et al., 1983).

## Later childhood

The inception of new cases of epilepsy falls off sharply from the age of 5 or 6 years and probably amounts to 2–4/1000 children of school age per annum (DHSS, 1969). Even those children who have had severe epilepsy in the early years of childhood may show improvement during the school years. However, as Taylor (1971a) has emphasized, the school years are also the period in which the child with epilepsy is exposed to society and its expectations for the first time. The limitations on activity and intelligence, the need for continuing medical care, the effects of drug therapy and of clinical and subclinical seizures on the child's ability to learn all begin to influence the extent to which the child can learn to live with and master his environment. Behaviour problems, formerly latent and private, become public and sometimes intolerable. Normal schooling may become impossible or, at least, severely disrupted.

## Adolescence

Adolescence brings its own share of emotional difficulties and readjustments under normal circumstances. When the extra burden of epilepsy is present, it may be difficult to know whether the moodiness, aggressiveness, irritability and emotional changeability are normal adolescent phenomena or largely due to the predicament of having epilepsy. If the epilepsy is not functionally disabling, it is more likely that the behavioural difficulties are due to adolescent turmoil. There is evidence that adolescents are often poorly informed about epilepsy and have many misconceptions about it, and that this correlates with poor psychosocial adaptation. Paradoxically, the adolescent whose seizures have been witnessed in public seems better able to adapt to them than are adolescents who still fear the day when seizures will occur outside the home. The reality seems easier to live with than the apprehension and the stigma of epilepsy is more easily tolerated when the condition is overt (Vining, 1989a). Poor self-esteem is another characteristic which is frequently present in the adolescent with epilepsy (Viberg, Blennow and Polski, 1987). Temporal lobe epilepsy becomes increasingly more common during adolescence and may be associated with particular behavioural difficulties (see Chapters 10 and 13). Taylor (1971a) pointed out that adolescents with temporal lobe epilepsy, in addition to the normal identity crisis associated with adolescence, may also have problems of personal identity deriving from the temporal lobe abnormality itself. Williams (1969) wrote that the most important function of the temporal lobe is the integration of sensations of all kinds. The temporal lobe enables an individual to appreciate himself as a unified being (i.e. the sense of 'I am') because it receives information from the special senses, the viscera and the higher centres. Disruption of this function may have serious psychological consequences. Surgical removal of the temporal lobe for epilepsy may be followed later by lonely, withdrawn, apathetic and passive behaviour and by the presence of hyposexuality (Taylor and Falconer, 1968, Toone, 1986).

## The role played by specific varieties of epilepsy

This particular aspect of the emotional disorders connected with epilepsy has already been discussed to some extent and the importance of temporal lobe epilepsy has been alluded to in the previous section (see Chapter 10). The way in which any child reacts to having a seizure disorder varies considerably depending on the personality of the child, the family psychopathology and the extent to which the epilepsy responds to medical treatment. There are, however, certain specific syndromes of abnormal behaviour which need description.

### The hyperkinetic syndrome

This is probably the best known of the abnormal behaviour syndromes and may be defined as a pathological excess of energy found in young children with mental defect and brain injury, particularly when epilepsy is present as an additional handicap. Ounsted (1955) used the term 'hyperkinetic syndrome in epileptic children' to describe such patients and found an incidence of 8% in a consecutive personal series of 830 children presenting with epilepsy. Apart from overactivity, the majority of the children showed evidence of distractibility, short attention span, wide scatter on test results when given formal intelligence tests, fluctuations of mood with euphoria as the abiding background, aggressive outbursts, diminution or absence of spontaneously affectionate behaviour, lack of shyness and lack of fear. The intelligence level in his patients ranged from high normal to severe mental handicap. These abnormalities, combined with overactivity sustained over months or years, made these children intolerable in both ordinary schools and hospitals and created for their parents and siblings emotional and practical problems of a serious and intractable nature.

The term 'hyperkinetic syndrome' has, in fact, been in use for over one hundred years (Hoffman, 1845) and has been applied to a syndrome which begins early in life, is more common in boys than girls and is characterized by hyperactivity, impulsivity, distractibility and excitability. Aggressive and antisocial behaviours, specific learning difficulties and emotional lability are often included as features of this syndrome. Terms such as 'brain damage syndrome', 'minimal brain damage' and 'minimal brain dysfunction' are often used synonymously with the term 'hyperkinetic syndrome' with unfortunate consequences. If the term 'brain damage' is used in its literal sense meaning structural abnormality of the brain, then 'brain damage syndrome' is an inaccurate and misleading term, since the majority of overactive children do not suffer from frank brain damage and most brain-damaged children do not present with the hyperkinetic syndrome (Rutter, Graham and Yule, 1970). The term 'minimal cerebral dysfunction' has been used to describe children with subtle defects in attention, coordination, perception or language development, but here again the symptoms and signs may only occasionally be associated with actual damage to the brain (Rutter, 1968). Moreover, many hyperkinetic children do not demonstrate these subtle neurological signs.

If we return to a consideration of hyperkinesis as a behavioural syndrome only, it should be realized that it has many different causes and that it always requires careful evaluation. Present evidence suggests that the term hyperkinetic syndrome describes a heterogeneous group of children with different aetiologies. In some cases the disorder may be due to structural abnormality of the brain, in others there may be an abnormality of physiological arousal of the nervous system, or there may be a genetic basis for the disorder (Goodman, 1989), while in many more no cause will be found. The reader is referred to the excellent reviews by Cantwell (1977) by Taylor (1986) and by Weiss (1990).

It is important to remember that, apart from the behavioural abnormality, learning difficulties are of major importance as an associated problem, whatever the cause of the overactivity. It was suggested by Ounsted (1971) that there is a disruption of exploratory learning in hyperkinetic children which disbars them from developing the basic mental structures which are the foundation of normal learning and intelligence. It should be remembered, as Bax (1972) stressed, that the overactive child, particularly the overactive schoolchild, may simply be reacting to stresses in his environment or may be suffering exposure to an inappropriate educational milieu. Children with neurotic or antisocial psychiatric disturbances or who have specific learning difficulties may also demonstrate overactivity, and much of it may be reaction to the predicament in which they find themselves. Furthermore, there are normal children (and adults) who are temperamentally restless, unable to sit still, and who become excited easily over minor matters, demonstrating their emotion by the use of motor activity.

Returning to the question of hyperkinesis in children with epilepsy, it is now realized that its incidence in epileptic children generally is much lower than the 8% mentioned by Ounsted (1955). The reason for this is that it has now become clearly apparent that overactivity can be produced or potentiated by related drugs such as phenobarbitone and primidone, and that other drugs such as clonazepam may have a similar effect. Withdrawal of these drugs should always be the initial treatment when a patient taking them for epilepsy becomes overactive. Another important point which should be emphasized is that in a child with epilepsy, of whatever kind, the overactivity may be generated by anxiety, which in turn may be related to a frightening aura or may be a reflection of parental anxiety about the child's epilepsy.

There is no doubt that hyperkinetic behaviour can occur in children with temporal lobe epilepsy. Ounsted, Lindsay and Norman (1966) found it present in one-quarter of their sample of 100 children. It was commoner in males and in those who had suffered an early brain insult or who had had status epilepticus. They concluded that cerebral damage acquired in the course of an initiating illness may be more important in the causation of the hyperkinetic behaviour than is the temporal lobe epilepsy itself. They also found that age was a critical factor, and very early onset of the epilepsy was a feature of their hyperactive children. They also found that the intellectual devevelopment of their hyperactive children was significantly retarded compared with other groups of children with only temporal lobe epilepsy. Pond (1961) showed that the behavioural syndrome of overactivity occurred in brain-injured children of low intelligence, particularly males, who did not also have epilepsy. Again, however, he stressed that many of these children did not come from normal homes and, of course, the possible adverse effects of drugs must always be remembered in the mentally handicapped with or without epilepsy. In the more recent monograph describing experiences with the original cohort of 100 children observed from 1948 to 1986, Ounsted, Lindsay and Richards (1987) noted that the classic hyperkinetic syndrome in association with temporal lobe epilepsy had become rare. They ascribed this to improved therapy for acute severe childhood infection, especially meningitis and to declining use of barbiturates as antiepileptic drugs in brain-damaged children.

## Rage and temper outbursts

Ounsted, Lindsay and Norman (1966) reported outbursts of catastrophic rage in approximately one-third of their children with temporal lobe epilepsy. However, these rage outbursts are not peculiar to children with temporal lobe epilepsy but seem to represent a general biological reaction, of an intermittent kind, to frustrating situations in brain-damaged people. The Oxford workers suggested that these rage outbursts, although occurring in many different kinds of brain syndrome, might nevertheless be released from specific centres in the hypothalamus. Lindsay (1972) regarded the outbursts as a form of 'fail-safe' device, i.e. the rage occurred when the child had been overloaded with emotional stimuli of one sort and another. She gave as an example a child who had been confined in an overcrowded room or school or hospital from which there was no escape route away from the ambient circumstances. She pointed out that phenobarbitone and related compounds might potentiate the rage phenomenon. Unlike the hyperkinetic syndrome, which is limited to the early years of life, children with temporal lobe epilepsy may manifest rage outbursts at any age and unexpectedly. This can lead to complications in older patients and may take the form of murderous assaults and the infliction of bodily injury on others. However, the argument that all adolescents and adults with temporal lobe epilepsy have psychopathology is no longer tenable. These individuals suffer social rejection and discrimination as a consequence of their unexpected and embarrassing attacks and are likely to react aggressively to these attitudes at times (Treiman and Delgado-Escueta, 1983). Those children in the Oxford series (Ounsted, Lindsay and Norman, 1966; Ounsted, Lindsay and Richards, 1987) who had had an early brain insult were more likely to develop the rage phenomenon, and those who had had an episode of status epilepticus were the next group most likely to do so. The age of onset of seizures was earlier in the group manifesting rage outbursts and this phenomenon occurred in children of both high and low intelligence and equally in both sexes. There was an overlap between rage outbursts and the hyperkinetic syndrome, but the two could occur independently of each other. The combination of the two in an individual child virtually guaranteed his or her exclusion from a normal school. As already noted in the case of the hyperkinetic syndrome, the incidence of severe rage outbursts is also declining in children with temporal lobe epilepsy.

Reference is made in the next chapter to the study by Stores (1977) on behaviour disturbance and on the type of epilepsy in children attending ordinary school. In this study he found that, in general, the children were significantly more anxious, inattentive, overactive and socially isolated than were normal children, and also that boys appeared to be more affected than girls. His EEG investigations showed that anxiety, inattentiveness and (with the exception of the 3 Hz spike-wave subgroup) social isolation particularly characterized each male subgroup, but the left temporal spike subgroup of boys emerged as the most disturbed of all and were also significantly more active when compared with normal boys. Neither the sex nor the subgroup differences were explicable on the basis of seizure frequency or type of drug therapy.

## The factor of structural or organic brain abnormality

The factors that tend to increase psychiatric morbidity in epilepsy are an early age of onset and chronicity, a disturbed family background, specific kinds of epilepsy such as temporal lobe epilepsy and evidence of structural or organic brain abnormality. The classic study on the part played by the last in causing psychiatric disorders in children with epilepsy is that organized by Rutter in the Isle of Wight (Graham and Rutter, 1968; Rutter, Graham and Yule, 1970). The total population of children of compulsory school age (total 11 865) was studied to determine the prevalence of epilepsy, cerebral palsy and other neurological disorders. The association between organic brain dysfunction and psychiatric disorder was examined by comparing the neurological and psychiatric findings in the children with epilepsy or with lesions above the brain-stem (cerebral palsy and similar disorders) with those in the following:

1  A random sample of the general population.
2  Children with lesions below the brain-stem, such as muscular dystrophy and paralyses following poliomyelitis.
3  Children with other chronic physical handicaps not involving the nervous system, such as asthma, heart disease or diabetes.

The prevalence of psychiatric disorder in the general population of children aged 10 and 11 years was 6.8%. Psychiatric disorder was nearly twice as common (11.5%) among children with chronic physical disorders not involving the brain, including those due to disease or damage at or below the brain-stem. However, the rate of psychiatric disorder among children with neuroepileptic disorders was very much higher; in fact over a third (34%) showed psychiatric disorder – a rate five times that in the general population sample. The rate was highest in children with neurological disorders accompanied by seizures (58.3%) and lowest in those with uncomplicated epilepsy (28.6%). In those with neurological lesions above the brain-stem but no seizures the rate was 37.5%. It was concluded, on the basis of a study of factors associated with psychiatric disorders, that the high rate of psychiatric disorder in the neuroepileptic children was due to the presence of organic brain dysfunction rather than just to the existence of a physical handicap, although the latter also played a part. Moreover, organic brain dysfunction was not associated with any specific type of psychiatric disorder, thereby dispelling any lingering doubts about the existence of a specific 'epileptic personality' disorder. Within the neuroepileptic group the neurological features and the type of seizure, intellectual and educational factors, and sociofamilial factors all interacted in the development of the psychiatric disorder.

The implication of these findings is that an organic brain disorder puts the individual at special risk of developing psychiatric disorders, both directly as a result of the brain disorder and indirectly as a result of the failure to adapt to the handicap, and that the psychiatric disorders are no different in kind from those of the population at large whether physically handicapped or not. Epilepsy is associated not only with high rates of psychiatric disorder but also, as we have already seen, with many other interrelated indicators of personal and social handicap which are likely to set individuals apart as a disadvantaged group.

## The influence of drugs

The effects of various antiepileptic drugs in causing behavioural disturbances in children with epilepsy have already been referred to on several occasions, and the adverse effects of antiepileptic drugs generally are dealt with in detail in Chapter 26. The possibility that behavioural and personality disorders may be due to the chronic toxic effects of the patient's medication should constantly be in the physician's mind (Reynolds, 1981). Some drugs, and particularly phenytoin, may cause a progressive encephalopathy due to chronic drug intoxication (Vallarta, Bell and Reichert, 1974). Higher rates of major depressive disorders have been reported in children on treatment with phenobarbitone, and depression did not invariably remit when the drug was withdrawn (Brent et al., 1990). Patients may demonstrate progressive psychomotor deterioration which is indistinguishable from that due to a degenerative disease of the central nervous system. Behavioural abnormalities have also been reported, including stubborness, aggressiveness, destructiveness, confused withdrawn behaviour, and an abnormal degree of lethargy and inattention to personal needs. Psychotic manifestations, including hallucinations, abnormal interpersonal relationships and thought disorders, may also occur. Bizarre gestures and choreoathetoid movements may be observed. All these disorders may be further complicated by impaired intellectual performance. Paradoxically, an increased frequency of seizures and even status epilepticus may be associated with chronic drug intoxication with phenytoin. This may lead to yet another increase in dosage by the unwary physician. Recognition of the problem and the monitoring of blood serum levels of drugs are essential to detect it because this type of encephalopathy is usually reversible if the drugs are withdrawn. Since some of the symptoms, and especially the psychomotor regression, are probably related to interference with folic acid metabolism, measurement of blood serum folate levels is mandatory and should lead to the prescription of folic acid supplements if low levels are detected (Reynolds, 1983).

## The relationship to serious psychiatric disorders, particularly psychosis

It will be evident from the preceding sections of this chapter that while children with epilepsy are more prone to neurotic or behavioural disorders than normal children, the clinical manifestations of these disorders are no different from those occurring in other disturbed children who do not have epilepsy. However, children with epilepsy may have ictal experiences peculiar to their complaint and some of these resemble transient adult psychotic states, for example hallucinations, depersonalization, derealization, delusions, nameless dread, confused speech and interference with rational thought processes. In the nineteenth century writers on epilepsy liked to categorize the mental peculiarities of people with epilepsy into peri-ictal disorders, interictal disorders and long-term psychoses, and it is still valid to look at epilepsy in this way today (Taylor, 1973b). The peri-ictal disorders can include prodromal mood changes (e.g. sullenness, listlessness, irritability and aggressiveness) preceding an attack and can last for hours or even days; various aurae may occur, including some so bizarre that they resemble the phenomena of schizophrenic psychosis; some epileptic attacks include automatic behaviour with wandering and apparently purposeful but inappropriate actions; and confusional states often coloured by vivid hallucinations may complicate the postictal period, especially after a series of attacks. Changes of mood, often reversing the preictal mood and including feelings of extraordinary well-being and relaxation, may be noticed by parents after a major attack.

The interictal disorders have already been dealt with in detail in this chapter and, in this respect, modern writers have abandoned the pejorative concept of an 'epileptic personality'. They have realized that no particular single form of personality could emerge from different degrees and types of cerebral damage occurring at different ages and stages of development in individuals with dissimilar genetic endowments, suffering from different types of epilepsy of varying severity and raised in contrasting environments.

A *psychotic breakdown* in a child with epilepsy is rare before puberty. Conversely, epilepsy is very rare in the syndrome of early infantile autism. Creak and Pampiglione (1969), in a carefully selected group of 35 autistic and withdrawn children who were followed up for between 5 and 19 years, found a rate of EEG abnormalities which was above that found in the general population. However, no evidence of any specific abnormality was detected. There may be an increased incidence of epilepsy developing during adolescence in autistic children (Rutter, 1977). In the phenocopy of autistic behaviour which occurs in some children who have had infantile spasms and who are subsequently mentally handicapped and often hyperkinetic, chronic epilepsy and an abnormal (and epileptic) EEG are usual (Ounsted, 1970).

The word psychosis implies a qualitative change from normal behaviour which is understandable neither in ordinary human terms nor in terms of the patient's life experience and environmental circumstances. The classic study of Slater, Beard and Glithero (1963) confirmed that there was an association between epilepsy and a paranoid-schizophrenia state, and that it was greater than that predicted by chance association through the frequency of each condition independently; it was shown that the psychosis occurred in individuals with temporal lobe epilepsy. Flor Henry (1969) demonstrated that there was a relationship between the hemisphere affected by temporal lobe epilepsy and the psychological and social sequelae. Left temporal lobe lesions tended to be associated with psychopathic behaviour and psychosis, including a schizophrenia-like state, whereas right temporal lobe lesions were associated with neuroses and depressive psychoses. Although mesial temporal sclerosis was found in half of the material obtained at the operation of temporal lobectomy, Falconer and Taylor (1968) reported that temporal lobe epilepsy due to this neuropathological lesion was rarely accompanied by chronic psychosis. This observation was further elaborated by Taylor (1971b) when he showed that, in individuals with temporal lobe epilepsy who did not develop psychosis, the period of maximum inception of the epilepsy was largely located in early childhood, whereas in those with temporal lobe epilepsy who developed psychosis the period of maximum inception of the epilepsy was around puberty. He also found a general relationship between the onset of epilepsies which lead to psychosis and the adolescent growth spurt in each sex, and that these epilepsies tended to begin earlier in the growth spurt period in girls than in boys. The occurrence of psychosis in relation to lesions of the temporal lobes is not surprising when one remembers the significance of the integrative functions of these parts of the brain in achieving the essential sense of personal identity or 'I am'. Another important factor is the close association between the temporal lobes and the limbic system – that phylogenetically old ring of cortex which loops under the corpus callosum and which has connections with the cerebral cortex, the brain-stem and the hypothalamus (see *Figure 10.1*). It has been argued (Taylor, 1977) that schizophrenic symptomatology may result from disorganization of the structures subserving language and thought (and hence also socialization) which are normally compactly located in the left side of the brain. In the brains of some individuals a tenuous and precarious balance may be temporarily disrupted by a variety of stresses, of which epilepsy is one, and in others this disruption may be more or less total and irreversible. Trimble (1991) has written the definitive monograph on this difficult subject.

## Summary

In this chapter an attempt has been made to provide an orderly and coherent account of the emotional and psychiatric aspects of epilepsy in childhood and adolescence. It is hoped that it is apparent to the reader that this is a difficult and often confusing subject and that the physician confronted with these problems in the epileptic individual will need help from several different disciplines if he is to evaluate the situation successfully. For example, the findings of Rutter, Graham and Yule (1970) that children with epilepsy and an organic or structural disorder above the brain-stem have a one in three chance of having an additional psychiatric disability and an equal likelihood of intellectual or educational retardation makes it clear that paediatricians and neurologists dealing with such children need to have considerable expertise in these related subjects. Despite the frequent need for a multidisciplinary approach, there is no substitute for the interested and concerned physician who is both experienced and skilled in the care of children and sympathetic towards the problems of children with epilepsy especially. He or she should be prepared to give time, encouragement, advice, education and support to the patient and his family, if necessary for many years (Vining, 1989b). He or she will be in a position to recognize emotional difficulties early before such problems worsen and become more difficult to manage. This is real preventative psychiatry in action and the reward will be a family which is well adjusted to the predicaments occasioned by having a child with epilepsy, and able to look forward to a stable and rewarding adult life for the patient in the future.

Finally, it should be emphasized that each child with epilepsy and his/her family will be different and that psychosocial problems are certainly not invariable. Many children will have few seizures, will respond well to medication and live perfectly normal undisturbed lives. Many children outgrow epilepsy completely. It is essential that the physician should understand the diversity and complexity of the epilepsies and try to educate the family involved accordingly so that undue pessimism and even despair about the condition may be avoided.

## References

BAGLEY, C. (1972) Social prejudice and the adjustment of people with epilepsy. *Epilepsia*, 13, 33–45

BAX, M. (1972) The active and the over-active school child. *Developmental Medicine and Child Neurology*, 14, 83–86

BRENT, D. A., CRUMRINE, P. K., VARMA, R. *et al.* (1990) Phenobarbital treatment and major depressive disorder in children with epilepsy: a naturalistic follow-up. *Pediatrics*, 85, 1086–1091

CANTWELL, D. (1977) Hyperkinetic syndrome. In *Child Psychiatry: Modern Approaches* (eds, M. Rutter and L. Hersov), Blackwell Scientific, Oxford, London, Edinburgh, pp. 524–555

CLARE, M., SMITH, J. A. and WALLACE, S. J. (1978) A child's first febrile convulsion. *Practitioner*, 221, 775–776

CREAK, M. and PAMPIGLIONE, G. (1969) Clinical and EEG studies on a group of 35 psychotic children. *Developmental Medicine and Child Neurology*, 11, 218–227

DHSS (1969) *People with Epilepsy. Report of a Joint Sub-Committee of the Standing Medical Advisory Committee on the Health and Welfare of Handicapped Persons.* HMSO London

ERIKSON, E. (1966) *Childhood and Society.* Penguin, London

ERIKSON, E. (1977) *Childhood and Society.* Triad/Paladin, London

FALCONER, M. A. and TAYLOR, D. C. (1968) Surgical treatment of drug resistant temporal lobe epilepsy due to mesial temporal sclerosis: etiology and significance. *Archives of Neurology*, 19, 353–61

FLOR HENRY, P. (1969) Psychosis and temporal lobe epilepsy – a controlled investigation. *Epilepsia*, 10, 363–395

GOODMAN, R. (1989). Genetic factors in hyperactivity. *British Medical Journal*, 298, 1407–1408

GRAHAM, P. and RUTTER, M. (1968) Organic brain dysfunction and child psychiatric disorder. *British Medical Journal*, 2, 695–700

GREEN, M. and SOLNIT, A. J. (1964) Reactions to the threatened loss of a child: a vulnerable child syndrome. *Pediatrics*, 34, 58–66

HACKNEY, A. (1976) Child epilepsy: the fight against prejudice. *The Sunday Times*, January 11, London

HOARE, P. (1984) Psychiatric disturbance in the families of epileptic children. *Developmental Medicine and Child Neurology*, 26, 14–19

HOFFMAN, H. (1845) *Der Struwwelpeter: Oder lustige Geschichten und drollige Bilder.* Insel Verlag, Leipzig

LENNOX, W. G. and MARKHAM, C. H. (1953) The sociopsychological treatment of epilepsy. *Journal of the American Medical Association*, 152, 1690–1694

LINDSAY, J. (1972) The difficult epileptic child. *British Medical Journal*, 2, 283–285

LIVINGSTON, S. (1972) *Comprehensive Management of Epilepsy in Infancy, Childhood and Adolescence.* Charles C. Thomas, Springfield, Illinois

LOISEAU, P., PESTRE, M., DARTIGUES, J. F. *et al.* (1983) Long-term prognosis in two forms of childhood epilepsy: typical absence seizures and epilepsy with Rolandic (centrotemporal) EEG foci. *Annals of Neurology*, 13, 642–648

OUNSTED, C. (1955) The hyperkinetic syndrome in epileptic children. *Lancet*, 2, 303–311

OUNSTED, C. (1970) A biological approach to autistic and hyperkinetic syndromes. In *Modern Trends in Paediatrics* (ed. J. Apley) Butterworths, London, pp. 286–316

OUNSTED, C. (1971) Some aspects of seizure disorders. In *Recent Advances in Paediatrics* (eds. D. Gairdner and D. Hull) J. and A. Churchill, London, pp. 363–399

OUNSTED, C., LINDSAY, J. and NORMAN, R. (1966) *Biological Factors in Temporal Lobe Epilepsy*, Clinics in Developmental Medicine, No. 22, Spastics Society/Heinemann Medical, London

OUNSTED, C., LINDSAY, J. and RICHARDS, P. (1987). Temporal lobe epilepsy 1948–1986. A biographical study. *Clinics in Developmental Medicine*; No. 103. Blackwell Scientific Publications, Oxford

POND, D. (1961) Psychiatric aspects of epileptic and brain-damaged children. *British Medical Journal*, **2**, 1377–1382, 1454–1459

REYNOLDS, E. H. (1981) Biological factors in psychological disorders associated with epilepsy. In *Epilepsy and Psychiatry* (eds. E. H. Reynolds and M. R. Trimble), Churchill Livingstone, Edinburgh and London, pp. 264–290

REYNOLDS, E. H. (1983) Mental effects of antiepileptic medication: a review. *Epilepsia*, **24**, Suppl. 2, S85–S95

RUTTER, M. (1968) Lésion cérébrale organique, hyperkinésie et retard mental. *Psychiatrie de l'Enfant*, **11**, 475–492

RUTTER, M. (1977) Infantile autism and other child psychoses. In *Child Psychiatry: Modern Approaches* (eds. M. Rutter and L. Hersov), Blackwell Scientific, Oxford, London, Edinburgh, Melbourne, pp. 717–747

RUTTER, M., GRAHAM, P. and YULE, W. (1970) *A Neuropsychiatric Study in Childhood*. Clinics in Developmental Medicine, Nos 35/36, Spastics International/Heinemann Medical, London

SILLANPÄÄ, M. (1973) Medico-social prognosis of children with epilepsy. *Acta Paediatrica Scandinavica*, Suppl. 237

SLATER. E., BEARD, A. W. and GLITHERO, E. (1963) The schizophenia-like psychoses of epilepsy. *British Journal of Psychiatry*, **109**, 95–150

STORES, G (1977) Behavior disturbance and type of epilepsy in children attending ordinary school. In *Epilepsy: The Eighth International Symposium* (ed. J. K. Penry), Raven Press, New York pp. 245–249

TAYLOR, D. C. (1969) Some psychiatric aspects of epilepsy. In *Current Problems in Neuropsychiatry*. Special publication No. 4. *British Journal of Psychiatry*

TAYLOR, D. C. (1971a) Psychiatry and sociology in the understanding of epilepsy. In *Psychiatric Aspects of Medical Practice* (eds M. G. Gelder and B. M. Mandlebrote), Staples Press, London, pp., 161–186

TAYLOR, D. C. (1971b) The ontogenesis of chronic epilepsy psychosis: a reanalysis. *Psychological Medicine*, **1**, 247

TAYLOR, D. C. (1973a) Aspects of seizure disorders. II. On prejudice. *Developmental Medicine and Child Neurology*, **15**, 91–94

TAYLOR, D. C. (1973b) Epilepsy, brain and mind. *British Journal of Hospital Medicine*, **9**, 187–91

TAYLOR, D. C. (1977) Epilepsy and the sinister side of schizophrenia. *Developmental Medicine and Child Neurology*, **19**, 403–407

TAYLOR, D.C. (1987) Epilepsy and prejudice. *Archives of Disease in Childhood*, **62**, 209–211

TAYLOR, D. C. and FALCONER, M. A. (1969) Clinical, socioeconomic and psychological changes after temporal lobectomy for epilepsy. *British Journal of Psychiatry*, **114**, 1247–1261

TAYLOR, E. A. (ed.) (1986) The overactive child. *Clinics in Developmental Medicine*; No 97. Blackwell Scientific Publications, Oxford

TEMKIN, O. (1971) *The Falling Sickness*, Johns Hopkins Press, Baltimore and London, p. 44

TOONE, B. (1986). Sexual disorders in epilepsy. In *Recent Advances in Epilepsy* No 3. (eds T. A. Pedley and B. S. Meldrum), Churchill Livingstone, Edinburgh, London, pp. 233–260

TREIMAN, D. M. and DELGADO-ESCUETA, A. V. (1983) Violence and epilepsy: a critical review. In *Recent Advances in Epilepsy, No. 1* (eds J. A. Pedley and B. S. Meldrum), Churchill Livingstone, Edinburgh and London, pp. 179–210

TRIMBLE, M. (1991) *The Psychoses of Epilepsy*, Raven Press, New York

VALLARTA, J. M., BELL, D. B. and RETCHERT, A. (1974) Progressive encephalopathy due to chronic hydantoin intoxication. *American Journal of Diseases of Children*, **128**, 27–34

VI BERG, M., BLENNOW, G. and POLSKI, B. (1987) Epilepsy in adolescence: implications for the development of personality. *Epilepsia*, **28**, 542–546

VINING, E. P. G. (1989a) Psychosocial issues of children with epilepsy. *Cleveland Clinic Journal of Medicine*, Supplement to Vol **52**, Part 2, S214–S220

VINING, E. P. G. (1989b) Educational, social and life-long effects of epilepsy. *Pediatric Clinics of North America*, **36**, No 2, 449–461

WEISS, G. (1990) Hyperactivity in childhood. *New England Journal of Medicine*, **323**, 1413–1415

WILLIAMS, D. (1969) Man's temporal lobe. *Brain*, **91**, 639–654

# Learning disorders in children with epilepsy. The acquired aphasia with epilepsy syndrome

## Learning disorders

The problem of learning disorders in children with epilepsy is a confused and controversial one and the author is particularly indebted to the work of Stores (1971, 1973, 1975, 1978, 1981; Stores and Hart, 1976) in trying to clarify the various issues involved. Many of the early writers were pessimistic about cognitive function in children with epilepsy, and up to the 1940s and even beyond, the concept of progressive 'epileptic dementia' was popular and was attributed by some to the cerebral dysfunction itself and by others to brain damage sustained during attacks. However, as Stores (1971) pointed out, the groups studied were often heterogeneous with respect to age, type and duration of attacks, treatment and associated physical handicaps, and assessment was almost exclusively restricted to 'IQ testing' (*see* Chapter 24), the educational bias of which put many epileptic patients at a disadvantage, especially epileptic children who had lost time at school. However, in recent times psychologists have moved away from the assessment of global intelligence towards the assessment of specific cognitive functions, and groups of children with well defined types of epilepsy and with other factors in common have been studied.

## Poor school progress

The fact that a problem does exist is beyond doubt. Holdsworth and Whitmore (1974a) studied a random group of children with epilepsy attending normal schools. They found that barely one-third were making wholly satisfactory progress. Half the children were achieving a very indifferent performance in the classroom (holding their own at a below-average level), one in six was falling appreciably behind in work and one in five presented with a behaviour problem. These authors emphasized that, even in ordinary schools, children with epilepsy were an educationally vulnerable group. In an earlier survey (Whitmore and Holdsworth, 1971) of children with epilepsy attending normal schools, 42% were described by their teachers as being 'markedly inattentive'. The children were described as lethargic, absent-minded, sleepy, lacking in concentration or otherwise unresponsive to what was happening in class. Inattentiveness was found to be associated with unsatisfactory educational progress and with difficult behaviour. Seidenberg *et al.* (1986), in similar studies in the United States, found that, as a group, children with epilepsy were making less academic progress than expected for their age and IQ level. Academic deficiencies were greatest in arithmetic, followed by spelling, reading, comprehension and word recognition. In their classic monograph on temporal lobe epilepsy, Ounsted, Lindsay and Norman (1966) had asked why so many children with seizure disorders who had at least normal overall intelligence and good control of attacks failed to come up to academic expectations. There are probably many reasons for this failure but at least one of them could be the effects of medication.

## Effects of antiepileptic drugs

Antiepileptic drugs may have adverse effects on both cognitive function and behaviour. The former may be defined as the ability of a person to use information about his or her environment in an adaptive way and the latter as the ability to adapt or otherwise to interpersonal relationships. Stores (1975) reviewed the possible harmful effects of antiepileptic drugs on the learning process and emphasized that there is a widespread belief among teachers that children treated with these drugs are inevitably handicapped and that this belief contributes to the underexpectations which teachers generally have about children with epilepsy, underexpectations which, unfortunately, parents may also share. Phenobarbitone and primidone have often been incriminated in the learning difficulties of children with epilepsy, and Hutt *et al* (1968) found that phenobarbitone had an adverse effect on intellectual tasks involving sustained effort. The paradoxical effect of phenobarbitone in young children which results in overexcitement and overactivity may also interfere with any sort of sustained attention and concentration. Vining *et al.* (1987) compared phenobarbitone and valproic acid with reference to their effects on cognition and behaviour in children being treated for epilepsy and found that phenobarbitone produced more adverse side-effects. Brent *et al.* (1990) have written that phenobarbitone increases the risk for major depressive illness in children with epilepsy.

Chronic intoxication with phenytoin can lead to intellectual deterioration, and this is discussed in Chapter 26. Stores and Hart (1976), in a study of factors associated with the progress of children with epilepsy attending normal schools, found that the reading skills of those children who had taken phenytoin for at least 2 years were significantly inferior to those who had taken other antiepileptic drugs over a similar period. Andrews *et al.* (1986) found that phenytoin particularly affected tasks involving short-term memory, and Vining (1987) mentions its adverse effects on attention, problem solving ability, and performance of visuomotor tasks.

Ethosuximide has been linked occasionally with adverse effects on learning in children, mainly as a cause of global mental impairment, but Browne (1983) has shown that the psychosocial effects of ethosuximide are minimal while its effectiveness in reducing absences and spike-wave EEG discharges greatly improves intellectual function, behaviour and school performance. Sodium valproate is much less detrimental to cognitive function than either phenytoin or phenobarbitone and such effects as it has appear to be dose-related (Trimble and Thompson, 1984). Behavioural changes, including irritability, hyperactivity, lassitude and drowsiness, also seem to have a relationship to high levels of that drug (Herranz *et al.* 1982). Clonazepam is likely to produce both behavioural disturbances and cognitive impairment but clobazam is less likely to do so (Trimble, 1988).

Ever since its introduction, reports of the effect of carbamazepine on both cognitive function and behaviour have been consistently favourable. Thomson and Trimble (1983), in patients who had been given psychological testing using a battery of tests which included memory, attention and concentration, perceptual speed, decision-making speed and motor speed tasks, showed that those on monotherapy with either phenytoin or sodium valproate had impairments in performance at high serum levels which were approximately twice those observed at low serum levels of the drugs, even though both high and low serum levels were within the therapeutic ranges for the drugs. In contrast, carbamazepine-treated patients showed minimal changes in performance during both high and low serum level sessions (Thompson and Trimble, 1983). Furthermore, there is considerable evidence that carbamazepine is psychotropic in its effects, while phenobarbitone, and perhaps other drugs also, may sometimes exacerbate or even precipitate affective disturbances in adults and children (Trimble, 1988; Brent et al., 1990).

It is difficult, as yet, to assess the effects of the new antiepileptic drugs, vigabatrin and lamotrigine, on cognition and behaviour. Both are most frequently employed in polytherapy regimes for intractable epilepsy and this makes evaluation difficult. However, vigabatrin has been reported as causing sedation and memory problems in a small proportion of patients (Remy and Beaumont, 1989) and lamotrigine may also cause some drowsiness.

Finally, it must be emphasized that the effects on cognitive function of antiepileptic drugs are greatly amplified by their administration in polytherapy regimes. Drug-related cognitive dysfunction may often be reversed simply by changing to monotherapy, and such a change also facilitates more reliable monitoring of serum drug levels, an essential investigation in any child with behaviour and/or learning problems who is receiving medication for epilepsy (Stores, 1975; Vining, 1987).

Excellent reviews of the effects of antiepileptic drugs on cognition and intellectual function have been written by Reynolds (1983), Vining (1987), Trimble (1987) and Trimble and Cull (1988).

## Male preponderance

Many authors, including Holdsworth and Whitmore (1974a, b), have commented on the preponderance of males among the educationally retarded with epilepsy. Stores (1978), in a survey in which children with epilepsy attending normal schools were compared with non-epileptic children attending normal schools, found that epileptic boys were significantly more inattentive and overactive than non-epileptic boys according to their teachers and parents, and that they performed significantly less well on tests of sustained attention and perceptual accuracy. No such differences were found between epileptic and non-epileptic girls. This contrast between the epileptic groups was not attributable to drug effects or EEG abnormalities. In this context, of course, it should be remembered that epilepsy may coexist with mental subnormality of varying degree which, in its own right, may frequently be associated with defects of attention. Distractibility and overactivity may be other features of the mentally subnormal.

## Clues from EEG

The results of several investigations have suggested that certain features characterize the type of seizure discharge which is most disruptive of performance in tests of attention or of cognitive motor abilities. The more generalized, bilaterally synchronous and symmetrical the seizure discharge, the more regular and organized the spike-wave complexes (as exemplified by the 3 Hz pattern of juvenile absence epilepsy or true petit mal), and the longer the duration of the burst the greater is the effect on attention.

Browne *et al.* (1974) studied responsiveness before, during and after spike-wave paroxysms using an auditory stimulus (a sharp whistling noise), a response unit (a telegraph key) and a digital clock that measured time from the onset of stimulation to the closing of the circuit in the response unit. The 26 patients studied ranged in age from 5 to 20 years with a median age of 12 years and all were suffering from 'absence seizures'. They found that the reaction times during the 1 second before a paroxysm were within normal limits but only 43% of the reaction times were normal at the onset of a paroxysm. Responsiveness was recovered quickly after a paroxysm. They found that the degree of maximal impairment of auditory responsiveness was the same in paroxysms of both long and short duration, and they concluded that, if possible, therapy for absence seizures should aim at controlling all spike-wave paroxysms.

Hutt (1967) showed that both clinical and subclinical generalized spike-wave bursts could disrupt not only the registration of information but also its storage and recall, and that these effects depended upon the amount and complexity of the information as well as on the rate at which the child worked. It has been said that petit mal makes holes in the mind like a paper doyley (C. Ounsted, 1978, personal communication). That such transitory cognitive impairment can occur during subclinical EEG discharges has been known since the earliest days of electroencephalography, and the subject is comprehensively reviewed by Binnie (1988).

## Absences and defects of attention

The position with regard to absence seizures generally is a little more complicated when other types of absence seizure, apart from those due to true petit mal, are considered. Mirsky and van Buren (1965) reported a significant decrease in responsiveness to a visual and auditory continuous performance test in the seconds preceding a seizure. Their patients, however, had a mean age of 22 years, and studies were made during a number of types of EEG abnormality, including spike-wave, polyspike and wave and other forms. The defects of attention which occur with paroxysmal discharges of the spike-wave type may be less obvious in the absences seen in children with myoclonic epilepsy and in those occurring in some children with temporal lobe epilepsy. Furthermore, there may be a specific perceptual deficit present in each of these varieties. Another complicating factor is that some children with absences of various kinds may show attention defects between overt attacks and in the absence of EEG abnormalities, possibly because of a persistent disturbance of subcortical mechanisms (Stores, 1973).

## Concentration and attention factors: orientation reaction

Clinical experience shows that the occurrence of seizures is sometimes related to particular activities or experiences. Lennox, Gibbs and Gibbs pointed out, as long ago as 1936, that the frequency of seizures was lessened by tasks requiring some degree of concentration or arousal. Ounsted and Hutt (1964) demonstrated that seizure discharges occurred less frequently in circumstances which were neither boring nor excessively stressful. If the degree of attention required became too stressful the seizure discharges increased and performance declined.

Although defects of attention are usually associated with subcortical seizure discharges, there is reason to suppose that frequently occurring localized cortical discharges may adversely affect some aspects of attention and learning. Studies of focal epilepsy suggest that when a part of the brain is occupied by an electrical discharge it cannot perform its normal functions. A chronic epileptic focus may be associated with permanent alterations of postsynaptic membranes and with loss of dendritic spines, thereby causing deafferentation (Purpura, 1979). In general, it has been found that temporal lobe lesions in the hemisphere dominant for speech cause impairment of verbal abilities, including defects of retention and learning of verbal material, while lesions of the temporal lobe on the non-dominant side tend to impair visuospatial skills and to cause perceptual difficulties (Ounsted, Lindsay and Norman, 1966; Fedio and Mirsky, 1969).

It may be that a chronically discharging cortical focus, at least in some areas, disturbs the 'orientation reaction' either by increasing excitation of corticoreticular connections and maintaining a heightened arousal state or by interfering with the normal reactivity to novel stimuli and causing inattentiveness. The orientation reaction is defined as the total action of paying attention to important stimuli, and consists of a variety of physiological changes which increase the sensitivity of the sense organs and prepare the organism to deal with the situation. Characteristics of stimuli which elicit the orientation reaction include novelty, intensity, complexity, uncertainty and surprise (Lynn, 1966).

## Perceptual difficulties

Gastaut (1965), using comprehensive psychological testing on children with epilepsy, showed that as many as a third had perceptual difficulties which could cause a considerable handicap in learning to read and write. Rutter, Graham and Yule (1970), in their comprehensive study in the Isle of Wight, found that reading skills were substantially impaired in almost one-fifth of the children with epilepsy. Stores and Hart (1976) investigated the *reading skills* of children with epilepsy attending normal schools. Their conclusions were as follows:

1   The reading skills of children with electrographically generalized epilepsy and subclinical seizure discharges seemed to be no worse than those of non-epileptic matched controls.
2   In contrast, children with persistent focal spike discharges tended to have lower reading levels than their non-epileptic matched controls.
3   The inferior performance of the focal group was largely attributable to those children with left hemisphere focal spikes, and these were predominantly boys.
4   The reading skills of epileptic boys, whatever their type of epilepsy, were inferior to those of epileptic girls.

5   The long-term use of phenytoin was associated with lower levels of reading skills than were other forms of antiepileptic medication.

It should be pointed out that other authors have reported findings at variance with the above. Camfield *et al.* (1984) were unable to show any difference on cognitive testing between children with left and right temporal lobe foci. Giordani *et al.* (1985) found that overall intelligence was the same in children and young adults with generalized and with partial seizures but that those with primarily or secondarily generalized seizures did worse on tests related to attention, visuospatial orientation and sequencing ability. Seidenberg *et al.* (1986) did not find the site of the EEG focus to be significant in their test results.

## Factors at home and at school

Quite apart from the effects of structural brain abnormality, seizure discharges and drugs on attention and learning ability in the child with epilepsy, it seems likely that unfavourable environmental factors at home and at school may adversely affect the development of the child's cognitive and social skills. Indeed, Hartlage and Green (1972) suggested that the academic achievement of the epileptic child may be more closely related to environmental factors than to any specific disability of neurological origin. In their study they found that the academic and social underachievement of children with epilepsy could be attributed, at least in part, to inappropriate dependency on their parents. They did not feel that this overdependency was due to any single faulty attitude on the part of the parents (such as overprotectiveness), but rather to the direct impact of epilepsy and its treatment on the child's psychological development causing a delay in emotional growth. A further unfortunate consequence of epilepsy has been highlighted by the report of Britten *et al.* (1986), describing findings in a cohort of people born in Britain in 1946. People with idiopathic epilepsy who had shown no evidence of social handicap at the age of 26 were doing poorly economically at the age of 36 in comparison to controls. Adverse social and economic factors were thought to be responsible and the pervasive prejudice against people who have epilepsy of whatever type (Taylor, 1987) was certainly implicated.

Holdsworth and Whitmore (1974b), in a study of the *attitudes of teachers* towards children with epilepsy attending normal schools, found that these have been improving in recent years and that head teachers and class teachers were now more sympathetic towards these children and were anxious to treat them as normally as possible in school. They also found that many teachers showed an increased willingness to retain a child with epilepsy in school if his seizures were not too severe or frequent. While they welcomed this improved tolerance on the part of the teachers, they felt that it may have misled the teachers into expecting a lower level of work from the children than they might have accepted had the children not been subject to epilepsy. This, in turn, led to underachievement by the children. However, they emphasized that it is not easy for teachers to maintain a balance between overprotection and underprotection where children with epilepsy are concerned. Ross and Tookey (1988) have stressed that doctors should encourage parents to share the problem of their child's epilepsy with the school and that doctors should contact the school by means of letters, telephone calls, and even visits, provided that the parents are agreeable to such a course of action.

It should be apparent from the foregoing discussion of this very complex problem that there may be many different factors concerned in the causation of learning difficulties in children with epilepsy. Furthermore, since it seems likely that cognitive defects may generate disturbed behaviour in these children, early recognition and treatment of these deficits may produce beneficial results both in the learning situation and in the personality development of the child. Stores reviewed the subject comprehensively in 1981 and emphasized the important contribution which ambulatory monitoring (*see* Chapter 23) was making to the better understanding of these difficult problems. Addy (1987) has reviewed the topic succinctly and comprehensively and the symposium report, entitled 'Epilepsy, Behaviour and Cognitive Function', edited by Trimble and Reynolds (1988) is also strongly recommended to the reader.

## The acquired aphasia with epilepsy syndrome

It seems appropriate at this point to mention an unusual disorder first described by Landau and Kleffner in 1957 which they called a 'syndrome of acquired aphasia with convulsive disorder in children'. It is now sometimes known as the Landau–Kleffner syndrome. They described six children who, after apparently normal acquisition of speech and language, developed aphasia for periods ranging from days to months or longer. Worster-Drought (1971) described a further 14 cases seen over a period of 10 years in which an acquired receptive aphasia was the outstanding symptom. Temporary aphasia is known to occur in association with certain types of epilepsy, particularly temporal lobe epilepsy, and usually follows a seizure or a series of seizures. In general, such aphasia recovers after a variable interval but may recur after further seizures. Temporary aphasia may also follow a head injury in childhood (so-called cerebral shock) or may be seen after an acute vascular accident such as an arterial thrombosis involving the dominant hemisphere, but slow recovery usually ensues in both instances. Speech may also be permanently lost in certain cerebral degenerative disorders, for example, in Addison–Schilder's disease (Forsyth, Forbes and Cumings, 1971; Monaghan *et al.*, 1987). However, in the syndrome of acquired aphasia, previously normal children become aphasic, usually completely, without any evidence of other neurological abnormalities or a known focal brain pathology. At about the same time, or shortly afterwards, between 60 and 80% of the patients are reported as developing clinical epilepsy (Dulac, Billard and Arthuis, 1983), which may consist of generalized or partial seizures with predominantly motor components. The patients usually display paroxysmal EEG abnormalities. Typically there are bilateral, asymmetrical, paroxysmal discharges, mainly over the post-central areas, with a lateralization which is not necessarily to the dominant hemisphere. Deonna *et al.* (1977) noted focal slow spikes, sometimes followed by a slow wave, either isolated or occurring in long bursts or even continuously. In addition to the focal abnormalities, there may be bursts of multifocal slow spikes, either isolated or occurring in bursts, and usually bilateral but asynchronous. Sleep records may show discharges while the waking record is normal and, because the focal findings vary in time and intensity, frequent records may be necessary for diagnosis.

The onset of the disorder has been reported as occurring from the age of 3 years up to 9 years and it may be abrupt or gradual. The evolution of the condition is also variable. The onset may be rapid and a prompt recovery may ensue but subsequently recurrences and fluctuations may follow. In this type there may be a close association with the occurrence of clinical epilepsy.

In another variation of the disorder, there is no recovery of language function after repeated seizures or episodes of acute aphasia. Sometimes, a very slow and imperfect recovery takes place, perhaps because the contralateral hemisphere assumes some aspects of the language function. In the type of this disorder which corresponds most closely to the syndrome as described by Landau and Kleffner (1957) there is a progressive loss of language comprehension. Recovery is very variable and seizures are infrequent or do not occur at all.

The defect in language function is usually a verbal–auditory agnosia with an inability to comprehend language because of a defect in decoding phonologically, as emphasized by Worster-Drought (1971) in his classic paper on the disorder. Loss of comprehension is soon followed by loss of the ability to execute speech. A remarkable feature of the condition is that intelligence is usually unimpaired. Behavioural disturbances may coincide with the onset of the disorder and are usually due to the acute anxiety generated in a child rendered incapable of understanding spoken language. The differential diagnosis is from acquired deafness, elective mutism, autism, disintegrative psychosis, Rett syndrome, and severe personality disorder. Clinical neurological examination is normal and CT scans show normal appearances. The author is unaware of any MRI studies in the acute stage of the disorder. The history, EEG findings and examinations by a skilled psychologist, a speech therapist and an audiometrician will usually confirm the diagnosis.

The aetiology of the syndrome is still unknown. Landau and Kleffner (1957) suggested that persistent epileptic discharges in parts of the brain concerned with linguistic communication result in a functional ablation of these areas as far as normal linguistic behaviour is concerned. It is axiomatic that parts of the brain affected by epileptic activity cannot be used for normal function as, for example, in the case of Todd's paralysis after prolonged febrile seizures. Gordon (1964), writing about so-called central deafness, drew attention to the work of Geschwind and Kaplan (1962) in cases of adult dysphasia, and postulated a disconnection syndrome in which one part of the brain was isolated from others by reason of disease or functional abnormality. In a recent review, Gordon (1990) has developed this hypothesis as follows in order to explain the acquired aphasia with epilepsy syndrome. When a skill is being acquired, anything that interferes with cerebral integration is likely to have disastrous effects. Learning, and the maintenance of a skill, largely depend on the ability to integrate information from various sensory input channels with memories, particularly those of past experiences and their emotional content and with the motor performance necessary for the execution of the skill. Recently acquired skills are particularly vulnerable to any disturbance of function. If this is the result of abnormal neuronal discharges preventing normal activity and the spread of impulses from one part of the brain to another (which is an essential mechanism for the development of language), then not only will development be impaired but regression will occur. Since there appear to be optimum periods for learning in children, if the formation of intracerebral connections is prevented for any reason during certain periods of life, then such connections may never develop. This could explain why language function may not improve when seizures and EEG discharges have ceased. Studies of affected patients by means of EEG topographic mapping suggest that widespread electrophysiological dysfunction of the fronto-central-parietal areas, associated with markedly unstable paroxysmal discharges, is a striking feature of the disorder (Nakana, Okuno and Mikawa, 1989).

Worster-Drought (1971) speculated that the underlying cause of the syndrome in some cases might be a form of low-grade selective encephalitis affecting particular parts of the brain but there is no definite evidence for this possibility, although in one of the author's cases, the aphasia developed in a setting of what might have been an encephalitic illness. Another suggestion is that there may be an isolated cerebral arteritis which may be responsive to the calcium antagonist group of drugs (Pascual-Castroviejo, 1991). It is possible that, at least in part, the cause may be due to a developmental failure of some kind rather than to an acquired condition. There is no doubt that the degree of recovery depends on the child's stage of development as well as the severity of the disturbance. The older the child at the time of onset the better the prognosis, which is the opposite to what occurs in childhood aphasia resulting from structural lesions of the brain. With onset before the age of 5 years, the outcome is poor with little chance of full recovery. Presumably at this critical developmental stage for speech and language development, impairment of high-level auditory processing is catastrophic in its long-term effects. Older children are less severely affected, since much of language function has already been learnt, and there is more likely to be a restoration of previously acquired skills.

Seizures, which may be generalized or partial and which are not usually severe, occur in about two-thirds of cases. Treatment with antiepileptic drugs may be of benefit and they should be tried (Deonna, Peter and Ziegler, 1989). Carbamazepine and sodium valproate have been those usually employed. Lerman, Lerman-Sagie and Kivity (1991) advise that, in acute cases, a course of ACTH or prednisolone should be given early and in adequate dosage and that this therapy may be effective in reversing the aphasia and may also work well in relapses of the condition. In a personal case, ACTH also had a very beneficial effect on seizure frequency during a relapse.

The literature indicates that the long-term prognosis for full recovery from the aphasia is not good and that it becomes permanent in about 40% of cases. The seizures are usually infrequent and remit, as do the EEG abnormalities, before the age of 15 years. In Worster-Drought's (1971) series of 14 cases observed over a long period, 6 children recovered more or less completely, 3 recovered partially and, in the remaining 5, recovery was slight or very limited and the children were left with severe deficits in the comprehension and execution of spoken language. The author's experience with nine cases of the disorder, observed over many years, has been similar to that of Worster-Drought.

The correct and early diagnosis of this syndrome is essential, firstly, because treatment with ACTH or corticosteroids may reverse and/or arrest the disorder but also because, for severely affected children, special education linked to speech therapy is needed. This can best be provided in a unit for children with language disorders.

## References

ADDY, D. P. (1987) Cognitive function in children with epilepsy. *Developmental Medicine and Child Neurology*, **29**, 394–397

ANDREWES, D. G., BULLEN, J. G., TOMLINSON, L. *et al.* (1986) A comparative study of the cognitive effects of phenytoin and carbamazepine in new referrals with epilepsy. *Epilepsia*, **27**, 128–134

BINNIE, C. D. (1988) Seizures, EEG discharges and cognition. In *Epilepsy, Behaviour and Cognitive Function* (eds M. R. Trimble and E. H. Reynolds), John Wiley and Sons, Chichester, New York, pp. 45–49

BRENT, D. A., CRUMRINE, P. K., VARMA, R. *et al.* (1990) Phenobarbital treatment and major depressive disorder in children with epilepsy: a naturalistic follow-up. *Pediatrics*, **85**, 1086–1091

BRITTEN, N., MORGAN, K., FENWICK, P. B. C. and BRITTEN, H. (1986) Epilepsy and handicap from birth to age 36. *Developmental Medicine and Child Neurology*, **28**, 719–728

BROWNE, T. R. (1983) Antiepileptic drugs and psychosocial development: ethosuximide. In *Antiepileptic Drug Therapy in Pediatrics* (eds P. L. Morselli, C. E. Pippenger and J. K. Penry), Raven Press, New York, pp. 181–187

BROWNE, T. R., PENRY, J. K., PORTER, R. J. and DREIFUSS, F. E. (1974) Responsiveness before, during and after spike-wave paroxysms. *Neurology*, **24**, 659–665

CAMFIELD, P. R., GATES, R., RONEN, G. *et al.* (1984) Comparison of cognitive ability, personality profile and school success in epileptic children with pure right versus left temporal lobe EEG foci. *Annals of Neurology*, **15**, 122–126

DEONNA, TH., BEAUMANOIR, A., GAILLARD, F. and ASSAL, G. (1977) Acquired aphasia in childhood with seizure disorder: a heterogeneous syndrome. *Neuropädiatrie*, **8** 263–273

DEONNA, TH., PETER, CL. and ZIEGLER, A-L. (1989) Adult follow-up of the acquired aphasia-epilepsia syndrome in childhood. Report of 7 cases. *Neuropediatrics*, **20**, 132–138

DULAC, O., BILLARE, C. and ARTHUIS, M. (1983) Aspects électro-cliniques et évolutifs de l'épilepsie dans le syndrome aphasie-épilepsie. *Archives Française de Pediatrie*, **40**, 299–308

FEDIO, P. and MIRSKY, A. F. (1969) Selective intellectual deficits in children with temporal lobe or centrencephalic epilepsy. *Neuropsychologia*, **7**, 287–300

FORSYTH, C. C., FORBES, M. and CUMINGS, J. N. (1971) Adrenocortical atrophy and diffuse cerebral sclerosis. *Archives of Disease in Childhood*, **46**, 273–284

GASTAUT, H. (1965) Enquiry into the education of epileptic children. In *Epilepsy and Education: Report on a seminar in Marseilles, April 1964*, British Epilepsy Association and International Bureau for Epilepsy, p. 3

GESCHWIND, N. and KAPLAN, E. (1962) A human deconnection syndrome. *Neurology*, **12**, 675

GIORDANI, B., BERENT, S., SACKELLARES, J. C. *et al.* (1985) Intelligence test performance of patients with partial and generalized seizures. *Epilepsia*, **26**, 37–42

GORDON, N. S. (1964) The concept of central deafness. In *The Child Who Does Not Talk*, Clinics in Developmental Medicine, No. 13, Spastics Society/Heinemann Medical, London, pp. 62–64

GORDON, N., (1990) Acquired aphasia in childhood: the Landau–Kleffner syndrome. *Developmental Medicine and Child Neurology*, **32**, 267–274

HARTLAGE, L. C. and GREEN, J. B. (1972) The relation of parental attitudes to academic and social achievement in epileptic children. *Epilepsia*, **13**, 21–26

HERRANZ, J. L., ARTEAGA, R. and ARMIJO, J. A. (1982) Side effects of sodium valproate in monotherapy controlled by plasma levels: a study of 88 paediatric patients. *Epilepsia*, **23**, 203–14

HOLDSWORTH, L. and WHITMORE, K. (1974a) A study of children with epilepsy attending normal schools. I: Their seizure patterns, progress and behaviour in school. *Developmental Medicine and Child Neurology*, **16**, 746–758

HOLDSWORTH, L. and WHITMORE, K. (1974b) A study of children with epilepsy attending ordinary schools. II: Information and attitudes held by their teachers. *Developmental Medicine and Child Neurology*, **16**, 759–765

HUTT, S. J. (1967) Epilepsy and education. In *Proceedings of the 1st International Conference of the Association for Special Education*. Association for Special Education, Stanmore, Middlesex, p. 103.

HUTT, S. J., JACKSON, P. M., BELSHAM, A. and HIGGINS, G. (1968) Perceptual-motor behaviour in relation to blood phenobarbitone level: a preliminary report. *Developmental Medicine and Child Neurology*, **10**, 626–632

LANDAU, W. M. and KLEFFNER, F. R. (1957) Syndrome of acquired aphasia with convulsive disorder in children. *Neurology*, **7**, 523–530

LENNOX, W. G., GIBBS, F. A. and GIBBS, E. L. (1936) The effect on the EEG of drugs and conditions which influence seizures. *Archives of Neurology and Psychiatry*, **36**, 1236–1245

LERMAN, P., LERMAN-SAGIE, T., and KIVITY, S. (1991) Effect of early corticosteroid therapy for Landau–Kleffner syndrome. *Developmental Medicine and Child Neurology*, **33**, 257–260

LYNN, R. (1966) *Attention, Arousal and the Orientation Reaction*, Pergamon Press, Oxford

MIRSKY, A. F. and VAN BUREN, J. (1965) On the nature of the 'absence' in centrencephalic epilepsy: a study of some behavioural, electroencephalographic and autonomic factors. *Electroencephalography and Clinical Neurophysiology*, **18**, 334–348

MONAGHAN, H., TEMPANY, E., MCMENAMIN, J. and O'DONOHOE, N. (1987) Adrenoleucodystrophy: a review of nine cases. *Irish Medical Journal*, **80**, 142–144

NAKANA, S., OKUNO, T. and MIKAWA, H. (1989) Landau–Kleffner syndrome. EEG topographic studies. *Brain and Development*, **11**, 43–50

OUNSTED, C. and HUTT, S. J. (1964) The effect of attentive factors upon bioelectric paroxysms in epileptic children. *Proceedings of the Royal Society of Medicine*, **57**, 1178

OUNSTED, C., LINDSAY, J. and NORMAN, R. (1966) *Biological Factors in Temporal Lobe Epilepsy*, Clinics in Developmental Medicine, No. 22, Spastics International/Heinemann Medical, London; p. 110

PASCUAL-CASTROVIEJO, I. (1990) Nicardine in the treatment of acquired aphasia and epilepsy (letter). *Developmental Medicine and Child Neurology*, **32**, 930

PURPURA, D. P. (1979) Pathobiology of cortical neurons in metabolic and unclassified amentias. In: *Congenital and Acquired Cognitive Disorders*, Research Publications of the Association for Research in Nervous and Mental Disease, No. 57 (ed. R. Katzman) Raven Press, New York, pp 43–68

REMY, C., and BEAUMONT, D. (1989) Efficacy and safety of vigabatrin in the long-term treatment of refractory epilepsy. *British Journal of Clinical Pharmacology*, **27**, Supplement 1, 125 S–129 S

REYNOLDS, E. H. (1983) Mental effects of antiepileptic medication: a review. *Epilepsia*, **24**, Suppl. 2, S85–S95

ROSS, E. M. and TOOKEY, P. (1988) Educational needs and epilepsy in childhood. In *Epilepsy, Behaviour and Cognitive Function* (eds M. R. Trimble and E. H. Reynolds), John Wiley and Sons, Chichester, New York, pp. 87–96.

RUTTER, M., GRAHAM, P. and YULE, W. (1970) *A Neuropsychiatric Study in Childhood*, Clinics in Developmental Medicine, Nos. 35/36. Spastics International/Heinemann Medical, London

SEIDENBERG, M., BECK, N., GEISSER, M. *et al.* (1986). Academic achievement of children with epilepsy. *Epilepsia*, **27**, 753–759

STORES, G. (1971) Cognitive function in children with epilepsy. *Developmental Medicine and Child Neurology*, **13**, 390–393

STORES, G. (1973) Studies of attention and seizure disorders. *Developmental Medicine and Child Neurology*, **15**, 376–382

STORES, G. (1975) Behavioural effects on anti-epileptic drugs. *Developmental Medicine and Child Neurology*, **17**, 647–658

STORES, G. (1978) School children with epilepsy at risk for learning and behaviour disorders. *Developmental Medicine and Child Neurology*, **20**, 502–508

STORES, G. (1981) Problems of learning and behaviour in children with epilepsy. In *Epilepsy and Psychiatry* (eds E. H. Reynolds and M. R. Trimble), Churchill Livingstone, Edinburgh and London, pp. 34–38

STORES, G. and HART, J. (1976) Reading skills of children with generalised or focal epilepsy attending ordinary school. *Developmental Medicine and Child Neurology*, **18**, 705–716

TAYLOR, D. C. (1987) Epilepsy and prejudice. *Archives of Disease in Childhood*, **62**, 209–211

THOMPSON, P. J. and TRIMBLE, M. R. (1983) Anticonvulsant serum levels; relationship to impairments of cognitive functioning. *Journal of Neurology, Neurosurgery and Neuropsychiatry*, **46**, 227–233

TRIMBLE, M. R. (1987) Anticonvulsant drugs and cognitive function: a review of the literature. *Epilepsia*, **28**, Supplement 3, S37–S45

TRIMBLE, M. R. (1988) Anticonvulsant drugs: mood and cognitive function. In: *Epilepsy, Behaviour and Cognitive Function* (eds M. R. Trimble and E. H. Reynolds), John Wiley and Sons, Chichester, New York; pp 87–96

TRIMBLE, M. R. and CULL, C. (1988) Children of school age: the influence of antiepileptic drugs on behaviour and intellect. *Epilepsia*, **29**, Supplement 3, S15–S19

TRIMBLE, M. R. and REYNOLDS, E. H. (eds) (1988) *Epilepsy, Behaviour and Cognitive Function*. John Wiley and Sons, Chichester, New York:

TRIMBLE, M. R. and THOMPSON, P. J. (1984) Sodium valproate and cognitive function. *Epilepsia*, **25**, Supplement 1, S60–S64

VINING, E. P. G. (1987) Cognitive dysfunction associated with antiepileptic drug therapy. *Epilepsia*, **28**, Supplement 2, S18–S22

WHITMORE, K. and HOLDSWORTH, L. (1971) *Some Observations from a Study of Children with Epilepsy who were Attending Ordinary Schools*. Spastics Society Study Group on Medical Aspects of Children with School Difficulties, Durham, England:

WORSTER-DROUGHT, C. (1971) An unusual form of acquired aphasia in children. *Developmental Medicine and Child Neurology*, **13**, 563–571

# Chapter 22

# Diagnosis and differential diagnosis of epilepsy

Paediatric neurology may be defined as the application of the neurological sciences to the developing, learning and growing child. As a discipline, it has contributed significantly to the ways in which the neurological problems of children, including epilepsy, are evaluated.

## History taking

Careful and detailed history taking remains the essential cornerstone of accurate diagnosis (Brett, 1990). This will usually be obtained from the parents, and older patients may be able to contribute subjective information about their complaint. An eye-witness account of the attack by a parent, teacher or nurse, if the seizure occurs in hospital, is extremely useful in distinguishing the different types of epilepsy and in differentiating true epilepsy from other paroxysmal disorders. Attacks are often difficult to describe, and asking the informant to mimic the attack is sometimes useful. A sequential account of the clinical characteristics should be obtained in an attempt to determine if there are focal or lateralizing features present.

It should be remembered, however, that the young patient may be quite unaware of the reasons for his visit to the doctor. A child with true petit mal, for example, may only be made aware that something unusual is happening by the reactions of those close to him. The child who has had a major tonic–clonic attack will have complete amnesia of the event and will remember only the circumstances in which he found himself on recovery. He will, however, realize that something very dramatic has taken place because of the concern shown by his family to him. It is important, therefore, to bear these matters in mind while taking the history from the parents if the child is present.

A full history should include any complaint of subjective sensations preceding the seizure (although an account of these is rarely obtained in young children), the characteristics and duration of the seizure itself and the occurrence of any postictal phenomena such as confusion, headache, drowsiness and sleep. Denis Williams (1968), writing about adults, repeatedly emphasized the importance of asking about the circumstances in which the seizure or seizures occurred, remembering that anyone can have a seizure under exceptional circumstances and that everyday events such as fatigue, fever, illness and emotional upset may precipitate an attack in those with an inherent susceptibility to convulse. Writers, from Hughlings Jackson onwards, have emphasized that epilepsy is a paroxysmal and recurring disorder in which there are disturbances of consciousness, sensation or behaviour of any sort which are caused primarily by cerebral disturbances (Williams, 1968). Since anyone can have a seizure under exceptional circumstances, *the solitary seizure should not lead to a diagnosis of epilepsy* and all that implies for the patient. The problem of the solitary seizure is discussed more fully in Chapter 8.

The history should, of course, include a search for causes, and the family history, the mother's reproductive history, the circumstances of the pregnancy and birth, the events of the newborn period, the developmental milestones of the patient, and the history of any previous illnesses or injuries should all be taken into account. Paediatricians today have learned that early developmental aberrations are particularly relevant to the later progress of the child, and disorders of growth, including intrauterine growth retardation, have a similar significance. Inquiries should be made with regard to the child's emotional development and current behaviour, and about his school progress and learning ability. In younger children aspects of play and the learning of skills should be discussed.

## Clinical examination

Clinical examination of the child should include inspection for the external stigmas of diseases frequently associated with epilepsy, such as tuberose sclerosis and the Sturge–Weber syndrome. Posture, movements and adaptive behaviour are particularly important in infancy and, later on, gait, speech and language development and the acquisition of simple skills should be observed and assessed. Evidence of crippling disorders such as hemiplegia, in which the incidence of epilepsy may be as high as 50%, should be looked for; even a mild degree of asymmetry in the face and limbs may be a clue to the presence of cortical atrophy on the side opposite to that on which somatic atrophy is present. Most paediatricians today are familiar with schemes of examination designed to detect the *'soft' neurological signs* which may indicate the presence of neurological dysfunction (*Table 22.1*). Information about these can be found in the monographs by Paine and Oppé (1966) and Baird and Gordon (1983).

Formal neurological examination should include vital measurements (particularly of the head circumference); observation for any asymmetries in skull, face or limbs; auscultation for intracranial bruits; examination of the nervous system generally and, of course, examination of the fundi. A general physical examination should not be neglected; for example, enlargement of the liver and the spleen may be associated with certain degenerative disorders of the central nervous system resulting in seizures, and congenital heart disease may be complicated by cerebral thrombosis or cerebral abscess which may later be followed by the development of epilepsy. The assessment of the higher nervous activities probably comes under the heading of investigation, but the doctor experienced with children will usually be able to make a working estimate of the child's intellectual capacities without recourse to formal psychological testing which may, of course, be necessary later.

**Table 22.1 'Soft' neurological symptoms and signs**

Overactivity
Impulsiveness
Distractibility
Irritability
Emotional immaturity
General clumsiness
Poor visual motor function, e.g. in writing, drawing and catching a ball
Poor performance of skilled acts, e.g. in tying shoelaces and fastening buttons
Abnormalities of gait, e.g. limp and failure to swing arms normally
Positive Fog test, i.e. the child is asked to walk on the outer sides of the feet, when associated movements of arms appear, particularly supination. May identify hemiplegia
Jumping, there is an inability to do so over the age of 3 years
Hopping, there is an inability to do so over the age of 5 years
Difficulties in picking up small objects – absence of pincer grip, athetoid movements, ataxia and tremor
Presence of abnormal movements or tremor on extending upper limbs anteriorly and spreading fingers
Difficulties in imitating gestures carried out by the examiner
Difficulties in performing rapid alternating movements, e.g. pronation/supination
Persistence of mirror or synkinetic movements in older children, e.g. when performing rapid pronation/supination, opposing thumb and individual fingers or performing rapid clenching movements of one hand
Crossed laterality
Speech problems and abnormal tongue movements

# Syncopal attacks

Perhaps the commonest single error at all ages is to label *syncopal or fainting attacks* as epileptic. Syncope is exceedingly common and there are very few people who have not experienced this disturbance at some time during their lives. A typical faint usually has an apparent reason, such as standing still for a time (especially in school or in church), a warm and stuffy atmosphere, pain, emotional upset, the sight of blood or a lurid film or television presentation. Some people faint on exposure to cold which makes diving into the sea or swimming pools a risky business. A simple faint rarely happens without some warning and the onset is slower than in epilepsy. The usual premonitions are muscle weakness, tremor, nausea or a sinking feeling in the abdomen, sweating and lightheadedness. These feelings may persist after a return to full consciousness, in contrast to epilepsy where consciousness is clouded following the attack. Simple fainting usually occurs when the patient is standing or sitting and not when he is lying down. If the patient falls he tends to slump slowly to the ground or he may have time to reach a chair before failing, whereas falling in epilepsy is a sudden and dramatic event. An eye-witness account is invaluable because deathly pallor is the rule in fainting and the peripheral pulse is impalpable. If a deathly pallor does not occur and if unconsciousness lasts more than a few seconds, then the attack is unlikely to be a simple faint. Recovery of full consciousness is usually rapid following syncope compared with slow recovery after an epileptic seizure.

The immediate cause of syncope is cerebral ischaemia and anoxia and the attack may be aborted by lowering the head below the level of the heart or by lying down and, when that happens, consciousness is not lost. It is important to realize that patients in syncope may stiffen, jerk, be incontinent of urine or even bite their tongues by accident in falling during a simple faint. The jerky movements occur at the conclusion of the syncopal attack and are always clonic and few in number. They may be preceded by brief tonic stiffening, especially causing brief flexion of the upper limbs. The clonic movements never precede a simple faint. Such a seizure is properly entitled an anoxic seizure and is a direct result of the acute deprivation of blood and oxygen supply to the brain consequent on cardiac asystole (Stephenson, 1990). In the author's experience and that of others, syncope can occur at any age from babyhood onwards (Sheldon, 1952), although it is probably more common in later childhood and early adolescence and in females.

Illingworth (1956) drew attention to an uncommon cause of syncope in early life due to abnormality and fusion of the cervical vertebrae in the Klippel–Feil syndrome. The usual story is that the child faints after any sudden movement of the neck. The attack is usually brief and leaves no sequelae. It was suggested that the cause of the syncope might be sudden compression of an abnormally placed medulla oblongata. In one such personal case, the patient had been on unnecessary antiepileptic medication for several years.

EEG examination is usually not necessary in the diagnosis of syncope unless atypical features are present. It is important to stress that even physicians experienced in the diagnosis of epilepsy can be misled by apparent syncopal attacks at times and an EEG can be salutary. An ECG or even ambulatory ECG monitoring may be indicated when the diagnosis is in doubt or for suspected cardiac arrhythmias.

Parents should be reassured that syncopal attacks do no harm and, especially, that they do not damage the brain in any way. They should be advised that syncope may recur but that drug therapy is useless and pointless and even injurious to the patient. If the patient has already been put on a drug, usually phenobarbitone, then it should be stopped forthwith. One frequently obtains a family history of syncope in parents, so presumably an unstable vasomotor centre can be inherited.

## Breath-holding attacks

Another very common problem in early childhood, and one familiar to all paediatricians, is that of breath-holding attacks. These have been the subject of medical writing for centuries and the reader is referred particularly to the outstanding reviews by Lombroso and Lerman (1967) and by Stephenson (1990). The clinical story is that the child is, without warning, frightened, hurt, frustrated or angry; he cries vigorously for one or a few breaths and then holds his breath in the expiratory phase of respiration. After a few seconds he becomes more or less cyanotic, loses consciousness and falls limply. The limpness may be followed by a few jerks or even by a short period of stiffening. When such attacks occur frequently or are followed by longer periods of unconsciousness, or when apnoea and loss of consciousness supervene early after crying or even after a gasp only, or when marked stiffening or opisthotonos or even genuine convulsive movements develop then alarm and concern are aroused and it is not surprising that a diagnosis of epilepsy is suspected or misapplied to the patient. Although cyanosis is usual in breath-holding attacks, marked pallor may be present instead, and Lombroso and Lerman (1967) distinguished what they termed the cyanotic and pallid types of infantile syncope to cover these two types of attack.

The frequency of the attacks varies greatly, ranging from very occasional attacks to several times a day. Affected children soon outgrow their problem, and there is a sharp fall in frequency after the third birthday. In the Boston series (Lombroso and Lerman, 1967) 85% of the children were free of attacks by 5 years of age. No significant relationship to either mental retardation or later epilepsy was found. The only reported fatality in a breath-holding attack probably followed the aspiration of gastric contents (Paulson, 1963) and there is no convincing evidence at the present time to indicate that cyanotic breath-holding attacks are other than benign (Stephenson, 1991). One striking observation by the Boston group was that 17% of their cases went on to develop syncopal attacks later. Conversely, some adults suffering from syncope have a history of breath-holding attacks in early childhood.

Many different *mechanisms* for the attacks have been proposed. Emotional factors are certainly involved, and the attacks are most frequent during the normal developmental phase of negativism. Males predominate and many of those affected are described by their parents as being demanding and rather stubborn children. Heredity and familial factors are also important and, in the Boston series, a family history of breath holding was obtained twice as often among the patients compared with the controls (23% against 1.1%). The elements of surprise and unexpectedness in whatever triggers the attack have already been mentioned. Vulliamy (1956) suggested that the basic mechanism was an acute reduction in cerebral blood flow produced by a sharp rise in intrathoracic pressure or Valsalva-like manoeuvre caused by breath holding in the expiratory phase, similar to the mechanism of the 'fainting lark' to be described later (*see* page 219). The initial crying produced hypocapnia due to hyperventilation and this, it was suggested, caused cerebral vasoconstriction. Then, when the breath was held suddenly in expiration, the intrathoracic pressure rose suddenly, producing a decrease in the effective perfusion pressure in the cerebral arterial vasculature by increasing jugular venous pressure and/or decreasing carotid arterial pressure. It has proved difficult to confirm this hypothesis experimentally in patients, for obvious reasons.

Gastaut and Gastaut (1958) demonstrated that attacks similar to breath-holding attacks could be produced by ocular compression (the oculocardiac or oculovagal reflex) and they monitored ECG, EEG and respiration during these induced attacks. They demonstrated that the loss of consciousness in these reflexly induced episodes was due to acute cerebral hypoxia secondary to vagal cardiac arrest and respiratory arrest. They concluded that the basic pathological physiology of clinical breath-holding attacks was a 'familial hypervagotonia' which was reflexly triggered by emotional or external factors, such as a sudden unexpected blow on the head (particularly in the occipital region), and which resulted in cardiac and respiratory inhibition and sudden loss of consciousness due to cerebral hypoxia.

The Boston study (Lombroso and Lerman, 1967) also used the oculocardiac reflex test on their patients (with resuscitation equipment on standby) and used similar monitoring methods. They defined a positive result to the test as a period of cardiac asystole of 2 seconds' duration or longer. They divided their cases into three groups, as follows:

1  The first and largest group (62%) were children in whom the evolution of the attacks corresponded to the usually described pattern, i.e. a stimulus followed by vigorous crying, with apnoea and cyanosis preceding unconsciousness. Only one-quarter of this group had an asystole of 2 seconds' duration or longer.

2  The second group (19%) consisted of patients who lost consciousness much more quickly than the first group, with a minimum of crying and usually without cyanosis. Pallor was often described in this group and some went on to

have stiffening or opisthotonos and convulsive movements. Nearly, two-thirds of this group had a period of asystole lasting 2 seconds or more. Where periods of asystole of 8 seconds or more were recorded, clinical convulsive seizures developed at the end of the attack.

3  In this group (19%) clinical features of both types were present in the same individual.

Following this study, Lombroso and Lerman (1967) proposed that two types of attacks could follow a noxious stimulus, i.e. cyanotic and pallid. They suggested that they were caused by different mechanisms, both leading to acute cerebral anoxia, and that both mechanisms could occasionally operate in the same child at different times. In the more common cyanotic type, they agreed that the mechanism suggested by Vulliamy (1956) was probably responsible, whereas in the pallid type, they thought that the sudden circulatory failure secondary to asystole was clearly responsible. In both instances acute cerebral anoxia was the end-result and was responsible for the loss of consciousness. Lombroso and Lerman (1967) also demonstrated marked generalized slowing of activity in the EEG during the early hypoxic stage of the attack which was followed by flattening of the record (electrical silence) if the attack was prolonged and cerebral anoxia supervened. They suggested that the electrical silence in the EEG was probably due to cessation of cortical neuronal activity and that the stiffening, opisthotonos and tonic seizures occasionally seen in prolonged attacks were due to the release of brain-stem structures from control by corticoreticular inhibitory fibres consequent on acute deprivation of blood and oxygen to the cerebral cortex (an anoxic cerebral seizure).

Lombroso and Lerman (1967) also found differences in the description of precipitating factors in the cyanotic group when compared with the pallid group. Emotional stimuli leading to frustration and anger were more commonly reported in the former, whereas minor injuries and sudden frights were more common in the latter. In the pallid group, unexpected blows on the head, especially in the occipital region, were frequently provocative and were more likely to occur in toddlers learning to walk. This difference in triggering mechanisms seems to tally with the alternative causative mechanisms proposed. They were surprised, as indeed most paediatricians have been, by the innocuous nature of the attacks as far as the child is concerned, considering their dramatic nature and rather terrifying pathological physiology. Stephenson (1978, 1983, 1990) has written extensively on what he terms the reflex anoxic seizures, the type II of Lombroso and Lerman. Although a painful surprise is the usual precipitant, these episodes can also occur during febrile illnesses and, if vagal-mediated cardiac asystole is prolonged, a generalized convulsion may occur in a susceptible child and be mistaken for a true febrile convulsion. This type of febrile convulsive syncope, although very similar clinically to a febrile convulsion, has a different natural history and episodes may recur into adolescence or even adulthood. Investigation should attempt to define this entity by demonstrating the sensitive oculovagal reflex during combined ECG/EEG recording. It should also be remembered that an estimated 5–10% of children with febrile convulsions may, on other occasions, suffer afebrile convulsions consequent on this type of anoxic syncope (i.e. anoxic cerebral seizures).

In the Boston series (Lombroso and Lerman, 1967), 76% of patients commenced their breath-holding attacks between 6 and 18 months of age, and most observers have reported them as being most frequent between the first and second birthdays. An onset in the early weeks of life was reported in a small number of patients in the

Boston group, but Livingstone (1972) felt that transient airway obstruction by aspirated milk or mucus could stimulate a breath-holding spasm. The author has seen undoubted simple cyanotic breath-holding attacks in early infancy but the clinician should also be aware of the phenomenon of prolonged expiratory apnoea in infancy which is described below. An infant who shows abnormal breathing patterns, excess periodic breathing or short or prolonged apnoeic episodes should be observed closely and perhaps monitored as a potential sudden infant death syndrome (Avery and Frantz, 1983). Breath-holding attacks uncommonly begin after the age of 2 years.

As regards treatment, children with breath-holding attacks are often prescribed sedative or anticonvulsant drugs either because a mistaken diagnosis of epilepsy is made or because the attending doctor believes that these drugs prevent or reduce the frequency of the spells. There is absolutely no evidence to support this view and, as has been repeatedly stressed in this book, these drugs should be avoided in children unless they are genuinely indicated for conditions such as true epilepsy. McWilliam and Stephenson (1984) reported a very successful trial of atropine metho-nitrate (Eumydrin) in a small series of children with unusually severe or frequent reflex anoxic seizures, i.e the second group of Lombroso and Lerman, who had originally suggested the use of atropine in 1967. However, the frequency of attacks is often reduced after a correct diagnosis has been made and after advice and reassurance have been given, simply because parents worry less about the condition and the emotional temperature surrounding the problem is reduced.

Finally, parents have tried a large repertoire of counter-stimuli to abort or terminate the attack with varying degrees of success. These include hearty slaps on the thighs or buttocks, the application of cold water or a wet flannel to the face, depressing the tongue and lower jaw with a blunt object and even throwing the child up in the air. Since recovery is variable, the wise parent faced with a wrathful child might be better advised to avoid adding injury to insult and simply do nothing. The innocuous nature of breath-holding spells should be strongly emphasized to anxious parents (Gordon, 1987; Stephenson, 1991).

As with many other apparently completely benign disorders in medicine, there are some traps for the unwary in the matter of cyanotic breath-holding attacks. Southall and his colleagues (1985) drew attention to the occurrence of prolonged cyanotic breath-holding episodes or what they termed 'prolonged expiratory apnoea' in infancy and its association with the presence of various abnormalities. In infancy, such prolonged apnoea may culminate in sudden death. Such attacks have been observed in association with developmental problems, following surgical treatment to the upper and lower airways, or following respiratory distress syndrome. Abnormalities of respiratory control have been postulated and Hunt (1991) recently reviewed this difficult topic. Apnoea in infancy may also occur with complex partial seizures and prolonged apnoea has been reported with brain-stem neoplasms (see review by Gordon, 1987). Apnoeic episodes during sleep in association with upper airway obstruction (obstructive sleep apnoea syndrome) manifest themselves by snoring, attacks of apnoea, difficult breathing during sleep, mouth breathing, restless sleep, and daytime somnolence. Secondary cor pulmonale is a possible complication. Obstructive sleep apnoea is very uncommon in infancy, most sufferers being from 2 to 8 years of age. However, early symptoms of the condition may begin before the first birthday. Careful investigation to assess the nature and extent of the airway obstruction is essential (Gordon, 1988; Editorial, 1989).

## Apparent fainting and sudden death

The syndrome of apparent fainting and sudden death in children is fortunately very rare but needs to be described briefly. Three different syndromes have been described, as follows:

1   The syndrome of Jervell and Lange-Nielsen (1957) (also called the surdocardiac syndrome) is characterized by neurogenic deafness, attacks of ventricular arrhythmia and a prolonged Q-T interval in the ECG present between attacks.
2   The syndrome described by Ward (1964) and also by Romano, Gemme and Pongiglione (1963), in which children have normal hearing but suffer from attacks of ventricular arrhythmia with a prolonged Q-T interval in the ECG (Ward–Romano syndrome).
3   A syndrome with multiple extrasystoles and attacks of ventricular arrhythmia, a prolonged Q-T interval and normal hearing.

The attacks are essentially similar to Stokes–Adams attacks in adults, and in children they may occur after strenuous exercise. One of Ward's cases occurred in a girl who lost consciousness while swimming vigorously in a pool. Epilepsy, simple syncope and breath-holding attacks are often mistaken diagnoses. An ECG is mandatory in any child who has attacks of loss of consciousness after exercise. Prophylactic treatment with beta-blocking agents or with phenytoin (which shortens the Q-T interval) has met with limited success and, unfortunately, the life of a child with one of these syndromes often hangs by a thread (Rennie and Arnold, 1984).

A variant of the prolonged Q-T syndrome in which the Q-T interval is normal but where severe ventricular arrhythmias occur on exercise or emotion has been described and mistaken diagnoses of epilepsy have been made in these patients also (Rutter and Southall, 1985).

## The fainting lark and mess trick

The 'fainting lark' and 'mess trick' are still occasionally practised by schoolboys. Usually, the method employed is to squat on the haunches and take several deep breaths. The individual then rises to his feet, closes his nostrils with his fingers and blows hard. Alternatively, the trick is played on a victim by others who persuade him to hyperventilate and then somebody standing behind him suddenly compresses his chest. Sudden brief loss of consciousness results in both instances. The first method is called the 'fainting lark' and the latter the 'mess trick'. In both the physiological mechanism is similar to that described for the cyanotic type of breath-holding attack. Although usually harmless, occasional fatalities occur as happened in a 12-year-old boy who fell during a self-induced attack and sustained intracerebral bleeding (Murphy, Wilkinson and Pollack, 1981). Hysterical overbreathing in adolescents can also lead to loss of consciousness.

## Benign paroxysmal vertigo

The first mention of *benign paroxysmal vertigo*, like many other original observations in paediatrics, can be attributed to Still (1909). It was fully described by Basser in 1964. This condition is important because it is often confused with epilepsy, but a distinguishing feature is the absence of loss of consciousness. It occurs in children aged 1–5 years, who are bright and neurologically normal. There are multiple brief episodes of sudden onset and without warning and they may last for up to 30 seconds (but sometimes longer), during which the child is frightened, unsteady and may fall. He clings to his mother, may sweat or even vomit. If he is old enough to describe his symptoms, then he will refer to a sensation of rotation. He seeks something to support himself and if this is not available he will sit down or crawl. Nystagmus may be observed. There is no loss of consciousness, no amnesia for the attack nor any postical symptoms. The frequency of attacks varies from rare to several in a week; the EEGs are invariably normal, but caloric tests show abnormalities of vestibular function (Koenigsberger *et al.*, 1970). The evidence available points to a self-limiting peripheral lesion, but neither its precise location nor its nature is clear. The attacks wane with maturation and usually disappear by the age of 4 or 5 years. However, they may be succeeded, after an interval, by the development of classical migraine attacks and a family history of migraine in patients with benign paroxysmal vertigo should suggest this possibility (Koehler, 1980).

*Vestibular neuronitis* is a condition which occurs in adults a few days after an upper respiratory tract infection. It can also occur in children but is not a paroxysmal disorder as is benign paroxysmal vertigo.

*Vertigo* can manifest itself as a symptom of temporal lobe epilepsy, usually with clouding or loss of consciousness, but this is very rare in the author's experience despite a report to the contrary (Eviatar and Eviatar, 1977). It must always be borne in mind that the list of *drugs* which can cause vertigo as a chronic side-effect is endless, and acute accidental self-administered poisoning by drugs or alcohol producing vertigo is well known to those working in the admission departments of children's hospitals. In practice, the main problem with recurrent vertigo in young children is to be aware of the existence of benign paroxysmal vertigo, to apply reassurance and avoid unnecessary medication.

## Other disturbances

Young children, usually between $2\frac{1}{2}$ and $3\frac{1}{2}$ years of age, quite commonly engage in peculiar *ritualistic movements* when they are tired, particularly when they are put down to sleep. They may recur if the child wakens in the night. They may be seen while the child is sitting at table or in a highchair, particularly if he is bored. The usual pattern is one of slow squirming hand movements which are sometimes accompanied by lower limb movements. The eyes may appear blank or may turn up, the child may laugh or giggle in a rather inane fashion. The movements stop immediately when the child's name is called. The ritual is constantly being added to and may become quite prolonged. The remote withdrawn behaviour of the child alarms parents and it may be misdiagnosed as petit mal, in much the same way as daydreaming at school in older children may be similarly mislabelled. There can be no doubt that the child finds the movement patterns pleasant and relaxing and, at night, a means of dropping off to sleep.

At times, similar movements may be frankly *masturbatory*. Still (1909) wrote as follows: 'a girl of 5 years, was brought with a history that she would several times a day, when she thought herself not observed by her mother, rock herself backwards and forwards as she sat on her chair, at the same time turning red in the face, and perspiring, and then turning white as if exhausted. Inquiry showed that masturbation occurred at night also.' Masturbation in small children is more common in females. The parents should be told that it is a harmless habit, that the outcome will be favourable, that the condition has no connection with later adolescent or adult sexuality and that the child will suffer no ill-effects on his or her subsequent physical or mental development. The perineal area should be inspected for treatable causes of local irritation such as a rash and the possibility of threadworm infestation should be considered.

*Night terrors* (pavor nocturnus) afflict most children at some time, and adults are not immune from them either. They are often familial and show a strong concordance in monozygotic twins (Kales *et al.*, 1980). They usually occur in the first few hours of sleep while the child is in deep non-REM sleep which is associated with high voltage slow waves in the EEG. *Nightmares*, on the other hand, occur in the lighter REM sleep with which dreaming is associated and which is a feature later in the night or towards morning. In a night terror, a few strangled words or cries precede screaming and the child usually sits up staring and wide-eyed. He may stumble from his bed and appears terrified. He does not recognize his worried parents or respond to their comforting words. However, within minutes he settles down to a sound sleep again and remembers little or nothing of the event next morning. In a nightmare, the child will awake and give an account of the frightening dream experience. It must be clearly understood that neither are epileptic phenomena nor are they usually associated with any particular emotional disorder affecting the child at home or in school (Kales, Soldatos and Kales, 1987). Gastaut and Broughton (1965) polygraphically recorded episodes of night terror and, in every case, they demonstrated that the attack occurred during intense and sudden arousal from deep slow-wave sleep. The form of management required is also different in the two conditions. In general, it is appropriate and possible to comfort a child who has woken from a nightmare. Attempts to wake a child in a night terror may cause him/her confusion and distress. Calm reassurance and holding until the episode subsides and preventing self-injury are required (Stores, 1991). If the attacks are very frequent then diazepam, which significantly reduces the amount of non-REM sleep, may be prescribed at bedtime (2–4 mg orally). The doctor should firmly reassure the parents that the condition is common and benign and that the child will grow out of it.

*Narcolepsy*, in contrast to night terrors, is a disorder of sleep rather than a disorder of arousal. The characteristic symptom is recurrent daytime episodes of irresistible drowsiness and sleep. These may or may not be associated with the following:

1   Cataplexy, which is a sudden loss of muscle tone resulting in a fall to the ground while consciousness is maintained.
2   Sleep paralysis, which is a sudden awareness, while falling asleep or during sleep, that one cannot move or cry out.
3   Hypnagogic hallucinations which consist of vivid visual or auditory imagery occurring at the onset of sleep.

The irresistible sleep attacks are commonly the only presenting symptom in childhood and they may be followed by any or all of the other symptoms after a variable period of time, usually earlier rather than later in paediatric patients compared with adults (Young *et al.*, 1988). Cataplexy is the commonest associated phenomenon to develop. In those individuals with a history of cataplexy, sleep paralysis or hypnagogic hallucinations, investigations have shown that they are associated with the intrusion of REM sleep upon wakefulness. Loss of peripheral muscle tone is a normal physiological correlate of REM sleep, accounting for the cataplexy and sleep paralysis. The hypnagogic hallucinations resemble dreams recounted after awakening from normal REM sleep. In contrast to normal individuals who enter sleep through a prolonged non-REM period, people with cataplexy, sleep paralysis and hypnagogic hallucinations exhibit a prolonged initial REM period both in daytime attacks and in nocturnal sleep, and in this their sleep pattern resembles that of the neonate. Individuals who have only attacks of irresistible sleep without the other auxiliary features of the syndrome may not demonstrate this unusual transition to REM sleep but they show the normal descending pattern to non-REM sleep both in their daytime attacks and in nocturnal sleep. It has been suggested that the term narcolepsy should be restricted to those whose daytime attacks are characterized by the sudden transition from wakefulness to REM sleep and that, if this sequence is not present, some other condition is responsible for the attacks of involuntary sleep. Therefore, it seems wise to recommend careful EEG investigation in alleged cases of narcolepsy in order to determine the sequence of events. If available, the technique of polysomnography, in which multiple physiological events, including the EEG, are recorded, should be employed (Young et al., 1988).

The aetiology of narcolepsy remains obscure. Genetic factors are suggested by a positive family history in some cases. Emotional factors, particularly tension and anxiety, may precipitate attacks. In some children, the attacks may appear to be self induced and associated with emotional problems in the family or school situation, but these cases should be investigated to determine whether they have true narcolepsy. Drugs such as the amphetamines, methylphenidate hydrochloride and the monoamine oxidase inhibitors have been tried in treatment, and of these dextro-amphetamine, which reduces REM sleep while minimally interfering with other sleep stages, seems very successful. A suitable dose would be 5 mg given in the morning, but smaller doses may be effective or larger doses may be required in some cases.

Narcolepsy is in no sense an epileptic disorder, but it may be misinterpreted as one. The 'sleep jerks', which occur in many normal children and adults while dropping off to sleep, may alarm parents and be misdiagnosed as epilepsy by some doctors, but they are normal phenomena. Even nocturnal enuresis and somnambulism may be labelled epileptic occasionally, particularly, or so it seems to the author, by psychiatrists. There is no evidence to connect these disorders with epilepsy although, of course, the child having a true nocturnal seizure may wet his bed. The reader interested in sleep disorders in infants and children is referred to the reviews by Anders and Weinstein (1972) and Tassinari et al. (1977). Stores (1991) has published an excellent review detailing the problems which may arise in the differential diagnosis between sleep disorders and the childhood and adolescent epilepsies (also see Chapter 17).

It is worth noting that *delirium* during acute febrile illnesses and even rigors may be mistaken for epileptic attacks. Children are prone to run much higher fevers with acute infections than are adults and rigors may be mistaken for febrile convulsions. Shivering and the lack of any real loss of consciousness will help to identify the rigor although the distinction can sometimes be difficult. However, it is an important clinical distinction in view of the controversy about the necessity of drug prophylaxis for children with febrile convulsions. *Shuddering spells* in infancy and early childhood may be confused with myoclonic epilepsy (Holmes and Russman, 1986).

*Hypoglycaemia* may occasionally present a problem in differential diagnosis. Convulsions are one of the commonest presenting symptoms of hypoglycaemia at any age and have already been described in connection with neonatal hypoglycaemia. During infancy, rare metabolic disorders such as hypoglycaemia due to leucine intolerance and hereditary fructose intolerance may present with seizures.

Infants or young children may unexpectedly develop hypoglycaemia, associated with an acute disturbance of consciousness (drowsiness, lethargy leading to coma) and sometimes with generalized seizures, in a setting of an acute febrile illness complicated by anorexia, vomiting and diarrhoea. Up to 1975, such dramatic illnesses were described by the general term of 'ketotic hypoglycaemia'. Since then, remarkable advances have been made in the knowledge of inborn errors of mitochondrial fatty acid oxidation, several of which have now been defined (Vianey-Liaud *et al.*, 1987; Nyhan, 1988). Oxidation of fatty acids is an essential energy supply for the cell, especially when glucose availability is decreased, as it may be in acute childhood illnesses where fasting and increased metabolic demand consequent on high fever occur in addition to gastrointestinal symptoms. The consequences of any defect of fatty acid catabolism are dramatic when the glucose supply is diminished. They involve, firstly, lack of energy for vital tissues due to impairment of production of ketone bodies (hepatic hypoketogenesis) and, secondly, a blocking of gluconeogenesis. The resulting hypoglycaemia is non-ketotic, since the synthesis of ketone bodies is deficient. Ketonuria, if it occurs, may be absent or slight although in the commonest variety of defect, medium-chain acyl coenzyme A dehydrogenase deficiency (MCAD), ward tests for urinary ketones may sometimes be strongly positive. An important differentiating feature from Reye's syndrome is the absence of hyperammonaemia. The finding of hypoketonuria with severe hypoglycaemia is highly suggestive of a fatty acid oxidation defect. Blood and urine specimens should always be preserved for analysis for fatty acids (so-called dicarboxylic aciduria) in such a clinical situation since diagnosis largely depends on the identification of abnormal plasma and urinary metabolites during acute attacks. A similar situation may obtain in the child who fails to make the expected recovery from an anaesthetic or who is unusually drowsy, has a seizure or is found to be hypoglycaemic postoperatively. This was the sequence of events in a personal case of MCAD deficiency presenting in a 2-year old after a simple operation.

A more specific diagnosis is based on the identification of the enzymatic defects. This involves global assays which allow a localization of the 'level' of the defect (i.e. the oxidation of long, medium or short chain fatty acids) and specific measurement of enzyme activities. The precise identification of these disorders is of prime importance because of the severity of the clinical symptoms and because of the risk of sudden death in an attack.

Treatment of these disorders consists mainly of the use of dietary measures to decrease the endogenous production of harmful metabolites. With certain rare exceptions, a regime of a high carbohydrate intake to compensate for impaired gluconeogenesis and to decrease lipolysis can be generally recommended (Przyrembel, 1987). Additional fat restriction and the oral use of L-carnitine (a substance present in large amounts in skeletal muscle and involved in mitochondrial oxidation processes) may be necessary in some patients. Genetic counselling for families is mandatory in these disorders which are inherited in an autosomal recessive manner.

In any child with a hypoglycaemic tendency, the possible coexistence with epilepsy should be remembered, with the former precipitating the latter on occasions. The presence of persistent paroxysmal EEG abnormalities will usually clarify the situation. Phenytoin has a slight hyperglycaemic effect and may be a suitable choice as antiepileptic therapy.

It has long been apparent to clinicians that there are striking points of similarity between epilepsy and *migraine*. Both are common paroxysmal disorders and in both the patient may appear perfectly normal between attacks. Neither condition has any specific abnormal physical findings. Although there is no diagnostic test for migraine, nevertheless the EEG may be mildly abnormal in a majority of affected children and sometimes the abnormality may be epileptiform in type (Hockaday and Whitty, 1969). A further similarity between the two conditions is that hereditary factors in conjunction with environmental factors seem important in causation. The two conditions may co-exist; there is an increased incidence of epilepsy in migraineurs and of migraine in patients with epilepsy (Andermann and Andermann, 1987).

The distinction between migraine and epilepsy is usually easy. Prensky and Sommer (1979) list the following criteria for diagnosis in children: (1) nausea, vomiting or abdominal pain in association with headache; (2) localized or generalized hemicrania; (3) a throbbing quality of headache; (4) relief after sleep; (5) visual, sensory or motor aura; (6) a history of migraine in 1st or 2nd degree relatives. However at times, differentiation between the two conditions can be extremely difficult. Headache is a common postictal symptom after both generalized and partial seizures, although rarely after simple partial seizures. Classical migraine beginning with focal neurological signs may be mistaken for a simple partial seizure. During the aura which often precedes the migraine headache, scotomata, perceptual distortions, paraesthesiae, aphasia, or mood changes may be experienced and may be misinterpreted as an epileptic aura (Rossi, Mumenthaler and Vassella, 1980). Normally consciousness is retained during the migraine attack but, rarely, the condition may be manifested by an acute confusional state which may be unassociated with headache (Gascon and Barlow, 1970). This symptom-complex is particularly associated with basilar artery migraine in children, a condition also characterized by non-lateralized headaches, vertigo, ataxia, visual disturbances and sometimes by alternating hemiplegia (Hockaday, 1979). It is also worth noting that loss of consciousness due to syncope may occur during a migraine attack.

A special form of epilepsy entitled benign partial epilepsy of childhood with occipital spike-wave discharges was described by Gastaut in 1982 (see Chapter 9). Visual phenomena are followed by seizures and severe headache and vomiting are frequent postictally. This rare syndrome and other seizures associated with visual phenomena may present problems in differential diagnosis from migraine and the difficulties are well discussed by Deonna and Ziegler (1984). When both epilepsy and migraine co-exist in the same patient, the clinical phenomena of the two conditions are usually quite distinct. When the clinical phenomena are associated, the migraine is either the triggering factor for a seizure or else the severe migraine-type headaches follow the seizure as a prominent postictal feature. The comprehensive monograph on migraine in childhood by Hockaday (1989) is strongly recommended to the reader.

Migraine is often included in the group of recurrent disorders in childhood entitled *periodic syndromes*. Abdominal pain is a common periodic complaint in children and Apley and Naish (1958), in a survey of 1000 unselected schoolchildren, found that it occurred in 1 in every 9 of the children studied. Emotional causes are usually responsible and an organic cause is rare (Apley, 1975). Recurrent abdominal pain and vomiting in early childhood may presage the later development of migraine but attacks are not associated with impairment of consciousness.

Epilepsy is also a common recurrent disorder in childhood and, in the past, it has been suggested that, when brief episodes of abdominal pain, nausea and occasionally vomiting occurred without apparent gastrointestinal cause, they could be manifestations of an 'epileptic equivalent' entitled 'abdominal epilepsy'. This proposition was reviewed by O'Donohoe (1971). It now seems highly unlikely that such an entity exists. In the author's experience, the causes of recurrent abdominal pain in childhood are usually those so well described by Apley (1975) and O'Donnell (1985). However, there is no doubt that autonomic symptoms and signs may be associated with epileptic discharges arising in the medial temporal area, where there is central representation of abdominal sensation (Penfield and Jasper, 1954), and in the frontal lobe. The most common ictal autonomic symptoms are gastrointestinal, usually abdominal discomfort or nausea, often ascending to the throat (epigastric rising), epigastric abdominal pain, borborygmi, belching, flatulence and even vomiting. Other autonomic symptoms such as pallor, sweating, and alterations in heart rate and respiration may be associated with the foregoing. When such premonitory symptoms constitute the aura of a complex partial seizure, they are followed by impairment of consciousness as the actual ictal event ensues. Given the difficulty that children have in describing auras and the diagnostic difficulties presented by complex partial seizures at any age, it is not surprising that there has been confusion about the problem of so-called abdominal epilepsy. This should reinforce the view that the label of epilepsy should never be applied speculatively and that the diagnosis should be supported by other evidence including, in this particular instance, evidence of alteration of consciousness and specific EEG changes.

## Non-epileptic seizures

Some seizures have a psychogenic basis and distinguishing between epilepsy and non-epilepsy may be easy or difficult or even impossible. It should be remembered furthermore that the two may co-exist in the same patient. Conversion disorders can be regarded as a form of body language or as enactments of sickness that present in response to a predicament of which the resolution is beyond the patient's control (Goodyer and Taylor, 1985). The commonest of these are abdominal pain, limb pains and headaches, and these occur without apparent organic cause in up to 20% of school children. About 2% of paediatric neurological referrals are for conversion disorders and the most common presentations are episodic loss of awareness in the form of pseudoseizures, apparent fainting or swoons (eyes closed, sinking to the floor, lying inert with peculiar eyelid flickering), or following voluntary hyperventilation; motor disorders such as gait abnormalities and pareses; and sensory disorders such as pain and numbness and special sense disorders, especially diplopia. Conversion disorders are extremely rare in children younger than 6 years, the sex ratio is equal under 10 years and, in adolescence, girls predominate in a ratio of 3:1 (Editorial, 1991). In many cases an infection or some other incident seems to precipitate illness behaviour of this kind but the underlying predicament may be hard to identify. Family difficulties are often hidden, although family disharmony is a common feature. A grief reaction may be responsible and incestuous relationships and other forms of sexual abuse are said to be precipitants of pseudoseizures especially (Wyllie et al., 1990). Academic failure and peer conflicts may also be implicated.

As already indicated, differential diagnosis can be very difficult and may require lengthy acquaintance with and study of the patient. This is particularly so with pseudoseizures which may mimic true epileptic seizures to a remarkable degree. So-called hysterical seizures, on the other hand, are usually bizarre and uncoordinated, resembling what the patient thinks an epileptic seizure should be like, and usually occur before an audience. In children, they often closely resemble temper tantrums.

When a conversion disorder is suspected, combined psychiatric and neurological care and investigation offer the best prospect for a definitive diagnosis. Careful history taking and observation of the child during day-to-day activities are essential. Over-investigation should be avoided. EEG examination is, of course, essential and ambulatory or telemetred EEG may be necessary in difficult cases. Non-specific or specific EEG abnormalities present problems in some cases, however, especially in patients with both true and false epilepsy. Combined ictal video and EEG recording of an attack is the ideal for diagnosis (Wyllie *et al.*, 1990) but may not be easily available. Prolactin estimation after a suspect seizure can be very helpful but a baseline estimation is essential for comparison (Rao, Stefan and Bauer, 1989). It is crucial that a true organic disorder should not be overlooked in the investigation of neurological conversion disorders in children and adolescents. True epilepsy can, on occasions, be bizarre in its manifestations and disorders such as cerebral and spinal cord tumours and degenerative diseases of the central nervous system (especially juvenile neuronal ceroid lipofuscinosis and subacute sclerosing panencephalitis) are easily misdiagnosed.

The treatment of these disorders requires careful psychiatric management. Blunt confrontation of the patient with the diagnosis should be avoided. The underlying reasons for the attacks should be carefully explored and attack-free periods should be reinforced with praise while, at the same time, the patient is gently led to a recognition of the non-epileptic nature of the attack. The patient must not be rejected but allowed to save face. Intensive anxiety management and counselling may be necessary for victims of abuse, and relapses at times of stress should be expected (Betts, 1990).

*Epidemic or mass hysteria*, recorded in the medical literature for centuries, still appears regularly in newspaper reports. The condition shows a predilection for adolescents and preadolescents, usually females, and the rapid transmission of the illness is encouraged by sights and sounds such as the sight of blood and the wailing of ambulance and police sirens. Hyperventilation, weakness, dizziness, faintness and actual syncope are common. Rapid recovery is the rule (Small and Nicholi, 1982).

Meadow (1982) has described a condition as '*Munchausen syndrome by proxy*' where mothers consistently give fraudulent clinical histories and fabricated signs thereby causing needless hospital admissions, medical investigations and even treatment of their children over quite prolonged periods of time. Seizures have figured prominently among the spurious symptoms and actual loss of consciousness has been produced by carotid sinus pressure (Meadow, 1984). Recurrent apnoeic episodes, cyanotic attacks, seizures, and sudden death have occurred in infants as a result of repeated suffocation and strangling by parents (Meadow, 1990). The psychopathology in the parents in these special situations is complex and there are associations with the varieties of parental-induced non-accidental injury (Meadow, 1985, 1991).

# Conclusion

The differential diagnosis of epilepsy in children clearly involves a wide range of conditions (Pedley, 1983). Making a correct diagnosis is of paramount importance to the patient and the key to this is careful history taking. The label of epilepsy is a passport to prejudice and, if wrongly applied, it can have a disastrous and even permanent effect on the patient's life. Jeavons (1983) has estimated that 25% of the patients referred to his clinic did not have epilepsy and that this degree of misdiagnosis applied equally to children and adults. Doctors dealing with epilepsy should always look with suspicion at the phrase 'known epileptic' on the case-notes, and the word 'epileptiform' should be banished from the language of clinical description. These terms frequently indicate a reluctance on the part of the individual using them to take a detailed history of the patient's complaint and an additional lack of interest in or ignorance of the nature and clinical characteristics of epilepsy. The splendid monograph entitled 'Fits and Faints' by Stephenson (1990) is strongly recommended as a comprehensive account of the many 'funny turns' which complicate the differential diagnosis of epilepsy.

# References

ANDERMANN, E. and ANDERMANN, F. (1987) Migraine-epilepsy relationships: epidemiological and genetic aspects. In *Migraine and Epilepsy* (eds F. Andermann and E. Lugaresi), Butterworths, London, Boston, pp. 281–291

ANDERS, T. F and WEINSTEIN, M. S. (1972) Sleep and its disorders in infants and children: a review. *Pediatrics*, **50**, 312–325

APLEY, J. (1975) *The Child with Abdominal Pain*. Blackwell Scientific, Oxford

APLEY, J. and NAISH, N. (1958) Recurrent abdominal pains: a field survey of 1000 school children. *Archives of Disease in Childhood*, **33**, 165–170

AVERY, M. E. and FRANTZ, I. D. III (1983) To breathe or not to breathe: what have we learned about apnoeic spells and sudden infant death? *New England Journal of Medicine*, **309**, 107–108

BAIRD, H. W. and GORDON, E. C. (1983) *Neurological Evaluation of Infants and Children*. Clinics in Developmental Medicine, Nos 84/85. Spastics International/Heinemann Medical, London, J. B. Lippincott, Philadelphia

BASSER, L. S. (1964) Benign paroxysmal vertigo of childhood. A variety of vestibular neuronitis. *Brain*, **87**, 141–152

BETTS, T. (1990) Pseudoseizures: seizures that are not epilepsy. *Lancet*, **336**, 163–164

BRETT, E. M. (1990) 'It isn't epilepsy is it, doctor?' *British Medical Journal*, **300**, 1604–1605

DEONNA, T., and ZIEGLER, A. (1984) Paroxysmal visual disturbances of epileptic origin and occipital epilepsy in children. *Neuropediatrics*, **15**, 131–135

EDITORIAL (1989) Airway obstruction during sleep in childhood. *Lancet*, **334**, 1018–1019.

EDITORIAL (1991) Neurological conversion disorders in childhood. *Lancet*, **337**, 889–890.

EVIATAR, L. and EVIATAR A. (1977) Vertigo in children, differential diagnosis and management. *Pediatrics*, **59**, 833–838

GASCON, G. and BARLOW, C. (1970) Juvenile migraine presenting as an acute confusional state. *Pediatrics*, **45**, 628–635

GASTAUT, H. (1982) A new type of epilepsy: benign partial epilepsy of childhood with occipital spike-waves. *Clinical Electroencephalography*, **13**, 13–22.

GASTAUT, H. and BROUGHTON, R. (1965) A clinical and polygraphic study of episodic phenomena during sleep. In *Recent Advances in Biological Psychiatry*, Vol. 7 (ed. J. Wortis), Plenum Press, New York, p. 197

GASTAUT, H. and GASTAUT, Y. (1958) Electroencephalographic and clinical study of anoxic convulsions in children: their place in the framework of infantile convulsions. *Revue Neurologique*, **99**, 100–125

GOODYER, I. and TAYLOR, D. C. (1985) Hysteria. *Archives of Disease in Childhood*, **60**, 680–681

GORDON, N. (1987) Breath-holding spells. *Developmental Medicine and Child Neurology*, **29**: 811–814

GORDON, N. (1988) Nasal obstruction in childhood; the obstructive sleep apnoea syndrome. *Developmental Medicine and Child Neurology*, **30**, 261–265

HOCKADAY, J. H. (1979) Basilar migraine in childhood. *Developmental Medicine and Child Neurology*, **21**, 455–463

HOCKADAY, J. H. edit. (1989) *Migraine in Childhood*. Butterworth Scientific, Guildford.

HOCKADAY, J. H. and WHITTY, C. W. M. (1969) Factors determining the electroencephalogram in migraine: a study of 560 patients according to the clinical type of migraine. *Brain*, **92**, 769–788

HOLMES, G. L. and RUSSMAN, B. S. (1986) Shuddering attacks. *American Journal of Diseases of Children*, **140**, 72–73.

HUNT, C. E. (1991) Relationship between breath-holding spells and cardiorespiratory control: a new perspective. *Journal of Pediatrics*, **117**, 245–247

ILLINGWORTH, R. S. (1956) Attacks of unconsciousness in association with fused cervical vertebrae. *Archives of Disease in Childhood*, **31**, 8–11

JEAVONS, P. M. (1983) Non-epileptic attacks in childhood. In *Research Progress in Epilepsy* (ed. F. C. Rose), Pitman, London, pp. 224–230

JERVELL, A. and LANGE-NIELSEN, F. (1957) Congenital deafmutism and functional heart disease, with prolongation of the Q-T interval and sudden death. *American Heart Journal*, **54**, 59–68

KOEHLER, B. (1980) Benign paroxysmal vertigo of childhood: a migraine equivalent. *European Journal of Pediatrics*, **134**, 149–151

KALES, A., SOLDATOS, C. R., BIXLER, E. O. *et al.* (1980) Hereditary factors in sleep walking and night terrors. *British Journal of Psychiatry*, **137**, 111–118

KALES, A., SOLDATOS, C. R., and KALES, J. D. (1987) Sleep disorders: insomnia, sleep walking, night terrors, nightmares, and enuresis. *Annals of Internal Medicine*, **106**, 582–592

KOENIGSBERGER, M. R., CHUTORIAN, A. M., GOLD, A. P. and SCHVEY, M. S. (1970) Benign paroxysmal vertigo of childhood. *Neurology*, **20**, 1108–1113

LIVINGSTON, S. (1972) *Comprehensive Management of Epilepsy in Infancy, Childhood and Adolescence*, Charles C. Thomas, Springfield, Illinois, p. 35.

LOMBROSO, C. T. and LERMAN, P. (1967) Breath-holding spells (cyanotic and pallid infantile syncope). *Pediatrics*, **39**, 563–581

MCWILLIAM R. C. and STEPHENSON, J. B. P. (1984) Atropine treatment of reflex anoxic seizures. *Archives of Disease in Childhood*, **59**, 473–475

MEADOW, R. (1982) Munchausen syndrome by proxy. *Archives of Disease in Childhood*, **57**, 92–98

MEADOW, R. (1984) Fictitious epilepsy. *Lancet*, **2**, 25–28

MEADOW, R. (1985) Management of Munchausen syndrome by proxy. *Archives of Disease in Childhood*, **60**, 385–393

MEADOW, R. (1990) Suffocation, recurrent apnoea, and sudden death. *Journal of Pediatrics*, **117**, 351–357

MEADOW, R. (1991) Neurological and developmental variants of Munchausen syndrome by proxy. *Developmental Medicine and Child Neurology*, **33**, 267–272

MURPHY, J. V., WILKINSON, I. A. AND POLLACK, N. H. (1981) Death following breath-holding in an adolescent. *American Journal of Diseases of Children*, **135**, 180–181

NYHAN, W. L. (1988) Abnormalities of fatty acid oxidation. *New England Journal of Medicine*, **319**, 1344–1346

O'DONNELL, B. (1985) *Abdominal Pain in Childhood*. Blackwell Scientific Publications, Oxford, London

O'DONOHOE, N. V. (1971) Abdominal epilepsy. *Developmental Medicine and Child Neurology*, **13**, 798–800

PAINE, R. S. and OPPÉ, T. E. (1966) *Neurological Examination of Children*, Clinics in Developmental Medicine, Nos 20/21. Spastics Society/Heinemann Medical, London

PAULSON, G. (1963) Breathholding spells: a fatal case. *Developmental Medicine and Child Neurology*, **5**, 246–251

PEDLEY, T. A. (1983) Differential diagnosis of episodic symptoms. *Epilepsia* (Supplement 1), S31–S44

PENFIELD, W. and JASPER, H. (1954) *Epilepsy and the Functional Anatomy of the Human Brain*, Little, Brown, Boston, p. 422

PRENSKY, A. L. and SOMMER, D. (1979) Diagnosis and treatment of migraine in children. *Neurology*, **29**, 506–510

PRZYREMBEL, H. (1987) Therapy of mitochondrial disorders. *Journal of Inherited Metabolic Disease*, **10**, Supplement 1, 129–146

RAO, M. L., STEFAN, H., BAUER, J. (1989) Epileptic but not psychogenic seizures are accompanied by simultaneous elevation of serum pituitary hormones and cortisol levels. *Neuroendocrinology*, **49**, 33–39

RENNIE, J. M. and ARNOLD, R. (1984) Asystole in the prolonged QT syndrome. *Archives of Disease in Childhood*, **59**, 571–573

ROMANO, C., GEMME, G. and PONGIGLIONE, R. (1963) Aritmic cardiache rare dell' et' pediatrica. *Clinica Pediatrica*, **45**, 656–683

ROSSI, L. N., MUMENTHALER, M. and VASELLA, F. (1980) Complicated migraine (migraine accompagnée) in children. Clinical characteristics and course in 40 personal cases. *Neuropediatrics*, **11**, 27–35

RUTTER, N. and SOUTHALL, D. P. (1985) Cardiac arrhythmias misdiagnosed as epilepsy. *Archives of Disease in Childhood*, **60**, 54–56

SHELDON, W. (1952) Syncopal attacks in infancy. *Great Ormond Street Journal*, **3**, 20–22

SMALL, G. W. and NICHOLI, A. M. (1982) Epidemic hysteria among school children. *Archives of General Psychiatry*, **39**, 721–724

SOUTHALL, D. P., JOHNSON, P., SALMONS, S. (1985) Prolonged expiratory apnoea: a disorder resulting in episodes of severe arterial hypoxaemia in infants and young children. *Lancet*, **326**, 571–577

STEPHENSON, J. B. P. (1979) Reflex anoxic seizures ('white breath-holding'): non-epileptic vagal attacks. *Archives of Disease in Childhood*, **53**, 193–200

STEPHENSON, J. B. P. (1983) Febrile convulsions and reflex anoxic seizures. In: *Research Progress in Epilepsy* (ed. F. C. Rose), Pitman, London, pp. 244–252

STEPHENSON, J. B. P. (1990) *Fits and Faints. Clinics in Developmental Medicine*. No. 109., Blackwell Scientific Publications, Ltd., Oxford

STEPHENSON, J. P. B. (1991) Blue breath holding is benign. *Archives of Disease in Childhood*, **66**, 255–258

STILL, G. F. (1909) *Common Disorders and Diseases of Childhood*. Oxford University Press, Oxford. Also published as Still, G. F. (1938) *Common Happenings in Childhood*. Oxford Medical Publications, London

STORES, G. (1991) Confusions concerning sleep disorders and the epilepsies in children and adolescents. *British Journal of Psychiatry*, **158**, 1–7

TASSINARI, C. A., TERZANO, G., CAPOCCHI, G. *et al.* (1977). Epileptic seizures during sleep in children. In *Epilepsy: The Eighth International Symposium* (ed. J. K. Penry), Raven Press, New York, pp. 345–354

VIANEY-LIAUD, C., DIVRY, P., GREGERSEN, N., and MATHIEU, M. (1987) The inborn errors of mitochondiral fatty acid oxidation. *Journal of Inherited Metabolic Disease*, **10**, Supplement 1, 159–198

VULLIAMY, D. C. (1956) Breath-holding attacks. *Practitioner*, **177**, 517–519

WARD, O. C. (1964) A new familial cardiac syndrome in children. *Journal of the Irish Medical Association*, **54**, 103–106

WILLIAMS, D. (1968) The management of epilepsy. *British Journal of Hospital Medicine*, **2**, 702–707

WYLLIE, E., FRIEDMAN, D., ROTHNER, D. *et al.* (1990). Psychogenic seizures in children and adolescents: outcome after diagnosis by ictal video and electroencephalographic recording. *Pediatrics*, **85**, 480–484

YOUNG, D., ZORICK, F., WITTIG, R. *et al.* (1988). Narcolepsy in a pediatric population. *American Journal of Diseases of Children*, **142**, 210–213

# Chapter 23

# Investigation of epilepsy in childhood

In childhood epilepsy, as a general rule, investigations should be kept to the minimum necessary for making a firm diagnosis and for the exclusion of treatable causes. Linnett (1982), in an eloquent discussion on what he calls 'the burden of epilepsy' as seen from the standpoint of a general practitioner, emphasizes that, in the investigation of childhood epilepsy, a delicate balance has to be maintained between adding to parental anxiety by subjecting the child to a battery of interviews, tests and complex investigations, and the need to establish a firm diagnosis. He emphasizes that the latter may make parental fears less dreadful and formless in the relief of knowing what it is they have to face. It is important to remember that the child may not be aware of his complaint or he may be aware that something is wrong only as a consequence of the reactions of his parents and siblings. Therefore, a full diagnostic onslaught in hospital may bewilder and frighten the small patient. If possible, investigations should be performed on an outpatient basis or, at the very least, the period of hospitalization should be minimized. A close liaison should be maintained at all times between the specialist, the parents and their family doctor, and the medical personnel involved should allow adequate time for explanation to the parents of what is taking place.

The extent of the investigations will, of course, be determined to a large extent by the type of epilepsy being studied and will be based on the 'working' diagnosis reached after full history taking and physical examination. At all times the physician should resist the modern mania for excessive investigation. This is always expensive and time consuming and frequently in the worst interests of the patient. There are no 'routine' investigations: there are only those that are indicated by the specific diagnostic problem presented by the patient.

## Laboratory investigation

The investigation of epilepsy may, in certain cases, involve tests of renal function, serological tests (especially for viral infections), studies of the concentration of serum proteins and amino acids, chromosome analysis and even the highly elaborate studies involved in the differentiation of the various degenerative disorders of brain, nerve and muscle in childhood and of the rarer metabolic disorders. Establishing hypoglycaemia as a cause of first or recurrent seizures may require measurement of blood glucose at the time of the attack. Hypocalcaemia is rarely a diagnostic problem after the neonatal period but clinical signs of hypoparathyroidism may suggest its presence.

Specific neurological tests include diagnostic taps and plain skull radiography. Lumbar puncture should certainly not be regarded as a routine investigation. It is essential for the diagnosis of meningitis or encephalitis presenting with seizures or where seizures are associated with degenerative processes in the central nervous system such as metachromatic leucodystrophy or SSPE. In both conditions, a raised cerebrospinal fluid protein concentration may be found. Lumbar puncture should, of course, never be done where there is any suspicion of raised intracranial pressure.

## Radiography

Plain radiography of the skull may be revealing in the secondary generalized epilepsies of early childhood where calcification consequent on tuberose sclerosis, intrauterine cytomegalovirus disease or congenital toxoplasmosis may be seen. Characteristic intracranial calcification may also develop later in the Sturge–Weber syndrome. Cerebral lesions occurring in early childhood frequently exert an influence on the growth of the skull bones. This was studied by Miribel, Vieto and Favel (1963). They demonstrated that where hemiplegia follows a hemiconvulsive episode in the first 2 years of life, hemiatrophy of the cranium on the affected side followed almost invariably, and similar changes were frequent where the cerebral insult occurred between 2 and 4 years of age. From 4 years onwards the incidence of skull bone involvement decreased rapidly.

In temporal lobe epilepsy due to mesial temporal sclerosis, there may be associated bony changes in the ipsilateral middle cranial fossa, including flattening of the vault, elevation of the base and enlargement of nearby air cavities in bone. The overlying skull may also be thickened. These X-ray changes may be useful additional evidence for lateralizing the brain lesion when surgery is being contemplated. However, preoperative CT or MRI diagnosis of mesial temporal sclerosis is now considered more informative (Wyler and Bolender, 1983; Kuzniecky et al., 1987).

Epilepsy due to a condition such as a meningioma, so often associated with overlying hyperostosis of the skull or sometimes with bony erosion, is rare in childhood. Nevertheless, it is important to remember that indolent gliomas may be a cause of chronic epilepsy in childhood and adolescence and the overlying bony changes in the skull may easily be missed, even in a computed tomographic (CT) scan (Lee et al., 1989).

## Transillumination of the skull

It is worth remembering that simple *transillumination* of the skull in small children, using a torch fitted with a circular rubber extension applied to the skull, may be very informative in conditions such as hydrocephalus, porencephaly, hydranencephaly and localized brain atrophy. Fluid conducts light better than solid tissue and in a completely dark room one may clearly see the widespread diffusion of light through a fluid-filled area in the skull. Fibre-optic instruments now provide superior transillumination.

## Neuroimaging studies

The imagination and ingenuity of two men, Hounsfield (an engineer) and Ambrose (a neuroradiologist) led to the introduction of *computerized axial tomographic scanning* (CT scan, CAT scan; Ambrose and Hounsfield, 1973). Since then, the technique had revolutionized neuroradiology, clinical neurology and neurosurgery. Prior to the invention of CT scanning, paediatricians were conservative about the application of the various painful invasive and often dangerous methods which were available for imaging the nervous system. The image produced by CT represents brain structure, in contrast to electroencephalography which provides information about brain function. The use of contrast media, injected intravenously, was introduced early in the clinical experience with CT because they enhanced differences in tissue density. Although this technique increases visualization and improves clarity, it does carry a risk of adverse reactions to the contrast agent which, although infrequent, may very rarely be fatal. The average radiation dose from CT is within generally accepted values and is not thought to present somatic or genetic hazards.

Some concern has been expressed about the effects of multiple scans on myelin development and neuronal migration in the immature developing brain and caution should be exercised in using the technique in the very young.

Nuclear magnetic resonance has been used as a chemist's tool for determining the chemical composition of samples since 1952 and the development of the technique to create images was inspired by the work of Lauterbur (1973). With increasing use of the technique, it soon became clear that *magnetic resonance imaging [MRI]* could provide exquisite anatomical information that rivalled, and in many cases exceeded, the capability of CT imaging. Furthermore, it did this without the risks of ionizing radiation and with the minimum of discomfort to the patient. The basic principles of image production by MRI and the problems encountered with the technique are discussed by Armstrong and Keevil (1991a and b).

The two neuroimaging methods of CT and MRI complement electrophysiological studies by identifying structural disorders which may be causally related to the development of seizures. In the detection of a focal structural cerebral lesion there is now no doubt that MRI has significant advantages over CT because of higher sensitivity, superior image quality, lack of radiation exposure and capacity for multiplanar display. In particular, it is superior to CT in identifying abnormalities of cortical architecture, in visualizing the temporal lobes, and in detecting gliomas and cavernous malformations. In patients with complex partial seizures, typical lesions in the temporal lobe areas include arteriovenous malformations, subarachnoid cysts, hamartomas, old infarction, slow-growing gliomas and, commonest of all, mesial temporal sclerosis. MRI has been somewhat disappointing in detecting mesial temporal sclerosis but is still superior to CT in this respect (Kuzniecky *et al.*, 1987). It is essential that both axial and coronal values should be visualized by MRI when attempting to find mesial temporal sclerosis.

It must be recognized that CT scanning is much more widely available and less expensive than MRI scanning and is likely to be the neuroimaging technique most frequently employed for the foreseeable future. Yang *et al.* (1979), in a large study of CT findings in children presenting with all types of seizures, found an overall incidence of abnormalities of 33%. The presence of an abnormal neurological examination increased the incidence of CT abnormalities to 64%. In children with partial seizures of simple symptomatology, with partial seizures of complex

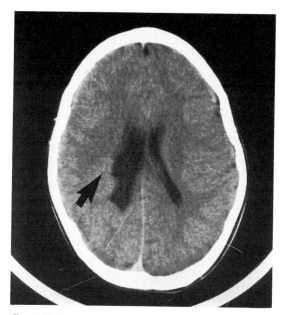

*Figure 23.1* CT scan with contrast in a child presenting with complex partial seizures. Scan shows presence of heterotopic grey matter located just lateral to the left lateral ventricle (arrow). (*Courtesy Dr Mary King*)

symptomatology and with generalized seizures of known aetiology, the scans were abnormal in 52% and 30% and 40% respectively. However, in patients with generalized seizures of primary type, CT was abnormal in only 8%. If mental handicap was the only neurological abnormality present, CT showed generalized atrophy, usually mild. If mental retardation was associated with a focal neurological abnormality, CT often demonstrated focal abnormality. When chronic seizure disorders began in the neonatal period and continued, CT was always abnormal, usually showing bilateral atrophy.

Gordon (1988), in a more recent study of a large number of children attending a special school for children with epilepsy (and therefore a selected group with chronic epilepsy and with associated handicaps in a proportion), again found an overall incidence of CT abnormality in about a third of cases. The usual abnormality found was some degree of generalized or focal atrophy. It is worth noting that, in children with chronic epilepsy who develop sudden changes in seizure pattern, neurological examination or EEG, a normal CT scan may be useful and reassuring in excluding a treatable condition or progressive disease. The role of CT in detecting the intracerebral lesions of tuberose sclerosis should also be remembered, especially in children with infantile spasms or with the myoclonic epilepsies.

The indications for neuroimaging (CT and MRI) in children with epilepsy have been defined by Scheuer and Pedley (1990) as follows: all children with partial seizures, except those with benign partial epilepsy of childhood, children with abnormal findings on neurological examination, and those with focal slow-wave abnormalities on the EEG. Patients with refractory seizures, even those of many years duration, should be considered for MRI scanning because of the possibility that a definable epileptogenic lesion may be present which may be amenable to resective surgery.

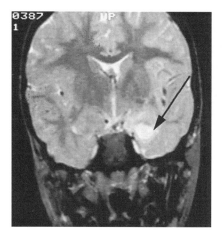

(a)

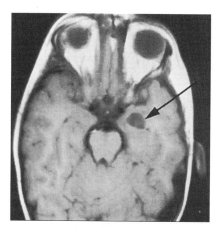

(b)

*Figure 23.2* Low grade astrocytoma in left temporal lobe. (a) Coronal $T_2$ weighted image shows small circumscribed mass in the region of the left hippocampus (arrow). (b) Axial $T_1$ weighted image shows the lesion (arrow) as low signal intensity with mild mass effect. The long $T_1/T_2$ characteristics suggest the lesion may have a cystic component. (*Courtesy of Dr Mary King*)

It must always be remembered that neuroimaging procedures are costly to perform and should be used with discretion in the child with suspected or established epilepsy. The evaluation of epilepsy remains as much an art as a science with history-taking still the cornerstone of diagnosis and electroencephalography as the primary diagnostic tool.

## Real-time ultrasonography

Non-invasive rapid evaluation of the neonatal and young infant's brain is now feasible with real-time ultrasonography through the anterior fontanelle. This has already been discussed in Chapter 3. Cerebral anatomy (including ventricles, parenchyma and vessels) is readily visualized in both coronal and sagittal planes. The procedure can be performed rapidly with a mobile real-time unit in the newborn nursery. Ventricular size, intracerebral haemorrhage, ventricular abnormalities, extracerebral fluid collections, cystic lesions and solid parenchymal lesions may be recognized. No sedation is necessary, and the examinations are usually performed without removing the infant from the incubator. Using the pulsed Doppler transducer with the ultrasound probe, it is possible to study cerebral blood flow velocity. One advantage of the ultrasound technique over CT in examining the infant brain lies in the avoidance of ionizing and possibly harmful radiation (Levene, 1990).

## Angiography

Angiography has a very limited use in paediatric neurodiagnosis today, perhaps most usually in the detection of arteriovenous malformations affecting the brain and spinal cord. However, even in this respect, MRI, with the addition of the agent gadolinium DTPA in order to enhance localized lesions, is proving very successful and is much less invasive (Faerber, 1991). A further new development is real-time magnetic resonance angiography which allows the display of vessels from any desired viewing angle without the use of intravenous contrast media.

## Other neuroimaging techniques

Seizures are associated with pronounced changes in cerebral blood flow and metabolism. During generalized seizures there is a global increase in cerebral blood flow while, during partial seizures, increases are more localized and may correspond to the area of the epileptogenic focus as defined by the EEG. Interictally, areas of reduced cerebral blood flow may be seen and, again, often correspond to the main focal EEG abnormality. Focal areas of hypometabolism also occur interictally in patients with partial seizures while, during seizures, striking increases in metabolic activity take place.

*Positron emission tomography* [PET] applies the imaging principles of CT to radioisotope brain scans in order to produce cross-sectional pictures displaying the functional activity of specific brain structures. Positron isotopes (which require the availability of a cyclotron for their production) are particularly well suited for tomographic imaging. The brain function displayed depends upon the positron-labelled compound used as a tracer substance. Specific brain functions which are studied with PET include glucose metabolism and oxygen utilization, blood flow and blood volume, protein synthesis, activity of neurotransmitter substances, and the distribution and breakdown of certain drugs. All of these measurements have real or potential application to the study of patients with epilepsy, not only in order to understand disturbances in specific functions, such as metabolism or blood flow, that may occur during the development of epileptic seizures, but also to obtain information about the actual brain mechanisms of human epilepsy. PET has also proved useful for localizing the area of brain responsible for generating epileptic seizures in patients who are candidates for surgical treatment, since glucose metabolism is usually reduced in such an area between seizures. A variety of abnormal patterns has also been demonstrated in syndromes such as the Lennox–Gastaut syndrome. However, PET scanning is complex, very expensive, and likely to remain restricted to major research centres for the foreseeable future (Engel, 1989).

Because of the limited availability and expense of PET, interest has grown in the potential of *single photon emission computerized tomography* [*SPECT*] for the study of brain function in epilepsy. In SPECT imaging, a radioisotope is given to the patient, either by inhalation or by intravenous injection, and carried to the cerebral circulation, where it crosses into the brain. A rotating gamma camera or multidetector scanner is then used to produce tomographic images of the distribution of the radiotracer. The images produced resemble PET scans, except that routine SPECT studies map only blood flow. SPECT findings in patients with generalized seizures have been variable but have been more consistent in the partial epilepsies. Interictally, areas of reduced blood flow can be demonstrated, corresponding to the epileptic focus as defined by EEG. During partial seizures, blood flow increases, again corresponding with the epileptic focus. Comparison with PET studies have shown that results with SPECT parallel these and that areas of reduced blood flow correspond well with regions of reduced glucose metabolism and oxygen utilization and that blood flow studies may be a more useful marker for epileptic foci. While SPECT may never be able to challenge PET in spatial resolution or in the capability for neurometabolic studies, it seems likely that, over the next decade, PET will contribute more to epilepsy research and SPECT more to the general investigation and management of epilepsy (Leading article, 1989).

## Electroencephalography

The investigation *par excellence* for epilepsy is, of course, the EEG. It has been said that the EEG was the glass slipper for the Cinderella disease of epilepsy. The story of Hans Berger's discovery of the human EEG in 1924 has never been better told than by Gloor (1974) at the Hans Berger Symposium which was held in Edinburgh in 1973 to celebrate the centenary of his birth.

Berger was the first to prove the correctness of Hughlings Jackson's hypothesis that an epileptic seizure was a manifestation of exaggerated discharges of grey matter taking place in an area of brain functionally related to the clinical symptomatology of the seizure although, as Gloor has pointed out, he was completely unaware of having done so, probably because his knowledge of English was poor and he was not familiar with Hughlings Jackson's writings. Berger was also the first person to record an absence attack in which he demonstrated the occurrence of regular rhythmic high-voltage slow waves at the rate of 3 per second. He failed to demonstrate the associated spikes and felt that he had recorded an artefact. The validity of his pioneering work was later confirmed in Great Britain by Adrian and Matthews (1934) and by workers in other countries.

The EEG measures differences in electrical potential arising between different parts of the head resulting from the spontaneous activity of the underlying brain. The growth of electroencephalography as a science since the 1920s has really paralleled that of its instrumentation, for when measured through the skull from electrodes placed on the unshaven scalp these potentials commonly show a voltage difference between the leads of only about 50 $\mu$V and only rarely in man do they exceed 200 $\mu$V. They are usually, therefore, about one-tenth or less of the magnitude of ECG potentials. Consequently they need considerable amplification before they can be recorded. The development of the modern thermionic valve made such amplification possible but the EEG machines using valves were large and cumbersome. The invention of the transistor in 1948 led to the development of the modern compact and often portable machines.

In the usual method of recording, potentials from several pairs of electrodes are led in through differential input stages and registered simultaneously, each pair of electrodes having its independent amplifying system and recording unit. Recordings between members of a pair of electrodes may be bipolar (i.e. from two electrodes which are over active brain) or unipolar (i.e. where one electrode is over active tissue and the other is over a distant and relatively inactive point; usually the mastoid process is used, although there is no truly inactive point anywhere on the head). The bipolar method of recording is in universal use today. Those seeking further information concerning the electrical activity of the nervous system should consult Brazier (1968).

The EEG has *limitations as an investigative tool*. It is a fussy technique requiring much attention to detail, particularly in the electrode placement and maintenance of apparatus in order to obtain good artefact-free recordings. It can pick up electrical signals from a limited area of the brain only, mainly from the convexity of the cerebral hemispheres. The small size of the potentials has already been mentioned and they are further attenuated by the distance of the electrode from the actual source of the activity. Perhaps most important of all, the abnormal patterns of electrical activity recorded are, except in very rare instances, non-specific with regard to pathology. This point will be discussed further. Also, it is important to remember that dead brain tissue does not produce abnormal electrical potentials. It is the surrounding and altered living cerebral tissue which undergoes changes of normal electrical activity which are then registered in the EEG recording.

*The advantages of the EEG examination* are that it is painless, fairly brief and relatively inexpensive. It is non-invasive, and even the invasive modifications employed in some adult examinations, such as the use of sphenoidal electrodes, are seldom used in childhood. Permanent records of the electrical activity of the brain are immediately obtained and easily stored for comparison, if necessary, with later recordings. The EEG can be studied during attention or at rest and also during sleep, and the degree of abnormality may vary from one state to another, particularly in the case of epilepsy.

## EEG techniques in childhood

As has been emphasized in other sections of this book, epilepsy is most common in the early years of life and it is in taking recordings from babies and young children that most technical difficulty is experienced. The author is convinced that such recordings are best done in an EEG department specializing in paediatric EEG and having the services of technicians with special experience in this particular field of electroencephalography. The technician should be able to allow time to play with the child and gain his or her confidence and cooperation. The recording room should be quiet and look as unclinical as possible. Soft furnishings, cheerful colours and plenty of toys, especially small toys for use during the recording, are essential. Sedation should rarely be necessary except for very disturbed children. In the department best known to the author, the product most commonly employed to placate rather than sedate is chocolate drops. The child should be given every opportunity to drop into a natural sleep if possible, since sleep is perhaps the most potent of all activating procedures in childhood epilepsy. Routine recordings are made either with the subject sitting or recumbent, or frequently the former followed by the latter, and activation by hyperventilation and intermittent photic stimulation, using a rapidly flickering light, is used where appropriate. The use of silver chloride disc electrodes rather than pad electrodes is essential in babies and young children if artefact-free records are to be obtained; in many paediatric EEG departments, stick-on electrodes are used exclusively.

## Interpretation of EEGs in childhood

The interpretation of EEG recordings from children, particularly infants and small children, requires special knowledge and experience on the part of the examiner and should preferably be done by an individual versed in the problems of neuropaediatrics. There are considerable differences from adults, and changes in the EEG, both in the waking state and during sleep, occur from infancy through early childhood and up to late childhood (Petersen and Eeg-Olofsson, 1971). In fact, the EEG may not reach a state indistinguishable from an adult record until the mid-teens.

Throughout the neonatal period, infancy and childhood the EEG pattern is much more easily disturbed by intercurrent metabolic and toxic changes than is an adult EEG recording. The normal response of the child's EEG to hyperventilation is an example of this. Cerebral lesions cause more widespread and marked abnormalities than would a comparable lesion in an adult. The EEG abnormalities seen in children suffering from epilepsy, whatever its type, are similar to those found in adults, but they are usually of larger amplitude, more widespread and are associated with a more generalized disturbance of brain rhythm than would be the case in an adult. There are also certain specific EEG patterns in children with diseases such as SSPE, neuronal ceroid lipofuscinosis (Batten–Vogt disease) and, of course, infantile spasms. As with paediatric neurology in general and childhood epilepsy in particular, the EEG of an infant or child is the result of a complex interplay of pathological, metabolic and maturational factors in the individual being studied.

Electroencephalography has precise but limited applications, and the study of the electrical activity of the brain should not be regarded with greater veneration than the study of any other function of the body, nor should an abnormal EEG be regarded as more significant than any other abnormal physical sign. Any neurological problem in a child or an adult should be assessed as a whole. An EEG may be able to tell us how the patient's brain appears to be working and whether the patterns present are within the normal range of maturity for his age. The responses to various stimuli can be assessed and differences in the function of the two hemispheres and between homologous areas of the brain can be studied. Essentially the EEG measures brain function whereas the newer imaging techniques such as CT and MRI define structure.

In general, clinicians unfamiliar with the EEG ask too much of the investigation, both in adults and in children, and are often disappointed by the results. It is appropriate to quote Denis Hill (1958) on this point. He wrote: 'The EEG is often used as a means of helping to decide whether a given patient's symptoms are epileptic or psychogenic or are due to some non-cerebral cause, such as syncope. I believe this is an improper use of the technique and that in fact the results of doing this can be misleading. A single routine normal EEG is not evidence against epilepsy, nor indeed is the finding of epileptic discharges in the EEG evidence that the patient's symptoms are necessarily epileptic in nature. Such discharges occur in the EEGs of some non-epileptic persons, in many with degenerative brain disorders, in some psychotics, and in cases of behaviour disorder. The prescription of anticonvulsants on the finding of such discharges in the EEG is unjustifiable and often illogical, and may lead the clinician to overlook more important issues for his patient. The recognition of the epileptic nature of any symptom or group of symptoms is, I believe, a clinical task and must remain so. When the clinician requests an EEG to confirm the diagnosis he is not so much interested in the question of whether the EEG demonstrates focal discharges in the expected area – he is merely disappointed but does not alter his diagnosis if it does not – as in the question of whether the EEG demonstrates the presence of a pathological process, either a local lesion or a diffuse one, which is of such importance for the prognosis.' Although these remarks concern adults and were written long before the development of techniques of long-term EEG monitoring, they remain valid and also largely applicable to children.

One happy circumstance for the paediatric electroencephalographer is that the interictal records of children with epilepsy are more likely to show abnormalities than those of epileptic adults, and these may include spikes, spike and wave complexes and other paroxysmal abnormalities. These EEG findings are not specific for epilepsy but they are vastly more common in those who have had seizures than in those who have not. The EEG will not usually tell us why the young patient has epilepsy although it is established that certain EEG patterns are associated with a predominantly inherited or genetic origin for the seizures while other EEG abnormalities are more likely to be caused by acquired brain damage. The EEG can be helpful in categorizing the type of epilepsy from which the child is suffering, and this aspect has been described in more detail in the chapters dealing with the particular varieties of epilepsy. In general, only clear EEG abnormalities should be regarded as significant in young people. This dictum has always applied to routine tracings and is even more applicable to the tracings obtained during various stimulation procedures and with the several sophisticated EEG monitoring techniques now available.

A widespread misconception about the EEG is that it will always or even usually tell the clinician if the patient's epilepsy is improving and, therefore, that it can be used to decide whether or not it is safe to stop treatment or even, at a later date, if it is safe for the patient to drive a car – this is not so. Epilepsy is a clinical state and consists of having seizures and not simply of having abnormal brain waves: assessment of improvement should be predominantly a clinical exercise. For example, in benign focal epilepsy of childhood, the frequency of the epileptic discharges in the centrotemporal areas bears no direct relationship to the severity or otherwise of the clinical epilepsy, and discharges may persist long after the epilepsy has remitted (Aicardi, 1979).

The EEG has much to contribute in deciding whether or not the patient is a suitable case for temporal lobectomy, but the techniques now employed in centres where the operation is done are much more elaborate than those of an ordinary EEG department. However, the consistent finding in routine recording of a unilateral temporal lobe focus in a patient with intractable epilepsy is a useful starting point.

## Non-specific nature of EEG abnormalities

The question of whether seizures are due to a space-occupying lesion is one that agitates the minds of parents and their doctors but, as discussed elsewhere, supratentorial tumours are very uncommon in childhood. It is important to emphasize, in this context, that the EEG never directly indicates a pathological process. A delta wave abnormality in the EEG may be caused by tumour or abscess, by infarct or haemorrhage, by a local area of demyelination or by many other lesions (Gloor, Ball and Schaui, 1977). A change in the abnormality, for better or worse, in serial recordings may be useful in differentiating the various diagnostic possibilities. It should be remembered, as mentioned previously, that the abnormal waves are not produced by the tumour or abscess or whatever, but by damaged brain cells in the vicinity. One further pitfall is that, since the brain appears to function by conveying electrical impulses from one area to another, abnormal activity can sometimes be recorded from areas which are relatively remote from their site of origin and 'mirror foci' may occur on the contralateral side from the area of primary abnormality.

In the early days of the EEG a great deal of emphasis was laid on the need for accurate electrical localization. Fortunately, the great advances in neuroradiology have rendered such accuracy unnecessary and the EEG should now be able to find its proper place in the scheme of neurological investigation. As Matthews (1964) wrote:

> There is a serious need to find a middle course between blind acceptance of the EEG as a routine investigation and the attitude summarized by dismissing an EEG department as 'another waste-paper store'. Change will be difficult while every doctor expects his epileptic patients' problems to be solved by the EEG, and every patient demands it. Under such demands few electroencephalographers can claim never to have written such futilities as 'the record is compatible with epilepsy', well knowing that this applies to every record ever taken.

## EEG and classification of childhood epilepsy

Attempts to classify epilepsy in childhood in relation to EEG criteria have not been successful, mainly because the younger the child the more diverse the EEG abnormalities which correspond with the variable clinical manifestations of epilepsy in the young.

The role of EEG investigation in the neonate with seizures is discussed in Chapter 3. The grossly disorganized EEG pattern called *hypsarrhythmia* is seen in infants with infantile spasms but is a non-specific reaction on the part of the brain to a variety of insults. Hypsarrhythmia can also occur in severely mentally handicapped children who may not have clinical epilepsy. Friedman and Pampiglione (1971) studied 105 children who had shown the EEG features of hypsarrhythmia in the first year of life and who were followed up for a minimum of 7 years. Irrespective of the presenting symptomatology, and to some extent regardless of therapy, mortality in the group was of the order of 25% and occurred mainly before the age of 3 years, and the incidence of mental subnormality in the survivors was 77%. Only 18 children attained fairly normal standards of mental development and could attend ordinary schools. They concluded that hypsarrhythmia was a physical sign of grave prognostic significance, whatever the clinical picture at the time. It is important to realize that the EEG in many of these patients may eventually show no abnormality at all, in spite of serious and permanent mental handicap. In those who continue to have epilepsy, the hypsarrhythmic pattern may change into generalized repetitive slow spike-wave complexes.

Aicardi (1973) has written comprehensively about the slow spike-wave patterns which are frequently but by no means invariably seen in the myoclonic epilepsies. The main features are triphasic slow spikes or sharp waves followed by a slow component of variable shape occurring in runs of several seconds or minutes bilaterally. The rhythm is between 1.5 and 2.5 complexes per second and is often irregular, as are the spacing, configuration and distribution of the complexes in various leads. There is a tendency for the slow spike-waves to be better defined in the frontal regions. This slow spike-wave pattern is usually interictal, usually insensitive to stimulation (hyperventilation, flicker stimulation) and is activated by sleep, during which it tends to reinforce and become continuous. There is a tendency to equate this particular type of EEG pattern with the most severe type of myoclonic epilepsy (the so-called Lennox–Gastaut syndrome) but, as Aicardi has pointed out, diffuse slow spikewaves may be seen not only in the Lennox–Gastaut syndrome but also in a wide array of epileptic phenomena including other myoclonic epilepsies, minor status epilepticus and in association with some of the clinical manifestations of temporal lobe epilepsy. The slow spike-wave pattern, when seen in association with severe myoclonic epilepsy of the Lennox–Gastaut type, is an indication of a poor prognosis for later intellectual development.

Aicardi and Chevrie (1973) studied a large group of children under 3 years of age who had *seizures and paroxysmal EEG abnormalities*, other than hypsarrhythmia and slow spike-waves, and they compared them with a control group in the same age range who had seizures but no paroxysmal EEG abnormalities. All types of seizure, including febrile convulsions, were considered. They showed that seizures in young children associated with paroxysmal EEG abnormalities belonged preferentially to certain types of epilepsy with a bad mental outcome and vice versa. Febrile convulsions, which have a favourable prognosis, were seldom associated with a paroxysmal EEG abnormality (at least not under 3 years of age). Conversely, seizures due to organic brain damage were characterized both by poor mental outlook and by the frequent occurrence of EEG paroxysms. However, they showed that patients with generalized spike-waves occurring at a rate of three complexes per second had a more favourable intellectual outcome than patients with paroxysmal patterns such as generalized or lateralized spikes. Patients with these regular spike-wave patterns were, on the whole, older when their epilepsy started, fewer had gross brain pathology and more had a positive family history of epilepsy. Aicardi and Chevrie pointed out, however, that under 2 years of age the spike-wave patterns at three complexes per second were usually associated with or heralded the epilepsies with myoclonic features, whereas in older children they were associated with primary generalized epilepsy of the absence (petit mal) type. They concluded that children with paroxysmal abnormalities in their EEGs, especially when these were discovered in the first 2 years of life, belonged to the more severe group of childhood epilepsy, while children without paroxysmal abnormalities under the age of 3 years tended to have a better prognosis for their seizures.

As discussed elsewhere, the *interictal EEG* in children who have had *febrile convulsions* is usually normal. However, if records are taken within a day of the attack, over three-quarters of the children will show slow wave disturbances which are often more marked over one hemisphere. These abnormalities persist in a third of cases for about 3–5 days. Focal slow wave disturbances following a febrile seizure increase the chance of subsequent spike foci developing later in the EEG, but such foci are less common than generalized bursts of spike and wave discharge of short duration which should not be confused with the EEG abnormality of the true petit mal absence, the classic spike-wave complexes occurring at the rate of three per second. Lennox-Buchthal (1973) found that neither of these findings had any predictive value with respect to the risk of developing epilepsy later, although all the children in her series who did develop epilepsy later had shown spikes or spike and slow wave complexes in earlier records.

*Focal spike discharges* have a limited value in localizing brain lesions in children. As already mentioned, they are usually accompanied by more widespread disturbances of electrical activity around the main epileptogenic area and by more general disturbance in the record than in adults. Trojaborg (1968) carried out follow-up studies over periods ranging from 3 to 15 years in 242 children who had spike foci in their EEGs. Of these children, 85% showed a change in spike location during the study, and in half the change was from one hemisphere to another. All who report on children's EEGs will be familiar with this common and sometimes embarrassing phenomenon. Trojaborg concluded that spike discharges alone are of limited value as an indication of focal cortical damage in children, and that electroclinical correlations are not reliable unless serial examinations over several years show consistent focal abnormalities. It is interesting to consider this feature in the light of what has already been said in Chapter 9 about benign partial epilepsy of childhood, where the spike discharges are considered to represent a functional disturbance of a part of the brain rather than actual localized damage.

The persistence of focal spikes for many years after a child has been free of seizures is also well known. Trojaborg found persistent spikes in 52% of his patients who had been free of seizures for more than 2 years, and some were followed up for as long as 10 years. This common observation again highlights the limitations of the EEG with regard to the clinical management of epilepsy. Seizures are clinical events to which the frequency and incidence of EEG spikes are sometimes poorly related. The EEG must be used in the problems of childhood epilepsy with discrimination. Excessive reliance on the so-called routine EEG as a diagnostic tool should be avoided and findings should be evaluated in the context of the patient's individual situation. It is important to realize that seizure discharges (whether generalized or focal, spontaneous or evoked) may be found in the EEGs of a proportion of normal children, i.e. children with no history of clinical epilepsy.

There is increasing interest in the accurate diagnosis of *temporal lobe epilepsy* in childhood. The difficulties of recording EEGs from the mesiobasal parts of the temporal lobes have been well known since Gibbs and Gibbs (1952) observed that in psychomotor epilepsy a standard EEG recording had only a 30% chance of demonstrating an abnormality whereas a record taken from a sleeping patient was about three times as likely to do so. A sleep EEG is now regarded as the standard minimum procedure in the investigation of any case of temporal lobe epilepsy. Indeed, it should be standard practice in any paediatric EEG department to encourage as many patients as possible to drift into sleep during the recording. The experienced technician, working in the right surroundings and with time to devote to the individual patient, will achieve this goal in a surprisingly large proportion of patients. Occasionally, in restless difficult patients, sleep records may be obtained following mild sedation with a barbiturate and/or a phenothiazine drug. Using sleep records in this way, 80–90% of the patients with temporal lobe epilepsy will show one or more temporal lobe foci and possibly other abnormalities. The use of sphenoidal electrodes, i.e. electrodes inserted to record from the undersurfaces of the temporal lobes anteriorly, should only be considered for use in children who are being investigated for possible neurosurgery. Nasopharyngeal electrodes, which are passed in through the nose, have been used in adults to record from the mesiobasal parts of the temporal lobes, and smaller modifications of these are available for use in children. It must always be remembered that an EEG abnormality over the temporal lobe does not make a diagnosis of temporal lobe epilepsy (see discussion on benign partial epilepsy of childhood in Chapter 9). The historical and behavioural data and the EEG and radiological data must all add up to a diagnosis of this type of epilepsy before such a diagnosis is accepted, and this is particularly important in differentiating various psychic aberrations which may be mistaken for the behavioural changes of temporal lobe or psychomotor epilepsy.

For the reader who wishes to obtain further information about the EEG and about epileptiform EEG patterns in childhood, two recent short but comprehensive accounts by Drury (1989) and Holmes (1989) are recommended.

## EEG findings and frequency of seizures

One particular problem with the EEG diagnosis of temporal lobe epilepsy, and indeed with other types of focal epilepsy, is that there does not seem to be any close relationship between the occurrence of focal spikes and seizure frequency. In fact, recordings of actual temporal lobe seizures have shown that the EEG spike and the epileptic seizure are not very closely related to each other, although they are both related in some way to the epileptic properties of the cerebral lesion. This is one reason why the frequency of spike discharges in the partial or focal epilepsies should not be used to assess the efficacy or otherwise of a particular anticonvulsant drug. On the other hand, the frequency of occurrence of short bursts of spikes and of spikewave complexes in children with generalized convulsive seizures and true petit mal is very definitely related to the frequency of actual attacks, and can provide a good index of possible therapeutic benefit from a particular drug. The medication may be given parenterally during an actual EEG recording and its effects, when given on a regular daily basis, may be monitored by serial EEG recordings at intervals. Milligan and Richens (1981) have reviewed the methods of assessment of antiepileptic drugs.

Apart from their possible effects on seizure discharges, *drugs* can have their effect on the EEG in other ways (Montagu and Rudolf, 1983). The barbiturates and benzodiazepines induce fast activity in the record under normal circumstances and a lateralized or focal deficit of fast activity may indicate localized cortical abnormality, e.g. atrophy (Pampiglione, 1952).

## Intensive EEG monitoring in paediatrics

The episodic nature of epilepsy is one of its most characteristic features. Most patients have to be treated without any seizures being witnessed by a skilled observer and very few have an attack while an EEG is being recorded. Interictal

EEG findings in epilepsy are variable and only a proportion of patients show epileptiform discharges in the routine EEG in the waking state. This often leads to a dismissive attitude towards EEG on the part of clinicians, some of whom may refer patients indiscriminately for EEG examination anyway. The problem of distinguishing true from pseudoseizures is also an important one, particularly during adolescence. For all these reasons, it is important to try to maximize the yield of diagnostically useful findings. Obtaining a 'positive' EEG depends on several factors, including the duration of the recording, the skill and experience of the technician, the circumstances under which the recording is made, and whether serial EEGs are obtained. Both sleep and sleep deprivation increase the frequency of epileptic abnormalities. Activating procedures such as hyperventilation and intermittent photic stimulation are essential. Taking patients with probable epilepsy in all age-groups, about 29–50% have epileptiform abnormalities in the first EEG (more in paediatric than in adult patients) and, if multiple recordings are obtained, the proportion increases to 59–92% (Scheuer and Pedley, 1990).

Because the duration of the EEG is normally between 30 and 60 minutes, which may be too short to pick up significant intermittent abnormalities, methods of prolonged EEG monitoring have been devised and their use is increasingly widespread. Recording with a conventional EEG recorder from a patient lying immobile or seated on a chair is hardly appropriate, especially for children, particularly if the investigation is expected to last more than an hour. Techniques have therefore been devised to overcome this problem and to allow prolonged recording while the patient pursues normal daily activities or is asleep at night. In *FM radiotelemetry*, the EEG is sent by FM radio signals from a lightweight transmitter worn by the patient. This technique may be combined with a simultaneous video display of the patient on a split screen, allowing the clinician to view clinical events simultaneously with EEG events. Since the distance that the signal will travel is limited, FM radiotelemetry studies are usually performed in hospital. In addition to FM telemetry, some laboratories record continuous EEGs through a long flexible cable extending from the ambulant patient to a conventional EEG machine but this technique is not widely used in paediatric practice.

Ives and Woods (1975) developed *ambulatory cassette EEG recording* using the Oxford Medilog cassette recorder originally developed for long-term ECG monitoring. A further advance was the development of a head-mounted preamplifier, which allowed high-quality recordings without movement artefact. The overall value of ambulatory monitoring can be improved by combining EEG recording with other physiological measurements, especially ECG and respiratory patterns. This is possible with newer systems which provide several channels for physiological information and a channel for marking clinical events and recording time. The electrodes and head-mounted preamplifiers can usually be concealed under the patient's hair and the recorder is worn on a belt and is battery powered. The visual replay system reviews tapes at up to 60 times recording speed, allowing 24 hours of data to be reviewed within 24 minutes on a 12-inch screen. Ambulatory cassette EEG technology has been reviewed by Ebersole and Bridgers (1986) and Stores (1984) reviewed intensive EEG monitoring in paediatrics.

Another type of monitoring which is gaining wide acceptance in the diagnosis and classification of seizure disorders is *intensive video/EEG monitoring*. In this technique, 16–64 channels of EEG are recorded continuously onto a magnetic or optical storage medium while the patient remains in front of a closed-circuit television camera (American Academy of Neurology, 1989b). The clinical behaviour of the patient and the EEG pattern are displayed simultaneously on the television screen. This technological advance is particularly useful for distinguishing epileptic from nonepileptic episodic disorders. Localization of the seizure focus is of paramount importance for patients being considered for surgical treatment of epilepsy and intensive EEG/video monitoring of seizures is crucial to such localization issues.

What is entitled 'EEG brain mapping' refers to several quantitative EEG techniques, including EEG frequency analysis and various computer based calculations derived from the EEG. These techniques can help to highlight or identify regional features of the EEG which may have escaped identification by traditional visual inspection of the polygraph EEG alone (American Academy of Neurology, 1989a). EEG brain mapping cannot diagnose epilepsy but may help to differentiate primary generalized discharges from secondary bilateral synchronous discharges or to determine the localization of a focus. This technology is available in only a very few centres and has a very limited application in paediatric electroencephalographic diagnosis.

# References

ADRIAN, E. D. and MATTHEWS, B. H. C. (1934) Berger rhythm: potential changes from occipital lobes in man. *Brain*, **57**, 355–385

AICARDI, J. (1973) The problems of the Lennox syndrome. *Developmental Medicine and Child Neurology*, **15**, 77–81

AICARDI, J. (1979) Benign epilepsy of childhood with Rolandic spikes (BECRS). *Brain and Development*, **1**, 71–73

AICARDI, J. and CHEVRIE, J. J. (1973) The significance of electroencephalographic paroxysms in children less than 3 years of age. *Epilepsia*, **14**, 47–55

AMBROSE, J. and HOUNSFIELD, G. (1973) Computerized transverse axial tomography. *British Journal of Radiology*, **6**, 148

AMERICAN ACADEMY OF NEUROLOGY (1989a) Assessment: EEG brain mapping. *Neurology*, **39**, 1100–1101

AMERICAN ACADEMY OF NEUROLOGY (1989b) Assessment: intensive EEG video monitoring for epilepsy. *Neurology*, **39**, 1101–1102

ARMSTRONG, P. and KEEVIL, S. F. (1991a) Magnetic resonance imaging – 1: Basic principles of image production. *British Medical Journal*, **303**, 35–40

ARMSTRONG, P. and KEEVIL, S. F. (1991b) Magnetic resonance imaging – 2: Clinical uses. *British Medical Journal*, **303**, 105–109

BRAZIER, M. A. B. (1968) *The Electrical Activity of the Nervous System*, 3rd edn. Pitman Medical, London

DRURY, I. (1989) Epileptiform patterns of children. *Journal of Clinical Neurophysiology*, **6**, 1–39

EBERSOLE, J. S. and BRIDGERS, S. L. (1986) Ambulatory EEG monitoring. In *Recent Advances in Epilepsy* No. 3. (eds T. A. Pedley and B. S. Meldrum), Churchill Livingstone, Edinburgh, London, pp. 111–136

ENGEL, J. (1989) Positron emission tomography. In *Seizures and Epilepsy*. F. A. Davis Company, Philadelphia, pp. 328–330

FAERBER, E. N. (1991) Imaging of the central nervous system in infants and children. *Current Opinion in Paediatrics*, **3**, 4–11

FRIEDMAN, E. and PAMPIGLIONE, G. (1971) Prognostic implications of electroencephagraphic findings of hypsarrhythmia in first year of life. *British Medical Journal*, **4**, 323–338

GIBBS, F. A. and GIBBS, E. L. (1952) *Atlas of Electroencephalography*, Vol. 2: *Epilepsy*. Addison-Wesley, Cambridge, Mass

GLOOR, P. (1974) Hans Berger – psychophysiology and the discovery of the human electroencephalogram. In *Epilepsy: Proceedings of the Hans Berger Centenary Symposium* (eds P. Harris and C. Mawdsley), Churchill Livingstone, London, New York and Edinburgh, pp. 353–373

GLOOR, P., BALL, G. and SCHAUL, S. (1977) Brain lesions that produce delta waves in the EEG. *Neurology*, **27**, 326–333

GORDON, N. (1988) Computed tomography in childhood epilepsy. *Archives of Disease in Childhood*, **63**, 1114

HILL, D. (1958) Value of the EEG in diagnosis of epilepsy. *British Medical Journal*, **1**, 663–666

HOLMES, G. L. (1989) Electroencephalographic and neuroradiologic evaluation of children with epilepsy. *Pediatric Clinics of North America*, **36**, 395–420

IVES, J. R. and WOODS, J. F. (1975) 4-channel 24 hour cassette recorder on long-term EEG monitoring of ambulatory patients. *Electroencephalography and Clinical Neurophysiology*, **39**, 88–92

KUZNIECKY, R., SAYETTE, V. DE LA ETHIER, R. *et al.* (1987) Magnetic resonance imaging in temporal lobe epilepsy: pathological correlations. *Annals of Neurology*, **22**, 341–347

LAUTERBUR, P. C. (1973) Image formation by induced local interactions: examples employing nuclear magnetic resonance. *Nature*, **242**, 190–191

LEADING ARTICLE (1989) SPECT and PET in epilepsy. *Lancet*, **333**, 135–137

LEE, T. K. Y., NAKUSA, Y., JEFFREE, M. A. *et al.* (1989) Indolent glioma: a cause of epilepsy. *Archives of Disease in Childhood*, **64**, 1666–1671

LENNOX-BUCHTHAL, M. A. (1973) Febrile convulsions: a reappraisal. *Electroencephalography and Clinical Neurophysiology*, Suppl. 32

LEVENE, M. A. (1990) Cerebral ultrasound and neurological impairment: telling the future. *Archives of Disease in Childhood*, **65**, 469–471

LINNETT, M. J. (1982) People with epilepsy – the burden of epilepsy. In *A Textbook of Epilepsy*, 2nd edn (eds J. Laidlaw and A. Richens), Churchill Livingstone, Edinburgh and London; pp. 1–15

MATTHEWS, W. B. (1964) The use and abuse of electroencephalography. *Lancet*, **2**, 577–579

MILLIGAN, N. and RICHENS, A. (1981) Methods of assessment of antiepileptic drugs. *British Journal of Clinical Pharmacology*, **11**, 443–456

MIRIBEL, J., VIETO, N. and FAVEL, P. (1963) Value of simple radiography of the skull in epilepsy. *Epilepsia*, **4**, 261–284

MONTAGU, J. D. and RUDOLF, N. DE M. (1983) Effects of anticonvulsants on the electroencephalogram. *Archives of Disease in Childhood*, **58**, 241–243

PAMPIGLIONE, G. (1952) Induced fast activity in the EEG as an aid in the location of cerebral lesions. *Electroencephalography and Clinical Neurophysiology*, **1**, 79

PETERSON, I. and EEG-OLOFSSON, O. (1971) The development of the electroencephalogram in normal children from the age of 1 through 15 years. Non-paroxysmal activity. *Neuropädiatrie*, **2**, 247–304

SCHEUER, M. L. and PEDLEY, T. A. (1990) The evaluation and treatment of seizures. *New England Journal of Medicine*, **323**, 1468–1474

STORES, G. (1984) Intensive EEG monitoring in paediatrics. *Developmental Medicine and Child Neurology*, **26**, 231–234

TROJABORG, W. (1968) Changes of spike foci in children. In *Clinical Electroencephalography of Children* (eds P. Kellaway and I. Petersen), Aimqvist and Wiksell, Stockholm, pp. 213–225

WYLER, A. R. and BOLENDER, N. F. (1983) Preoperative CT diagnosis of mesial temporal sclerosis for surgical treatment of epilepsy. *Annals of Neurology*, **13**, 59–64

YANG, P. J., BERGER, P. E., COHEN, M. E. and DUFFNER, P. K. (1979) Computed tomography and childhood seizure disorders. *Neurology*, **29**, 1084–1088

# Chapter 24

# General management of childhood epilepsy

To have a correct outlook on the general management of epilepsy and its problems, one should constantly remember that seizures are symptoms and not diseases in their own right. Caring for the patient with epilepsy means much more than prescribing antiepileptic drugs in an attempt to control the attacks. In the broad context of childhood epilepsy, probably the minority of the patients will suffer from epilepsy alone; the rest will have, in addition, intellectual difficulties and defects of cognitive function, behavioural problems or perhaps some other neurological deficit. Surveys in various countries support these observations (Green and Hartlage, 1971; Pazzaglia and Frank-Pazzaglia, 1976; Stores, 1978), and they are discussed in detail in Chapter 21.

## Correct diagnosis is essential

The management of epilepsy cannot be started until a correct diagnosis has been made. It is difficult to overemphasize this point, and for this reason a great deal of attention was devoted to diagnosis and differential diagnosis in Chapter 22. Modern drug therapy is semispecific in its effects and therefore an accurate diagnosis of the type of epilepsy from which the patient is suffering is mandatory. Similarly, since the circumstances of each patient's epilepsy tend to be highly individual and are important for the establishment of a comprehensive plan of management, diagnostic study implies not only an investigation of the type of seizure, its frequency and severity, but also a determination of any conditioning or precipitating factors which may be present. The identification of any localizing factors is of importance and may be suggested by the case history, by the neurological examination or by special investigations.

The writer has chosen to adopt the International Classification of Seizures (Commission on Classification, 1981) for the purpose of categorizing the various seizure types described in this book. It is much easier to classify epileptic seizures based on symptomatology than it is to classify the epilepsies on an aetiological basis. Taylor (1979) has emphasized the dangers of classifying illnesses as opposed to diseases. One danger is that the categories, being arbitrary, can develop a valid existence which is nevertheless independent of physical reality. As he points out, symptoms such as fever, cough, pain or seizures can all be studied at a phenomenonological level, but simply cannot be contained within independent categories. Therefore, it is essential that an attempt be made to identify the epileptic syndromes of which individual seizures are but one feature but which draw attention to the existence of syndromes. To this end, the proposals of the Commission on Classification (1989) concerning classification of the epilepsies and epileptic syndromes have been adopted in this book. It is essential for the proper clinical approach to the management of childhood epilepsy that these classifications should be employed as far as is possible in such a diverse condition. Apart from their clinical usefulness, they have the virtues of being acceptable on an international level and of facilitating the exchange of information about epilepsy.

## Diseases, illnesses and predicaments

If we accept the advantages and limitations of classification as applied to epilepsy, we can then consider epilepsy, as Taylor (1979) has suggested, under the separate headings of disease, illness and predicaments.

### Diseases

In epilepsy, as with other symptoms, the physicians seeks *diseases* which are known to be relevant to the presenting symptom. These will include congenital abnormality, acquired brain injury, infections of the central nervous system and new growths of various kinds. Possible genetic influences will also be considered. Disease diagnosis includes both specifying structural and functional changes and providing a description of the causal mechanisms involved.

Knowledge of diseases grows with research, and in the case of epilepsy, it has grown dramatically in recent years as a result of discoveries in genetics and molecular biology and following the advent of neuroimaging by CT and MRI scanning. This may be of crucial importance for the illness of epilepsy because diseases allow scope for specific remediation by attacking and possibly eliminating or arresting the disease process involved. However, in the case of many of the known diseases of which epilepsy is a symptom nothing can be done or, alternatively, needs to be done, and the treatment of the symptoms alone is adequate therapy.

### Illnesses

'This is the process of declaration of disease in its symptomatic form . . . Unless it is predicated that all is already known about all diseases it has to be accepted that the concept of illness is valid without discoverable disease' (Taylor, 1979). This leads to an acceptance of a classification of epilepsy based on clinical symptomatology. Knowledge of disease is enhanced by classification, provided that we never allow ourselves to become hide-bound and the captives of our own classifications. Diagnosis of illness consists of description and, as has been seen, this is particularly true of epilepsy. Taylor reminds us that in the absence of disease definition all therapy is empirical, which again has been true of the drug therapy of epilepsy from the introduction of bromides onwards although recent advances in our understanding of central neurotransmission, particularly in relation to inhibitory and excitatory amino acids, are providing a rational basis for the search for new antiepileptic drugs (Meldrum, 1983). The recent addition of vigabatrin and lamotrigine to the therapeutic armamentarium is clear evidence of this.

**Predicaments**

Taylor (1979) uses the word 'predicaments' to mean the complex of psychological and social difficulties which bear on the individual as a result of having a chronic illness. He further emphasizes that people are expected to 'get well soon' and if they fail to do so they lose the status of being ill. People who are normally well and who develop acute illnesses tend to get more sympathy than those who have a chronic disorder. Illness which persists is not so supportable socially as is acute illness, particularly if, as happens with epilepsy, there is no definite underlying disease.

The predicament of an individual is more personal than environmental – it is how the individual is placed in his particular environment. As Taylor so beautifully puts it, the predicament of an individual with a chronic illness is much less that of a textbook description of the illness and much more of an up-to-date chapter in his personal autobiography. Predicaments are influenced by social *mores* and by the expectations of affected individuals and their families and friends. The diagnosis of a predicament requires time and discernment, and knowledge of the predicament grows with understanding (Taylor, 1979). Anyone who has looked after children with epilepsy over many years will be very familiar with this fact. It is one of the reasons why an affected child who sees the same physician over a period of years is likely to do far better than one who sees a succession of interns, residents or registrars at a hospital. The single physician, while he may produce little change in the disease or even the illness, may be able to influence the patient's predicament in all sorts of ways, i.e. psychological, social or otherwise.

In summary, if diagnosis is crucial for the proper management of epilepsy, then the diagnostic task should be to discover the disease (if possible), describe the illness and discern the predicament. This diagnostic triad is dependent on different philosophies, has different purposes and demands the development of separate skills. The attending physician will certainly have to call on people from other disciplines to help him complete the task. As with so many chronic diseases in childhood, a multidisciplinary approach is used. Successful therapy depends on having a broad approach to the physical, neurological and psychological aspects of each patient's problem. These points will be mentioned again when special centres for epilepsy are discussed.

## Acceptance and the term epilepsy

The acceptance of any chronic disorder and its limitations is difficult. It depends not only on factors such as the severity of the illness and the degree to which it handicaps the patient, but also on the inherent personality of the affected individual and on the understanding of the illness itself by the patient and/or his family. In the case of epilepsy, acceptance is particularly difficult because the afflicted individual and his family must acclimatize themselves not only to his illness and its associated hazards and complications, but also to the unfortunate adverse attitudes of society towards the entire epileptic population. Because of this dual difficulty, epilepsy is especially a disorder in which understanding and insight are exceedingly important factors in helping the patient and his family to learn acceptance. It should always be remembered that few experiences can be more frightening for parents than to see their child in a convulsion, and the basis of management must be sympathetic and knowledgeable advice, bearing in mind that epilepsy is still a word which causes misunderstanding and fear. Some physicians and clinics have adopted the policy of concealing the word 'epilepsy' from the patient and his parents and a variety of other more euphemistic terms have proliferated. The author agrees with Livingston (1972) that it is better not to withhold the term 'epilepsy' from the parents and the older patients. He points out that it is impossible to hide the word 'epilepsy' because it is used in medical textbooks, is seen in newspapers and magazines and is heard on radio and television. He believed that alternative terms are likely to create confusion and puzzlement for the patient and his parents, and that it is better to face the problem honestly and to explain that the word 'epilepsy' is derived from a Greek word 'epilepsia' meaning to be seized.

## Parents' reactions

Livingston (1972), in an excellent account of the general management of the epileptic child, described the first reaction of many parents to a diagnosis of epilepsy as being one of horror and frequently of disbelief. Many parents have a feeling of guilt stemming from the belief that they have brought a child into the world with a 'horrible disease'. He emphasized that there is a general belief that epilepsy is a shameful disease, and that the physician should, with tact and understanding, make the following points to them:

1   There is no definite proof that epilepsy is unquestionably an inherited disease.
2   There is no reason why epilepsy should carry a stigma.
3   They should look upon epilepsy as a disease differing in no way in its social implications from other diseases such as rheumatic fever, tuberculosis or diabetes.

Livingston also pointed out that the parents must be made to realize that nothing they have done has contributed to the development of epilepsy in their child. Parents may believe that the condition has resulted from some error of omission or commission on their part or even that the development of epilepsy is a 'punishment for their sins'. Such feelings may affect their attitude towards the child leading to either overprotection or rejection. Ward and Bower (1978) have dealt with these problems in detail in their excellent study.

Parents will want to know how much to tell the child. Obviously this will vary between patients, depending on the severity of the illness, the age of the child and the likelihood of his understanding the situation. Livingston (1972) believed that explanations of the illness are probably best given to the child by the parents after they themselves adequately understand the disorder, and that the doctor should indicate to the child that he understands how the child feels as a seizure comes on and after it is over. He emphasized that the term 'epilepsy' should not be concealed from the child as he gets older, and he believed that generally the time when the child can best accept and understand the full implications of epilepsy is when he reaches his early teens. A child who is not kept informed in this way may end up by being enlightened by outsiders and may then feel resentment against his parents because they concealed the information. The handicapping nature of epilepsy should not be minimized and, for the epileptic child or adolescent, this is usually related to what he can or cannot do.

In general, patients who are having seizures or who have been free from them for only a short time should be prohibited from climbing to any dangerous height and from participating in unsupervised swimming. Activities such as team sports and gymnastics are to be encouraged if feasible, because they tend to encourage feelings of normality, independence and wellbeing in the child. The question of bicycling may present difficulties and may have to be prohibited for a short time until the frequency of the attacks and the response to treatment are better defined (*see* Appendix 2). In adolescence, the patient will want to know about the likelihood of driving a car and about possible employment. In general, it is best for the patient to accept certain limitations in living imposed by the epileptic disorder while at the same time maintaining the highest degree of normal activity as possible. He should be taught 'to live with his epilepsy' and to disregard, as far as possible, society's prejudice and ignorance about the condition.

## Teachers and schooling

The question of telling teachers and school authorities about the child's epilepsy usually arises. While attitudes about this point will vary from case to case, it is best to inform teachers, particularly if the child's attacks are likely to occur at school.

It is essential that student teachers be informed about the nature of epilepsy and encouraged to have an enlightened and optimistic attitude towards the condition. They should be taught about the emergency treatment of a child having a major seizure in the classroom.

The teacher is the key to the school situation in much the same way as the parents are the key to the family situation. A capable teacher who can handle a seizure in the classroom with composure and who can then calmly explain the situation to the other children will contribute enormously towards improving attitudes about the disorder. This is a positive contribution not only to the afflicted child but also to the social education and development of desirable attitudes of the class as a whole. Furthermore, the teacher is often in the best position to evaluate the educational needs of the children with epilepsy with whom he deals and should be consulted on this matter.

Nowadays, it should be possible in cases of uncomplicated epilepsy to control seizures sufficiently for them not to disrupt a child's schooling unduly. In fact, many epileptic children never have seizures at school (Henderson, 1953), probably because their attention is engaged in class.

It is generally agreed that the child with epilepsy should be raised in circumstances, both at home and at school, which approximate to normal as nearly as possible. Extremes of neglect and overprotection should be avoided. Children with epilepsy are no less children because of their epilepsy, but they are children at a disadvantage and this is a fact which must be grasped if they are to develop their capabilities fully.

The question of the need for special residential schools for children with epilepsy needs consideration here. There are now four such schools in England. It is important to realize that, while special educational methods are required for the blind, deaf and mentally handicapped, no such methods are required for children with epilepsy. Most children with epilepsy are appropriately educated in normal schools. The child with severe epilepsy who also has another specific handicap such as mental handicap is more suitably looked after by the mental handicap service. A very small sub-group, representing about 1% of children with epilepsy, may require special schooling because of epilepsy alone. However, Kurtz (1983), reporting on a study to determine the reasons for referral to residential schools for children with epilepsy, found that the principal reasons were difficult behaviour, breakdown in the home situation and breakdown in the school situation in the majority of cases and that the seizures were the reason in only a small minority.

Besag, who has written extensively from his experiences as Medical Director of St. Piers Hospital School at Lingfield, Surrey, has listed the possible reasons for referral to such a school as follows (Besag, 1987):

1  Difficult epilepsy.
2  Other medical problems.
3  Cognitive problems.
4  Behaviour problems.
5  Peer group problems.
6  Family and social problems.
7  Psychiatric problems.
8  Multiple problems.

Many teachers find epilepsy a frightening and disruptive condition to deal with in the classroom and, although counselling of teachers and students may ameliorate this problem, nevertheless very frequent seizures may making teaching of the child in a normal classroom impossible. Major tonic–clonic seizures and drop attacks cause concern about the risk of head injury and wearing of protective headgear may be necessary. Teachers worry about their legal responsibility in such a situation. The risk of a prolonged seizure may require urgent medication with rectal diazepam: teachers may be unwilling to administer this and it is not always effective. Post-ictal drowsiness and abnormal behaviour may present problems in the classroom. The side-effects of drugs may also cause difficulties. The recognition of absence attacks of whatever type is difficult at the best of times. Such subtle seizure activity in the classroom may lead to inattention and to a major disruption of the learning process.

Epilepsy may be associated with other major disorders such as congenital heart disease or diabetes mellitus, or it may be a consequence of hydrocephalus or head injury or follow neurosurgical procedures. These children often experience difficulties in mainstream schooling and residence at a hospital school may provide an answer. Cognitive problems (see Chapter 21) may need assessment and advice from a multidisciplinary team which has had the opportunity of observing the child in the classroom. Problems of behaviour, problems with peer groups and, occasionally, severe psychiatric problems may necessitate schooling in a special setting.

The degree of mental stress between parents of a child with difficult epilepsy is high and marriage breakdown is also correspondingly high. There are problems of overprotection and rejection of the child, of sibling interaction and resentment.

The special residential school for children can provide both education and medical management. Besag (1987) points out that parents often express hopes that their child will develop confidence, maturity and independence at the school and that these qualities have been impossible to develop at home. He stresses that the inculcation of these qualities is part of the philosophy of the residential epilepsy school where there is emphasis on independence training, contact with the community and extensive work experience. Most will share his view that the aim of all these concerned with the education of children with epilepsy is to limit their lifestyle as little as possible and to encourage them to develop both intellectually and socially to the best of their abilities. For some children, this aim is greatly facilitated by educating them in one of the special schools for epilepsy.

## Intelligence levels and testing

The parents of children with seizure disorders and their doctors are always concerned with the prognosis for intellectual development and academic attainment, and the child with epilepsy should, ideally, have a full psychometric assessment. If possible, this should be carried out by an experienced and skilled psychologist who is familiar with and sympathetic to the problems of epileptic children. It appears that too often, in the author's experience, psychologists seem to harbour the same preconceived ideas and prejudices about epilepsy as society in general. It is not adequate simply to perform a battery of IQ tests. The possible effects of drugs and of subclinical discharges mean that a single IQ estimation, particularly if low, should be interpreted with caution. Ounsted (1971), in his review of some aspects of seizure disorders, emphasized that the responses to intelligence tests fluctuate unpredictably in children with seizures. This fact was established as early as 1924 by Fox, who showed that there were remarkable fluctuations, both upwards and downwards, in the levels of intelligence attained by these children. Furthermore, these fluctuations are often independent of the factors of medication and frequency of seizures although these factors may influence the results of testing at times, particularly in those children subject to episodes of minor epileptic status (Brett, 1966).

Another point which emerges from a study of the literature on intelligence in children with epilepsy is that opinions vary enormously, presumably depending on the particular sample of epileptic children the author has studied. Indeed, Rodin (1968) felt that the problem of intelligence in children with epilepsy was far from settled and that the answer must await 'more long-term interdisciplinary work between neurologists, psychiatrists, psychologists, and electroencephalographers'. It is probably fair to generalize to the extent that the mean IQ is likely to be average in children whose epilepsy is uncomplicated by organic brain disorders such as mental subnormality and cerebral palsy.

Rutter, Graham and Yule (1970) produced an IQ figure of 102 on the Wechsler's intelligence scale in children with epilepsy which was uncomplicated by organic brain disorders. Their very careful study of children in the Isle of Wight showed clearly the dangers of using unrefined averages when studying the intelligence levels of children with epilepsy. Many previous studies which had included children who derived their epilepsy from organic brain disorders, such as mental subnormality and cerebral palsy, had suggested that the IQ distribution in epilepsy generally was skewed towards the lower end of the scale. Taking cognisance of this fact, Rutter, Graham and Yule (1970) showed that the intelligence of children with such organic brain disorders arising above the brain-stem and associated with epilepsy was well below average. When the 28% of children with these disorders were considered together with the 72% of children with epilepsy uncomplicated in this way, the IQ level of their entire epileptic child population was also well below average. Considered separately, however, the remaining children with uncomplicated epilepsy were found to have the same IQ distribution as the general population of children and many children were of above average and even superior intelligence. Thus, while one of the underlying causes of epilepsy may also be a cause of low intelligence, the fact of having seizures is not in itself an indicator of low intelligence. It is probably reassuring for parents to hear the long list of famous epileptics in history, which includes Socrates, Julius Caesar, Alexander the Great, Dante, Byron and Dostoevski.

One may also look at this problem in another way, i.e. by considering the intelligence level in different types of childhood epilepsy. Normal intelligence is usually found in patients with primary generalized epilepsy of the childhood absence or idiopathic grand mal type and in the partial epilepsies with elementary or simple symptomatology as for example in benign focal epilepsy of childhood. Ounsted, Lindsay and Norman (1966), in their study of temporal lobe epilepsy in childhood, found that 68 of their series of 100 children had intelligence test results within the range required for normal schooling, but they also found that many of these children had learning difficulties. Fedio and Mirsky (1969) found specific patterns of intellectual impairment in children with unilateral temporal lobe abnormalities and epilepsy. Within the first decade of life, they found that involvement of the left temporal lobe imposed limitations on the development of verbal intelligence and on the learning and/or memory capacity for verbal material. Non-verbal functions were spared. The converse was true for children with right temporal lobe epilepsy; these were more likely to have perceptual difficulties related to visuospatial learning. The authors pointed out that the results were similar to those obtained in adults with comparable cerebral dysfunction, and that they supported the view that cerebral differentiation of intellectual processes was established in childhood and that early and late cerebral injury produced comparable results in childhood and adult life. As was emphasized in early chapters of this book, the serious types of epilepsy which commence in infancy and early childhood, such as infantile spasms and the severe varieties of myoclonic epilepsy, are very frequently associated with mental handicap, which is often profound. Many authors have stressed the close association between the early onset of epilepsy and later intellectual impairment (Chevrie and Aicardi, 1978; Cavazzuti, Ferrari and Lalla, 1984). Others, particularly those concerned with the follow-up of children suffering febrile convulsions, were unable to attribute a higher risk of mental retardation (defined as an IQ less than 70) to early appearance of seizures (Ellenberg, Hirtz and Nelson, 1984). Children with the early onset of frequent or intractable seizures tend to gravitate to special centres and adversely affect results for overall prognosis. However, when allowance is made for this, the writer agrees with those who prefer to give a guarded prognosis for those children who present with seizures before their first birthday, including those with febrile convulsions.

The possible association between frequency of seizures and later intelligence is also controversial. It seems, however, that the aetiology of the epilepsy is more important in determining the level of intelligence than is the actual number of seizures. No correlation was found between frequency of febrile convulsions and IQ at 7 years, for example (Nelson and Ellenberg, 1978). Children with frequent seizures, whatever the variety of epilepsy, are more likely to be taking more medication for a longer period of time with possible side-effects on cognition and later intellectual ability. The possible effects of status epilepticus on intelligence are discussed in Chapters 11 and 15.

It is widely accepted that there is a connection between complicated epilepsy and lower social class, although this is by no means a clear-cut association. It may be that lower standards of medical care together with an adverse environment could lead to a higher incidence of disorders which result in epilepsy. The theory of what is called social drift may also be relevant. According to this theory, persons with some form of handicap are unable to maintain their position in the social hierarchy and drift downwards to the lower social class occupations. In the case of epilepsy, however, incidence of new cases is highest in the formative years before employment is sought, so it may be more characteristic for people with epilepsy to tend to find jobs with a lower social status than their parents early in life.

# Precipitating factors

The identification of possible precipitating or conditioning factors in the causation of seizures in the individual patient is important in the management of epilepsy. Some people with epilepsy, for example, have all or most of their attacks during *sleep*. The association between sleep and epilepsy is dealt with in Chapter 17. The relationship of epilepsy to *menstruation* is also well known and refers to the fact that in some females seizures are observed to occur immediately before or shortly after the beginning of the monthly period, or they are more frequent and severe at that time. This type of epilepsy is called catamenial epilepsy. The phenomenon may reflect hormonal changes with associated changes in antiepileptic drug levels and, in addition, water retention may be a factor prior to and during menses (Rosciczewska *et al.*, 1986). Acetazolamide 250 mg or 500 mg daily, beginning 10 days prior to the expected onset of menses and continuing until bleeding stops, can be effective adjunctive therapy. Antiepileptic drug medication may need to be increased at this time to provide higher blood levels.

*Hyperventilation* may precipitate epileptic attacks and this is probably a specific effect in true petit mal. Curiously enough, however, the overbreathing associated with normal physical exertion rarely, if ever, causes absence attacks (*see* Appendix 2). *Photic stimulation* as a trigger mechanism of seizures is discussed with other causes of reflex epilepsy in Chapter 12.

*Emotional disturbances* such as excitement, fear, frustration, tension and anxiety may act as precipitants of attacks in some patients, particularly in older children and teenagers (Gastaut and Tassinari, 1966). However, as Livingston (1972) pointed out, the physician should be wary of overemphasizing this point to parents in case they respond by overprotecting the child and shielding him from the normal and often emotionally exciting circumstances of everyday life. This in turn may lead to a neurosis connected with his epilepsy and a deep sense of being different from his peers. Livingston (1972) also believed that a change of environment may favourably affect the course of epileptic seizures, particularly in children, and he cited some interesting case histories to prove his point. He quoted Hippocrates who in the fifth century BC stated: 'Epilepsy in young persons is most frequently removed by changes of air, of country and of modes of life.'

*Fever* is, of course, an important cause of convulsions in early childhood but illness and high temperature may also cause a convulsion in an older child with epilepsy. *Lack of sleep, chronic fatigue and alcohol* may act as precipitants, particularly in adolescence. Sometimes a combination of factors may operate; for example, one of the author's adolescent patients, at a time of great emotional stress in the family, developed partial seizures of complex symptomatology with the EEG showing a temporal lobe focus. He was described by his mother as 'sitting up most of the night talking to his friends, smoking French cigarettes and drinking black coffee'. Advice about a more orderly way of life, an improvement in the emotional climate and the prescription of carbamazepine for some months led to a complete and permanent cessation of his epilepsy and the EEG returned to normal.

The sudden *withdrawal of anticonvulsant drugs* is a common cause of an increase in the frequency of seizures or even of status epilepticus. The barbiturates and, to a lesser extent, phenytoin are particularly important in this respect. There is no justification for withdrawing anticonvulsant medication suddenly prior to an EEG examination, and happily this deplorable and dangerous practice seems to be dying out. Occasionally, where there is doubt about the diagnosis of true petit mal and the patient is already taking ethosuximide, it is reasonable to withdraw the drug slowly prior to an EEG examination. Sometimes, drug therapy has to be discontinued abruptly because of untoward reactions caused by the drug. In some instances it may be wise to protect that patient by the administration of a different anticonvulsant. The reader is also referred to the section on non-visual precipitating factors in the chapter on reflex epilepsy (page 144).

## Drug therapy and the patient

The following chapters will be devoted to the drug therapy of epilepsy and the adverse effects of such treatment. Treatment with anticonvulsant drugs is likely to remain the cornerstone of therapy in the foreseeable future. It is salutary, therefore, to consider that among adults with epilepsy it has been estimated that 30% of those suffering from repeated seizures never consult a doctor at all (Janz, 1976). A field survey among adults in Warsaw by Zielinsky (1974) disclosed that 37% of all patients who had had more than two epileptic attacks had never taken an anticonvulsant drug and that, at the time of the survey, only 35% were being given drug treatment. Admittedly, of the patients in the Warsaw study who had never been treated, most were suffering from mild forms of epilepsy; only a quarter of them had consulted a doctor and one-third had been free of seizures for more than 5 years. Among the untreated patients, many were subject to focal attacks or absences which they did not regard as requiring treatment, and major seizures were infrequent. Other patients, including those with major attacks, simply did not want to be treated, or thought that epilepsy was untreatable or refrained from consulting a doctor because they were afraid of being admitted to hospital and subjected to diagnostic procedures. Others had been treated and discontinued their medication because of side-effects or had discontinued their drugs because they considered them ineffective or they had become free of attacks.

While these observations are not directly applicable to children with epilepsy, they do, nevertheless, provide food for thought where the efficacy or otherwise of drug therapy is concerned. The reasons why these observations are less likely to apply to children are apparent from a commentary by Janz (1976) on his own work and on Zielinsky's findings. He points out that epilepsy differs from most other illnesses in that it is not the epileptic attacks which entail suffering for the patient, but rather their repercussions *vis-a-vis* society. The manifestations of epilepsy which make the strongest impression upon the onlooker – the sudden cry, the fall and the muscle contractions of the clonic stage – are suffered by the patient but are not really experienced by him. What actually impinges upon the patient's consciousness during an attack is in no way comparable with the shock experienced by the on-looker, usually parents, guardians or teacher in the case of a child. As Janz (1976) says: 'patients with epilepsy experience their illness chiefly as mirrored in the reactions of their fellow men.' Where children are concerned, the latter are likely to seek medical help in order to try to prevent a recurrence of the shocking event they have witnessed. Therefore, we can conclude that the motivation to seek treatment for epilepsy occurring in children is far greater than it is among adults with epilepsy.

Before prescribing antiepileptic drugs for a child with suspected epilepsy, one should establish a firm diagnosis, categorize the seizure type or types, attempt to identify the epileptic syndrome present, and try to make an aetiological diagnosis (O'Donohoe, 1991). The initiation of treatment needs to be considered on a risk *versus* benefit basis (Freeman, 1987). The nature of the epileptic syndrome present will influence the decision. For example, in benign partial epilepsy with rolandic spikes, up to a quarter of patients may have only one seizure and approximately half have fewer than five seizures (Beaussart and Faou, 1978). It should be remembered that single seizures may occur in any individual and do not necessarily mean a diagnosis of epilepsy. Studies of recurrences after a first unprovoked seizure in a child (Hirtz, Ellenberg and Nelson, 1984; Shinnar *et al.*, 1990) have shown that between 50 and 65% of children may remain seizure-free with or without medication. Key risk factors for recurrence are the aetiology (idiopathic versus a remote symptomatic cause) and the EEG. This matter is discussed in greater detail in the section in the single or solitary attack (Chapter 8).

It must also be remembered that antiepileptic drugs are potent substances which may cause side-effects, including idiosyncratic side-effects, and acute and chronic toxicity (see Chapter 26). The overall benign nature of much of childhood epilepsy must also be appreciated. Between 70 and 75% of children who remain seizure-free for 4 years on treatment remain so when treatment is stopped (Emerson *et al.*, 1981) and similar results have been reported after 2 years' treatment (Shinnar *et al.*, 1985). All these matters should make us pause and consider before embarking on long-term drug therapy. If we do use drugs, we should give as much as is needed but as little as is necessary to control the seizures, avoiding polytherapy if possible, and using drug level monitoring wisely.

## Patient compliance

The only absolute indication for drug therapy is chronic epilepsy, i.e. the repeated occurrence of seizures at fairly frequent intervals. The problems of the individual with the single seizure are dealt with in Chapter 8. The question of using prophylactic anticonvulsant medication is discussed in connection with the dangers arising from repeated febrile convulsions (see Chapter 6) and also where the prevention of post-traumatic epilepsy is concerned (see Chapter 14). When anticonvulsant medication is prescribed in any situation, it is only likely to be successful if the patients take their drugs conscientiously, regularly and in adequate doses over prolonged periods of time. Such a degree of patient compliance is essential if an unsatisfactory response to therapy is to be avoided. The patients should be carefully instructed concerning the importance of regular medication and should be familiar with the names of the drugs being used and their dosage schedules. It is the author's practice to write out the patient's dosage schedules for the parents, since solely verbal instructions may easily be forgotten or confused. The patient's drug serum level should be checked if noncompliance or poor compliance with instructions about treatment is suspected.

## Changing drugs

Changing from one drug to another should be done carefully, gradually withdrawing one drug and simultaneously introducing another in a stepwise fashion. Another method used for effecting a changeover of medication is to add the new drug to the old regimen, await the effects of the combined medication and then, if necessary, withdraw the original drug slowly. In this way one can assess the effect of the combined medication compared with monotherapy with either the old or the new drug. It is the author's practice to aim at twice daily medication if possible. Because the half-lives (i.e. the time taken for one-half of a given dose to be eliminated from the body) of most anticonvulsants are long, there is not much point in trying to adapt the daily dosage schedule to the time of day at which attacks are most likely to occur, although in certain mild types of epilepsy, such as benign focal epilepsy of childhood, the administration of medication at bedtime only may often be sufficient. Some parents become quite obsessional about giving the drugs at unsuitable times, such as 6.00 a.m. or 12.00 midnight, in the mistaken belief that this will prevent seizures occurring predominantly in the early morning or during sleep. However, this should be discouraged since it disrupts the child's normal day and is likely to be ineffective. In general, tablets are the desired form of medication because they provide an exact dose. Capsules have the same advantage for older children but cannot be divided. Liquid preparations of anticonvulsants are the least desirable because they are prone to provide inexact dosage. Drug boxes divided into compartments marked with the days of the week facilitate regular medication and prevent confusion between parent and child about omission of a dose (Gamstorp, 1983).

Quite apart from the precipitating or conditioning factors described earlier, children with epilepsy may inexplicably have good periods and bad periods, and parents should be discouraged from arbitrarily increasing the dosage of drugs in the bad periods because this may easily lead to overtreatment and its consequences. Similarly, with certain types of epilepsy associated with structural brain disease and mental and neurological handicap, parents should be instructed that seizures are unlikely to be controlled fully and that they should accept a certain 'inevitability of epilepsy' and learn to live with it, again without constant changes and increases in drug therapy.

## Special centres: the multidisciplinary approach

Because of the complexities of diagnosis and management of epilepsy, the question of the need for special centres and clinics for epilepsy needs consideration and has been reviewed in detail by Brown (1976). As he pointed out, there has been a veritable explosion of knowledge about the genetics, electrophysiology, neurochemistry and pharmacology of epilepsy in recent years making it difficult for anyone but the specialist to keep abreast of the changing epileptic scene. There has been a remarkable increase in knowledge of the adverse effects of anticonvulsant drugs (to be described later), including the recognition of various clinical syndromes, making it imperative that the physician dealing with epilepsy should have access to facilities for monitoring the levels of these drugs in the blood plasma. Something approaching a third of all epileptic children are mentally retarded to a greater or lesser degree (see Chapter 15) and many have behavioural difficulties. These include the hyperkinetic behaviour and other difficulties of the child with temporal lobe epilepsy, and the withdrawn autistic behaviour of the child who has had infantile spasms or severe myoclonic epilepsy and also a host of less severe reactions including enuresis, encopresis, phobias and anxieties. The educational and learning difficulties of the child of normal intelligence with epilepsy have already been discussed (see Chapter 21). Medicosocial problems are also common in the family with an epileptic child – the predicaments of the patient and his family.

It is clear that the child with epilepsy needs a multidisciplinary approach but, because of the way in which the growth and development of the child are so intimately linked with the type of epilepsy which may afflict him, in contrast to the relatively unchanging state of the adult, it seems unlikely that special centres for epilepsy are the answer as far as paediatric epileptology is concerned. The multidisciplinary approach to epilepsy in childhood should involve the participation of people with many different skills and interests, but not necessarily working under the same roof. The family doctor will have the closest contact with the family in their predicament, and the paediatrician will be involved when the child is first referred with epilepsy. The paediatrician is in the front line as far as the prevention of epilepsy is concerned, and this will be discussed in Chapter 29. The community physician, the teacher, the child psychiatrist and the psychologist may all be involved. A special outpatient clinic for children with epilepsy, based in a children's hospital or in the children's department of a general hospital and under the supervision of a paediatrician with a special interest in epilepsy or of a paediatric neurologist, is particularly valuable because it allows time to be allotted to the parents for discussion of their problems and also because it ensures continuing care by one concerned physician. The place of special schools for children with epilepsy has already been mentioned.

There is no doubt that there is a need for 'centres of excellence' to which intractable and difficult cases of childhood epilepsy may be referred for detailed study and where the psychotherapeutic management of the whole family in their predicament can be undertaken. An example of such a centre in the UK is the Park Hospital in Oxford where a distinguished group of specialists representing several disciplines has made many outstanding contributions to the understanding and management of childhood epilepsy (Ounsted, 1974). Guidelines for specialized epilepsy centres serving all age-groups have recently been published in the United States (National Association of Epilepsy Centres, 1990). 'Fourth-level' medical and surgical centres are recommended as regional or national referral centres, serving millions of people. These centres should provide intensive EEG and neuroimaging facilities, neuropsychological and psychosocial services and also facilities for surgical treatment or for referral to an appropriate surgical unit.

## References

BEAUSSART, M. and FAOU, R. (1978) Evolution of epilepsy with rolandic paroxysmal foci: a study of 324 cases. *Epilepsia*, **19**, 337–342

BESAG, F. M. C. (1987) The role of the special school for children with epilepsy. In *Epilepsy and Education* (eds J. Oxley and G. Stores), Education in Practice for the Medical Tribune Group, London, pp. 65–71

BRETT, E. M. (1966) Minor epileptic status. *Journal of the Neurological Sciences*, **3**, 52–75

BROWN, J. K. (1976) Special clinics for epilepsy. *Developmental Medicine and Child Neurology*, **18**, 809–811

CAVAZZUTI, G. B., FERRARI, P. and LALLA, M. (1984) Follow-up study of 482 cases with convulsive disorders in the first year of life. *Developmental Medicine and Child Neurology*, **26**, 425–437

CHEVRIE, J. J. and AICARDI, J. (1979) Convulsive disorders in the first year of life. Neurologic and mental outcome and mortality. *Epilepsia*, **19**, 67–74

COMMISSION ON CLASSIFICATION AND TERMINOLOGY OF THE INTERNATIONAL LEAGUE AGAINST EPILEPSY (1981) Proposal for revised clinical and electroencephalographic classification of epileptic seizures. *Epilepsia*, **22**, 489–501

COMMISSION ON CLASSIFICATION AND TERMINOLOGY OF THE INTERNATIONAL LEAGUE AGAINST EPILEPSY (1989) Proposal for revised classification of epilepsies and epileptic syndromes. *Epilepsia*, **30**, 389–399

ELLENBERG, J. H., HIRTZ, D. G. and NELSON, K. B. (1984) Age of onset of seizures in young children. *Annals of Neurology*, **15**, 127–134

EMERSON, E., D'SOUZA, B. J., VINING, E. P. et al. (1981) Stopping medication in children with epilepsy. Predictors of outcome. *New England Journal of Medicine*, **304**, 1125–1129

FEDIO, P. and MIRSKY, A. F. (1969) Selective intellectual deficits with temporal lobe or centrencephalic epilepsy. *Neuropsychologia*, **7**, 287–300

FOX, J. T. (1924) The response of epileptic children to mental and educational tests. *British Journal of Medical Psychology*, **4**, 235–248

FREEMAN, J. M. (1987) A clinical approach to the child with seizures and epilepsy. *Epilepsia*, **28**, Supplement 1, S103–S109

GAMSTORP, I. (1983) Co-operation between the physician and the patient and family. In *Antiepileptic Drug Therapy in Pediatrics* (eds P. L. Morselli, C. E. Pippenger and J. K. Penry) Raven Press, New York, pp. 303–308

GASTAUT, H. and TASSINARI, C. A. (1966) Triggering mechanisms in epilepsy: the electroclinical point of view. *Epilepsia*, **7**, 85–138

GREEN, J. B. and HARTLAGE, L. C. (1971) Comparative performance of epileptic and non-epileptic children and adolescents on tests of academic, communicative and social skills. *Diseases of the Nervous System*, **32**, 418–421

HENDERSON, P. (1953) Epilepsy in school children. *British Journal of Preventive and Social Medicine*, **7**, 9

HIRTZ, D. G., ELLENBERG, J. H. and NELSON, K. B. (1984) The risk of recurrence of non-febrile seizures in children. *Neurology*, **34**, 637–641

JANZ, D. (1976) Problems encountered in the treatment of epilepsy. In *Epileptic Seizures–Behaviour–Pain* (ed. W. Birkmayer), Hans Huber, Bern, Stuttgart, Vienna, pp. 65–75

KURTZ, Z. (1983) Special schooling for children with epilepsy. In *Research Progress in Epilepsy* (ed. F. C. Rose), Pitman, London, pp. 538–546

LIVINGSTON, S. (1972) *Comprehensive Management of Epilepsy in Infancy, Childhood and Adolescence*, Charles C. Thomas, Springfield, Illinois, pp. 123–166

MELDRUM, B. S. (1983) Pharmacological considerations in the search for new anticonvulsant drugs. In *Recent Advances in Epilepsy*, No. 1 (eds J. A. Pedley and B. S. Meldrum), Churchill Livingstone, Edinburgh, London, pp. 75–92

NATIONAL ASSOCIATION OF EPILEPSY CENTRES (1990) Recommended guidelines for diagnosis and treatment in specialized epilepsy centers. *Epilepsia*, **31**, Supplement 1, S1–S12

NELSON, K. B. and ELLENBERG, J. H. (1978) Prognosis in children with febrile seizures. *Pediatrics*, **61**, 720–727

O'DONOHOE, N. V. (1991) The epilepsies. In *Paediatric Specialty Practice for the 1990s* (eds J. Eyre and R. Boyd), Royal College of Physicians, London, pp. 51–63

OUNSTED, C. (1971) Some aspects of seizure disorders. In *Recent Advances in Paediatrics* (eds D. Gairdner and D. Hull), J. and A. Churchill, London, pp. 363–400

OUNSTED, C. (1974) A special care centre for children with seizures. *Health Trends*, **6**, 69–71

OUNSTED, C., LINDSAY, J. and NORMAN, R. (1966) *Biological Factors in Temporal Lobe Epilepsy*. Clinics in Developmental Medicine, No. 22, Spastics Society/Heinemann Medical, London

PAZZAGLIA, P. and FRANK-PAZZAGLIA, L. (1976) Record in grade school of pupils with epilepsy: an epidemiological study. *Epilepsia*, **17**, 361–366

RODIN, E. A. (1968) *The Prognosis of Patients with Epilepsy*. Charles C. Thomas, Springfield, Illinois, p. 154

ROSCISZEWSKA, D., BUNTNER, B., GUZ, J. and ZAWISZA, L. (1986) Ovarian hormones, anticonvulsant drugs, and seizures during the menstrual cycle in women with epilepsy. *Journal of Neurology, Neurosurgery and Psychiatry*, **49**, 47–51

RUTTER, M., GRAHAM, P. and YULE, W. (1970) A neuropsychiatric study in childhood. *Clinics in Developmental Medicine*, Nos. 35/36, Spastics International/Heinemann Medical, London, pp. 136–150

SHINNAR, S., VINING, E. P. G., MELLITS, E. M. et al. (1985) Discontinuing antiepileptic medication in children with epilepsy after two years without seizures. *New England Journal of Medicine*, **313**, 976–980

SHINNAR, S., BERG, A. T., MOSHÉ, S. L. et al. (1990) Risk of seizure recurrence following a first unprovoked seizure in childhood. A prospective study. *Pediatrics*, **85**, 1076–1085

STORES, G. (1978) School children with epilepsy at risk for learning and behaviour problems. *Developmental Medicine and Child Neurology*, **20**, 502–508

TAYLOR, D. C. (1979) The components of illness: diseases, illnesses and predicaments. *Lancet*, **2**, 1008–1010

WARD, F. and BOWER, B. D. (1978) A study of certain social aspects of epilepsy in childhood. *Developmental Medicine and Child Neurology*, **20**, Supplement 39

ZIELINSKY, J. J. (1974). Epileptics not in treatment. *Epilepsia*, **15**, 203–210

Chapter 25

# Antiepileptic drug therapy

The control of seizures is the essential and most important problem for all patients with epilepsy. Treatment with antiepileptic drugs is the standard form of therapy today and this situation is unlikely to change in the foreseeable future. The use of such drugs began with the discovery of the effectiveness of bromides in 1857, followed by the introduction of phenobarbitone in 1912 and phenytoin in 1938. Since then, there has been a steady expansion in the therapeutic armamentarium.

The most significant advance in the drug therapy of epilepsy in recent times has been the application of *pharmacokinetic principles* to the use of antiepileptic drugs. Pharmacokinetics encompasses the absorption, distribution and elimination of drugs from the time the drug is given until it is excreted. These processes are affected by factors such as age and by genetic and environmental influences. The development of techniques for measuring serum levels of drugs in low concentration has made it possible to study their pharmacokinetics accurately and scientifically and to study the relationship between drug dosage and serum levels. As a result, the era of the empirical management of epilepsy by drugs has passed and, furthermore, there has been a steady accumulation of new knowledge about the ill-effects of drugs on patients. Often, in the past, these ill-effects outweighed the benefits conferred by seizure control. Until the 1970s, polypharmacy with antiepileptic drugs was the accepted practice in the treatment of epilepsy. However, with refinements in diagnosis and drug monitoring and with the availability of new drugs, there has come the realization that *monotherapy* is a superior therapeutic practice (Reynolds and Shorvon, 1981).

It is as illogical today to treat epilepsy without the availability of serum levels as it would be to use anticoagulants without prothrombin times or antidiabetic agents without determining blood glucose levels. Nevertheless, it should always be remembered that the clinical response of the patient to drugs is still of paramount importance and that there is more to treating epilepsy than the dispensing of pills. The disadvantages of the routine use of drug assays will be considered later.

## Metabolism of antiepileptic drugs

Antiepileptic drugs are usually administered orally. To act effectively, they must be absorbed from the gastrointestinal tract, be disseminated in the circulation, diffuse into the brain's extracellular space and then act on the cell membrane or within the neurone. Most of the commonly used drugs are absorbed rapidly, carbamazepine and phenytoin rather more slowly than the others. After absorption, the various drugs are bound reversibly to plasma proteins, primarily albumin, to a greater or lesser degree. Phenytoin, carbamazepine and sodium valproate are bound to the greatest degree, phenobarbitone is partially bound and primidone and ethosuximide are bound hardly at all. The protein-bound drug serves as a reservoir to maintain the level of free drug in the plasma at a constant level and also to prolong the effects of the drug. The rates at which drugs diffuse across the blood–brain barrier depends on the availability of unbound or free drug in the plasma. This concentration of free drug creates a gradient across the blood–brain barrier. Most antiepileptic drugs are lipid soluble and distribute rapidly in brain tissue after crossing over from the plasma. The action of an individual drug on the brain is determined by the concentration of free drug in brain tissue. It is generally accepted that the estimated total serum concentrations of the various drugs are, for practical purposes, representative of their concentrations in the brain.

The duration of activity of antiepileptic drugs is dependent on their rate of *biotransformation* in the body. The metabolic stages of this process mainly take place in the liver and are mediated by microsomal enzymes located in the endoplasmic reticulum. A process of hydroxylation followed by conjugation with glucuronic acid or sulphate occurs. This leads to the inactivation of the compound and to its increased water solubility which is necessary for excretion via the kidneys. The metabolites produced by biotransformation are inactive, although occasionally, as for example with primidone, active metabolites may be produced which are usually of lower potency than the parent compound. The rate at which antiepileptic drugs are metabolized is governed by the activity of the microsomal enzymes and this activity is under genetic control and varies from individual to individual. It is also affected by age, sex, diet and by other drugs. The physiological changes of maturation affect drug metabolism in the child. In general, the process is relatively prolonged in newborns, whether premature or full-term, but this is soon followed by accelerated metabolism in infants (Dodson, 1983). Children under 5 years of age generally require larger doses of antiepileptic drugs relative to body weight than do older children. Individual variability in the biotransformation of drugs is an additional problem in young patients. For these reasons, more frequent drug level monitoring and adjustments of dosage may be necessary in this age group. As children grow and increase their body mass, there is a progressive decline in relative drug clearance. This offsets the effects of increasing size, with the result that many children do not need to increase their drug dosage during the midchildhood years. This means that they do not necessarily outgrow their dosage as they get older, despite the often expressed anxieties of parents that this may be happening. With the onset of puberty, drug utilization patterns reduce further to those of an adult (Dodson, 1983, 1987a,b, 1988).

As soon as absorption of a drug commences, biotransformation begins in the liver. In the case of the majority of antiepileptic drugs, the rate of biotransformation increases linearly with increasing concentration of the drug. This type of relationship between dosage and serum level is referred to as 'first-order kinetics' (*Figure 25.1a*). When biotransformation is independent of the concentration (or quantity administered) of the drug, it is said to be governed by 'zero-order kinetics' and in this situation, the relationship between dosage and serum level will not be linear (*Figure 25.1b*). Among the antiepileptic drugs, only phenytoin has nonlinear kinetics.

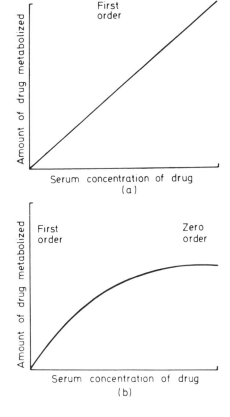

*Figure 25.1* Kinetics of drug metabolism. With first-order kinetics (a) the amount of drug metabolized is proportional to the serum concentration, whereas with saturation kinetics (b) there is a ceiling to the amount of drug metabolized. (From Prof. A. Richens. *Drug Treatments of Epilepsy*, 1976, by courtesy of Henry Kimton, Publishers, London)

This is of paramount importance in the use of phenytoin. The drug is metabolized by first-order kinetics at low serum concentrations but, as the serum level reaches the therapeutic range, the enzyme system becomes saturated, reaches its maximum rate of action and is then governed by the laws of zero-order kinetics. The rate of action of the enzyme systems, when saturated, cannot be exceeded and consequently small increments in dosage produce a disproportionately steep rise in the serum phenytoin level. The clinical implication of this is that it is dangerously easy to pass from subtherapeutic dosage to clinical intoxication when adjusting phenytoin dosage and some children appear more susceptible to this hazard than others (Dodson, 1988). Monitoring of serum levels when using phenytoin is particularly important and increments in drugs should be graduated in small quantities (Richens and Dunlop, 1975).

## Optimal drug schedule

When an antiepileptic drug is given orally in a single dose, the concentration in the plasma will rise to a peak and thereafter decline at a rate dependent upon the speed of its elimination, i.e. metabolism and excretion. Absorption and distribution on the one hand and elimination on the other produce an exponential curve when drug concentration is studied in relation to time. The *plasma half-life of a drug* is the time taken for the plasma concentration to fall by one-half once the elimination phase has been reached. A steady state or plateau level is usually attained after four to five half-lives.

The optimal dosage schedule for any drug involves administration at intervals equal to its biological half-life if a sustained drug effect is to occur. The purpose of such a treatment règime is to maintain trough concentrations of the drug within the therapeutic range without allowing peak concentrations to reach toxic levels. Although there is considerable variation between the half-lives of the various anti-epileptic drugs, this does not usually lead to practical difficulties in administration. In general, it seems more convenient for the majority of patients to take their daily medication in two equally divided doses (morning and evening). The patients or their parents are more likely to remember to administer the drug on such a schedule. However, thrice daily or more frequent dosage may be necessary in babies and small children where biotransformation of the drug is rapid. Sodium valproate, which has a short half-life, should need frequent administration but, when the enteric coated preparation is used, slow absorption blunts the fluctuations in serum levels between doses and makes twice daily administration feasible. With drugs such as carbamazepine, in which there is a narrow margin between the therapeutic level and the toxic level, dosage intervals shorter than the half-life may be preferred. A slow release preparation of this drug is now available. Although phenobarbitone has a very long half-life (36–72 hours in children), the usual twice daily dosage does not usually cause problems, although a once daily schedule should be adequate.

## Drug actions and interactions

The effects of the drugs themselves on the microsomal enzymes are of two kinds. Some drugs increase the activity of these enzymes (enzyme induction) while others decrease their activity (enzyme inhibition). The most potent enzyme inducers are phenobarbitone, primidone, phenytoin and carbamazepine. Sodium valproate is an inhibitor of drug metabolism and, if added to the treatment regimen of a child already receiving phenobarbitone or phenytoin, may cause short-term rises in the concentrations of these drugs into the toxic range. In the case of phenytoin, the situation is further complicated by the fact that both it and sodium valproate are strongly protein bound and may displace each other from binding sites on protein.

Drug-drug interactions between the enzyme inducing drugs are not of great clinical significance. Possibly the only noteworthy one is that between carbamazepine and phenytoin. Carbamazepine reduces the half-life of phenytoin as a result of more rapid metabolism consequent on enzyme induction, and a fall in the blood level of the drug ensues although this only happens in some patients. It is noteworthy that some patients seem more susceptible to the effects of drug interaction than others, probably for genetic reasons (Kutt, 1984).

A slow decline in the steady state levels of many antiepileptic drugs occurs over a period of weeks or months following the establishment of steady state or plateau levels. This is due to accelerated biotransformation consequent on enzyme induction. This may lead to the erroneous impression that the drug is no longer effective whereas what is required to regain the effect is an increase in dosage. Eventually, an appropriate dosage/serum level stability will be achieved. This effect is particularly important in the case of carbamazepine whose clearance doubles between the first and sixth week of treatment. Fortunately, this autoinduction effect of carbamazepine is shortlived and a steady state is usually achieved after 4–8 weeks of therapy (Dodson, 1988). Adding another drug such as phenobarbitone or phenytoin will, however, induce further increases in enzyme activity, and carbamazepine levels will again fall.

The important clinical effects of these potent enzymes inducers on certain naturally occurring endogenous substances will be considered in the next chapter.

## Drug monitoring in epilepsy

The rational use of antiepileptic drug level monitoring plays an important part in the control of seizures today. Spectrophotometric methods have been available since the late 1940s, but have not been particularly reliable. Gas-liquid chromatography, high-performance liquid chromatography and radioimmunoassay are widely used, are accurate and specific for a wide range of drugs and are extensively employed in research. These methods require the services of a skilled biochemist if reliable and reproducible results are to be obtained. Radioimmunoassay methods are employed for drugs such as the benzodiazepines. The broader application of this method has been limited by its use of hazardous, expensive, unstable and radioactive chemicals and its use of complex expensive instrumentation. Enzyme immunoassay uses the selective affinity of antibodies for specific molecules to measure small amounts of chemical compounds in biological fluids. Different methods are available and are rapid, easily learnt and accurate, but rather expensive. Whatever method of assaying antiepileptic drugs is employed, it is essential that the particular laboratory involved belongs to a quality control scheme designed to monitor the accuracy of results obtained in different laboratories (Goldberg *et al.*, 1983).

For the purposes of comparing successive serum drug concentrations, each sample should ideally be drawn at the same time with respect to the dosage schedule. There is no agreement, however, about whether trough levels, estimated before the morning dose when the concentrations are lowest, or levels estimated at some other fixed time in the day and measured consistently at that time, provide more useful information. If the response of the patient to therapy is unexpected or aberrant, then it is valuable to determine a profile of serum levels during 24 hours (Wallace, 1990).

### Indications for monitoring

Antiepileptic drug levels may be measured in plasma, serum or saliva (*Table 25.1*). The serum and plasma levels are comparable and are a measure of protein-bound and free drug concentrations, while the levels in saliva relate to the amount of free drug in plasma. Adequate volumes of saliva are difficult to obtain from children and estimations in plasma or serum are the rule. Methods for the rapid assay of antiepileptic drugs by enzyme immunoassay or fluorescence polarization immunoassay have recently become available and will produce results within 15 minutes, using small amounts of blood (Houtman *et al.*, 1990). These methods have advantages for outpatient clinic practice, especially where assays of phenytoin and carbamazepine are concerned. Wallace (1990), in a paediatric neurology clinic, found that immediate knowledge of phenytoin levels was particularly valuable and that improved drug treatment strategies generally were made possible by such rapidly available information.

Richens (1976) listed the following indications for drug level monitoring in epilepsy:

1   Where there is interindividual variation in the rate of metabolism of drugs, as is the case in childhood.
2   Where the phenomenon of 'saturation kinetics' occurs, as it does with phenytoin.
3   Where the therapeutic index is low, i.e. when therapeutic doses are close to toxic doses.
4   Where signs of toxicity are difficult to recognize clinically, as may occur in children or in the mentally handicapped.
5   Where patients are on multiple drug therapy with the associated problem of drug interaction.
6   Where other diseases of the gastrointestinal tract, the liver or the kidneys are present which may interfere with drug absorption or elimination.
7   Where the patient's reliability in taking his medication is in doubt (so-called patient compliance).
8   Where the patient's seizures are refractory to treatment.
9   Where therapeutic trials of a drug are being conducted.

The monitoring of drug levels in serum is most useful in the case of phenytoin for reasons related to the drug's metabolism and also because the drug's therapeutic range and toxic level are close. Phenytoin intoxication usually occurs at a serum concentration of 100–120 $\mu$mol/l (25–30 $\mu$g/ml). The therapeutic range and toxic level are less well defined for phenobarbitone. It is usually recommended that the serum level should exceed 43 $\mu$mol/l (10 $\mu$g/ml) for a therapeutic effect to be obtained, and toxic symptoms occur at levels of 108–215 $\mu$mol/l (25–50 $\mu$g/ml). Primidone is metabolized into phenobarbitone and phenylethylmalonamide (PEMA) and all three substances possibly have anticonvulsant action. The consensus is that its major effect is through phenobarbitone and it is now the practice to monitor phenobarbitone levels solely. Carbamazepine has a short half-life and its levels tend to fluctuate during the day. Random sampling of serum levels is of limited value and sampling should preferably be related to the time of dosing. A 24-hour profile of serum levels may be useful in demonstrating peaks and troughs and in relating those to the occurrence of seizures. Adjusting the dosage schedule or using a slow-release preparation of carbamazepine may then produce improved seizure control.

Monitoring is of limited practical value in the case of sodium valproate. Levels of the drug fluctuate during the day as one might expect from its short half-life. The clinical efficacy of sodium valproate seems to be related to total daily dosage and the fluctuations in serum levels do not seem to be clinically important. Fluctuations are less marked when enteric-coated preparations are used. Although steady-state levels with valproate are quickly achieved, it is frequently observed that there is a cumulative increase in the number of patients achieving seizure control subsequently, suggesting that there is a delay between the time when the effective blood level is reached and the maximum clinical benefit to the patient (Collaborative Study Group, 1987).

Ethosuximide has a long half-life and serum levels at any time of day will provide a representative value. Regular estimations of levels are useful when control of absences by the drug proves difficult to achieve. Monitoring of benzodiazepines requires special methodology which is expensive and time-consuming and, in any event, the rapid development of tolerance to these drugs makes levels meaningless.

The availability of drug level monitoring has undoubtedly led to the more rational use of drugs and to improved seizure control during the past 20 years. The reader is referred to the excellent review by Wallace (1990). Brett (1977) emphasized the importance of reliability of the method used and was concerned about the necessity for repeated venepunctures in children attending outpatient clinics. However, the volume of blood obtained by capillary sampling can suffice for the estimations (Houtman *et al.*, 1990).

It should always be remembered, however, that, despite the availability of monitoring, it is the clinical response of the individual patient which is of paramount importance rather than an arbitrarily decided therapeutic level (Vajda and Aicardi, 1983). When we use antiepileptic drugs, we should give as much as is needed but as little as is necessary to control the seizures, we should avoid polytherapy, and we should use drug level monitoring as wisely and as selectively as possible (O'Donohoe, 1991).

## Drugs now commonly used

During the past 2 decades, clinicians have been using a smaller range of antiepileptic drugs and using them more effectively and with as few concessions to polypharmacy as possible in a condition as diverse and occasionally intractable as epilepsy (*Table 25.2*). The main arguments against polytherapy may be listed briefly as follows (Bourgeois, 1988):

1   Pharmacokinetic interactions occur and are associated with significant changes in blood levels at a given dose. Frequent drug level measurements and dosage readjustments are necessary.
2   Toxicity appears to be cumulative as more drugs are added and side-effects occur more frequently.
3   The therapeutic range of a drug seems to depend on whether the drug is taken alone or in combination, so that polytherapy confuses the interpretation of serum measurements.
4   The presence of more than one drug adds to the difficulty in evaluating the efficacy or side-effects of any single drug.

Furthermore, there are certain idiosyncratic drug interactions which may occur. Sodium valproate, taken in combination with other antiepileptic drugs, particularly barbiturates, may be associated with the rapid development of a stuporous state (Marescaux *et al.*, 1982). Hyperammonaemia is not a feature of this state and it is reversible when one or both drugs are withdrawn. Hepatotoxicity due to sodium valproate is more likely to occur with combined therapy, rather than with monotherapy (see Chapter 26).

The drugs in common use today are phenobarbitone, primidone, phenytoin, carbamazepine, the benzodiazepines, and sodium valproate for the generalized epilepsies, ethosuximide and sodium valproate for epilepsies associated with absence attacks, and carbamazepine, phenytoin, and occasionally barbiturates for the partial epilepsies. Acetazolamide has a limited use in the treatment of absences (Lombroso and Forsythe, 1960) and as an adjunct or 'helper' drug to carbamazepine in the treatment of refractory partial seizures (Oles *et al.*, 1989).

Further information about the use of individual drugs for different epilepsies is given in the appropriate chapters. The reader is also referred to the textbooks by

**Table 25.1  Effective therapeutic levels of anticonvulsant drugs in children. (Pippenger, Penry and Kutt, 1978)**

| | |
|---|---|
| Carbamazepine | 25–50 $\mu$mol/l (6–12 mg/ml) |
| Clonazepam | 0.095–0.190 $\mu$mol/l (0.03–0.06 $\mu$g/ml) |
| Ethosuximide | 283–708 $\mu$mol/l (40–100 $\mu$g/ml) |
| Phenobarbitone | 64–172 $\mu$mol/l (15–40 $\mu$g/ml) |
| Phenytoin | 20–80 $\mu$mol/l (5–20 $\mu$g/ml) |
| Primidone | 37–55 $\mu$mol/l (50–100 $\mu$g/ml) |
| Sodium valproate | 300–600 $\mu$mol/l (50–100 $\mu$g/ml) |

Morselli, Pippenger and Penry (1983), by Levy *et al.* (1989) and by Eadie and Tyrer (1989).

Drugs introduced for the treatment of epilepsy during the past 3 decades and now in common use as 'first-line' treatment include carbamazepine, sodium valproate, and the benzodiazepines.

## Carbamazepine

This is a tricyclic compound which is structurally related to imipramine. It was introduced in Europe in 1962 and has been available in the USA since the early 1970s. It is now established as one of the most important antiepileptic drugs available and has replaced phenobarbitone and phenytoin as a drug of first choice for the treatment of partial seizures and generalized tonic–clonic seizures in children. Its advantages compared with the older drugs are that it is well tolerated, has no cosmetic side-effects and does not significantly alter behaviour, mood or cognitive function. To avoid the acute side-effects of the drug, it should be introduced gradually over a period of 1–2 weeks. The autoinduction effect of carbamazepine on liver enzymes has already been mentioned but is short-lived. Because of the short half-life of the drug, the total daily dose should be divided into at least two doses. However, fluctuations in carbamazepine levels may be greater in children than in adults and, for the very young patient or those severely affected or difficult to control, the drug may be administered up to four times daily.

The side-effects of carbamazepine induce fatigue, dizziness, ataxia, diplopia, nausea and vomiting (Pellock, 1987). Diplopia is a useful clinical indicator of drug overdosage. A generalized morbilliform rash occurs in up to 5% of patients treated. It usually develops after 7–10 days on the drug and necessitates immediate withdrawal of medication lest the more serious Stevens–Johnson syndrome should ensue. A transient or persistent leukopenia is common after the introduction of carbamazepine but this is a benign phenomenon and rarely requires withdrawal of the drug (Henriksen, Johannessen and Munthe-Kaas, 1983). There appears to be no aetiological relationship between the benign leukopenia and the development of the very rare and potentially fatal aplastic anaemia. The latter is an idiosyncratic, non-dose-related effect, the risk of which is greatest in the early months of treatment. Although its exceptional rarity (the writer has not had a personal case in nearly 30 years of using carbamazepine) has tended to induce complacency about this complication, it is wise, nevertheless, to monitor the white cell count weekly for 1 month and biweekly for a further 2 months after initiating treatment with carbamazepine (Porter, 1987).

In the writer's experience, carbamazepine has been an outstanding and safe

**Table 25.2 Drugs in common use in the treatment of epilepsy in childhood and recommended therapeutic dosages**

| | |
|---|---|
| Phenobarbitone | 4–5 mg/kg per day up to 20 kg only |
| Phenytoin | 5–6 mg/kg per day up to 30 kg only |
| Primidone | 20 mg/kg per day |
| Carbamazepine | 20–25 mg/kg per day |
| Nitrazepam | 0.25 mg/kg per day |
| Clobazam | 0.5–1 mg/kg per day |
| Clonazepam | 0.25 mg/kg per day (also see text) |
| Sodium valproate | 20–30 mg/kg per day up to 50 mg/kg per day in certain cases |
| Ethosuximide | 20–30 mg/kg per day |
| Acetazolamide | 20–25 mg/kg per day |
| Vigabatrin | 50–150 mg/kg per day (also see text) |
| Lamotrigine | See text |

NB   This table of dosages is meant as a guide. Some patients will not tolerate even the minimum doses recommended. Where a range of dosage is given, treatment should commence at the lower dosage. Drugs should be introduced slowly.

antiepileptic drug and has withstood the test of time. It is an excellent drug for general use in paediatric patients because of the absence of cognitive or behavioural changes (O'Donohue, 1977; Dodson, 1987). It is well tolerated by children of all ages. There is some evidence that it may have a psychotropic effect with improvement in the patient's powers of attention and concentration. Garnstorp (1976) summarized 10 years of experience in the use of the drug in children. Approximately two-thirds of the children with focal seizures, including temporal lobe attacks, became seizure-free or were greatly improved on carbamazepine. Generalized major seizures also responded well. No serious toxic effects were encountered. Henriksen, Johannessen and Munthe-Kaas (1983) and Okuno et al. (1989) have reported similar experiences after long-term use of the drug.

Carbamazepine is available in 100 mg, 200 mg and 400 mg tablets and in a sugar-free liquid containing 100 mg/5 ml. There is also a controlled release preparation available as 200 mg and 400 mg tablets. Experience with this project is limited, especially in children (Ryan et al., 1990). The maximum dose of carbamazepine is 20–25 mg/kg per day in divided doses, and slow introduction is strongly recommended. Experience suggests that the appropriate therapeutic range is 25–50 $\mu$mol/l (6–12 $\mu$g/ml).

In certain circumstances, the introduction of carbamazepine into the treatment regime may cause an exacerbation of seizures, especially when it is used to treat generalized atypical absences of the kind seen in association with the multiple seizure types of the Lennox-Gastaut syndrome (Snead and Hosey, 1985). It is important to be aware of this phenomenon in order not to ascribe the change mistakenly to a deterioration in the natural history of the epilepsy.

**Benzodiazepines**

These drugs have been in use since the early 1960s and their use in childhood epilepsy has been reviewed by Farrell (1986). They appear to exert their central effects by binding to specific receptor sites in the brain and facilitating or enhancing the effects of neurotransmitter GABA (MacDonald, 1983). Their most dramatic success has been in the treatment of status epilepticus, where intravenous diazepam is the treatment of choice. Related drugs, lorazepam and clonazepam are similarly

**Table 25.3 Official names of antiepileptic drugs**

| International non-proprietary name | Trade names |
| --- | --- |
| Acetazolamide | Diamox |
| Carbamazepine | Tegretol |
| Clobazam | Frisium |
| Clonazepam | Rivotril, Clonopin |
| Diazepam | Valium |
| Ethosuximide | Zarontin |
| Lamotrigine | Lamictal |
| Lorazepam | Ativan |
| Nitrazepam | Mogadon |
| Phenobarbitone, phenobarbital | Luminal, Gardenal |
| Phenytoin | Epanutin, Dilantin |
| Primidone | Mysoline |
| Sodium valproate | Epilim, Depakine, Depakene |
| Vigabatrin | Sabril |

Abstracted in part from: *Epilepsia* (1978), **19**, 430

employed. The use of rectal diazepam in the treatment of febrile convulsions is discussed in Chapter 6.

Clonazepam and clobazam are used orally in the treatment of epilepsy and both are valuable drugs for use in children. Clonazepam has been criticized for producing side-effects in small children, notably tiredness, drowsiness or even somnolence and, sometimes, for causing irritability similar to that produced by phenobarbitone. These side-effects may be reduced or even prevented by introducing the drug extremely slowly and gradually increasing the dose over a period of weeks. A rather troublesome side-effect in babies and small children, is the occurrence of salivary or bronchial hypersecretion. This is more common in the relatively immobile developmentally retarded infant or child, and supervision of the airway may be necessary in hospital. However, this side-effect usually diminishes with time. Clonazepam, like the other benzodiazepines, has no serious toxic effects.

As has been discussed in earlier chapters, clonazepam is particularly valuable in the treatment of the most difficult varieties of epilepsy of early childhood, especially infantile spasms and the myoclonic epilepsies (see Chapters 4 and 5). In these serious epilepsies, it is usually given as adjunctive or 'add-on' therapy in addition to ACTH, sodium valproate, or other drugs. Nitrazepam has also been used in a similar way and some consider it superior to clonazepam. In contrast to other antiepileptic drugs, clonazepam is effective to some degree in controlling all types of seizures and it may therefore be tried as initial monotherapy in generalized or partial epilepsies, although it is likely to be more effective in the former. It can be effective in controlling simple absences which are unresponsive to ethosuximide or sodium valproate but side-effects and the development of tolerance limits its use in that situation (Dreifuss *et al.*, 1975).

It must be admitted that the sedative side-effects of clonazepam can sometimes necessitate stopping the drug and this may occur even after a very slow introductory phase. The drug is available in tablet form in 0.5 and 2 mg sizes, and in some countries, it is also available as a liquid containing 2.5 mg of clonazepam in 5 ml. The usual daily dosage is 0.5–1 mg in infants, 1–3 mg in young children and 3–6 mg in children of school age. As with other antiepileptic drugs, the dosage of clonazepam should be governed by the child's clinical response and tolerance, and must be adapted to meet individual requirements. A certain amount of tolerance to the anticonvulsant properties of clonazepam may develop with the passage of time, but to a lesser degree than with other benzodiazepines. The drug may be given on of weight per day basis using 0.25 mg/kg per day but care should be taken that this does not lead to excessive doses in some children. Most important of all, initial doses should not exceed 0.25 mg at night in infants and small children and 0.5 mg at night in older children. The determination of serum levels in man usually requires radioimmunoassay techniques; the therapeutic range is poorly defined but is probably of the order of 64–256 nmol/l (20–80 ng/ml). Steady-state concentrations may not be reached until approximately 6 weeks of continuous therapy have elapsed (O'Donohoe and Paes, 1977). Clonazepam is also available for intravenous use, commencing with an initial dose of 0.05 mg/kg given slowly. It has the same disadvantages as diazepam in respect of respiratory centre depression.

Most benzodiazepines used as antiepileptic drugs have nitrogen radicals in positions 1 and 4. Clobazam, an anxiolytic drug, is a benzodiazepine with nitrogen radicals in positions 1 and 5, while the rest of the molecule is similar to diazepam. The drug has anticonvulsant properties and only mild sedative side-effects. The main indication for its oral use is as adjunctive therapy in refractory epilepsy and it is more effective in controlling generalized than partial seizures. The anticonvulsant effect is manifest very rapidly but tolerance develops in about 40% of patients within 4 months of commencing treatment (Farrell, 1986; Robertson, 1986). However, the drug may prove effective again after a short break in treatment and such intermittent therapy may be employed in treating intractable seizures (Gastaut and Low, 1979). The sedative side-effects of benzodiazepines are less frequent and severe with clobazam than with related drugs and positive effects may include reduction in anxiety, decreased behavioural problems, and increased attention. Dosage in children ranges from 0.5 to 1 mg/kg per day, although doses as high as 2 mg/kg per day have been used (Farrell, 1986). The drug is available in 10 mg capsules.

### Sodium valproate

Valproic acid was first synthesized at the end of the nineteenth century and was used as a solvent for other compounds up to the discovery, by serendipity, of its anticonvulsant properties in 1963. The sodium salt was introduced as an antiepileptic drug in 1967 and was marketed in the UK in 1974. It differs markedly in structure from other antiepileptic drugs and is thought to act by inhibiting GABA breakdown and modifying GABA synthesis through effects on several enzymes. GABA itself acts by inhibiting the propagation of seizure discharges in the nervous system.

The drug is rapidly absorbed after oral administration and is strongly bound to serum proteins. It is quickly eliminated, metabolism to a glucuronide conjugate in the liver being followed by excretion in the urine. The plasma half-life is only 7–9 hours, and as a consequence, it may be necessary to give sodium valproate more often than twice daily, although this is a controversial point. A sustained release form of the drug has been developed. Levels in serum can be assayed by various methods, but there is still debate about an appropriate therapeutic range. It probably lies between 300 and 600 $\mu$mol/l (50–100 $\mu$g/ml).

Sodium valproate is relatively lacking in sedative side-effects. Gastrointestinal side-effects are more common but may be avoided by gradual introduction of the drug. It acts as a microsomal enzyme inhibitor, although probably only briefly. In high dosage, it may inhibit blood platelet aggregation with prolonged bleeding times and thrombocytopenia. It is still an expensive drug for long-term use.

The first report of its anticonvulsant properties came from France in 1963 (Meunier *et al.*, 1963) and it was widely used in Europe for several years before becoming available in the UK in 1974 and in the USA in 1978. Jeavons and Clark (1974) reported enthusiastically on its clinical efficacy in generalized epilepsies. The best results in the generalized epilepsies have been reported in those patients whose EEGs showed spike and wave discharges and in patients with idiopathic or primary convulsive and non-convulsive generalized epilepsies. It has proved as effective as carbamazepine or phenytoin in the management of generalized tonic–clonic seizures, achieving complete control in the great majority of patients (Collaborative Study Group, 1989). It will control about 80% of childhood absence seizures (Callaghan *et al.*, 1982), but the writer does not consider that it has superseded the cheaper, safer and equally effective drug ethosuximide in this condition. The two drugs may be effective in combination in resistant cases (Rowan *et al.*, 1983). Where both absences and tonic–clonic seizures are occurring, sodium valproate monotherapy is preferred to ethosuximide. It is also the drug of first choice for treating photosensitive epilepsy (Harding, Herrick and Jeavons, 1978) and for juvenile myoclonic epilepsy of Janz (Dreifuss, 1989).

In the myoclonic epilepsies of early childhood, sodium valproate seems most effective in those children who have normal neurological and mental status although secondary or symptomatic cases may also respond. Combined treatment with clonazepam may sometimes be superior to either drug alone in these difficult cases. Sodium valproate may be helpful in treating infantile spasms (Siemes *et al.*, 1988). It is highly effective in the prophylaxis of febrile convulsions (Ngwane and Bower, 1980) but carries the risk of hepatotoxicity in the young, especially under 2 years of age.

Sodium valproate is less effective in controlling partial seizures, either simple or complex, when carbamazepine must be considered the drug of first choice. However, it may be effective in certain cases, especially when partial seizures are followed by secondary generalization (Dean and Penry, 1988).

Sodium valproate has the advantage, in contrast to the older antiepileptic drugs, of not being sedative. However, like all drugs used in the treatment of epilepsy, it has its share of side-effects and also toxic and idiosyncratic reactions. These will be discussed in Chapter 26. It is unusual among antiepileptic drugs in not causing microsomal enzyme induction. Its inhibitory effect in that respect may lead to increases in the circulating concentrations of other antiepileptic drugs and the additional effect, in the case of phenytoin, of displacing it from plasma protein binding sites leading to significant increases in the circulating levels of phenytoin.

The drug is available in 200 and 500 mg enteric coated tablets and 100 mg crushable tablets. There is a syrup containing 200 mg sodium valproate in 5 ml and a sugar-free preparation is also available. There is an intravenous preparation which contains 400 mg of powder per vial. Introduction of the drug orally should be gradual and the full pharmacological effect may not be observed for some weeks after steady state concentrations have been attained. Initial dosage in children over 20 kg should be 400 mg daily irrespective of weight with gradual increase in dosage until control is obtained. This is usually achieved with a dosage of 25–30 mg/kg per day but in resistant cases, up to 50 mg/kg per day has been used. Possible effects on blood platelet function should be remembered at these higher dosage levels.

As already mentioned, there is little correlation between valproate concentration and its pharmacological effect so that routine monitoring of serum concentrations is unnecessary and misleading although it may help to uncover poor compliance on the part of the patient. When monitoring is undertaken, standardization of sampling against time of dosing is advisable. Concentrations of sodium valproate above 1050 $\mu$mol/l (150 mg/l) in the presence of continuing seizures suggest that the drug is ineffective (Leading article, 1988). As with all medical therapy for epilepsy, the individual response of the patient to treatment is of first importance and this, rather than laboratory indices, should guide management.

## New antiepileptic drugs

The neurochemical mechanisms underlying epilepsy are poorly understood, but a logical pharmacological approach to treatment is to try to develop drugs which either enhance synaptic inhibition or reduce excitatory neurotransmission. The former is largely mediated by GABA (gamma-aminobutyric acid). *Vigabatrin* (gamma-vinyl-gamma aminobutyric acid) is a synthetic derivative of GABA and acts as an irreversible inhibitor of GABA transaminase, the enzyme responsible for the breakdown of GABA. This leads to an increase of the inhibitory neuro-transmitter GABA at the synapse.

After oral administration, the drug is rapidly absorbed and peak levels in plasma are achieved within 1–2 hours. The half-life of the drug is 5–7 hours and 80% of the drug is excreted unchanged in the urine. No clear relationship between concentra-tions in the blood and the clinical effects of the drug has been demonstrated and drug level monitoring is not advised. As the drug is not bound to protein, is excreted unchanged in the urine, and is not influenced by enzyme-inducing drugs, interactions with other antiepileptic drugs are not a problem, although unexplained falls in serum phenytoin levels may occur. Side-effects include drowsiness, fatigue, dizziness, and behavioural changes including the development of acute psychosis (Sander and Hart, 1990). Excitement and agitation have been reported in children taking the drug.

Vigabatrin has so far been used as adjunctive treatment for chronic and intractable epilepsy in adults. About half the patients treated have shown a reduction in seizure frequency with marked improvement in about 15% (Reynolds, 1990; Ring and Reynolds, 1992). Patients with partial seizures with or without secondary generaliza-tion have shown the best response. These seizures account for 40% of seizures in children and about 70% in adults so clearly vigabatrin will play an important role in the treatment of resistant epilepsy in the future and may begin to be used as first-line rather than adjunctive treatment. Thus far, experience of its use in the epileptic syndromes of childhood is limited and confined to intractable cases but partial seizures appear to respond best while myoclonic syndromes do less well, although intractable seizures in West's syndrome associated with tuberous sclerosis may respond (Luna *et al.*, 1989).

There is some concern about the long-term safety of vigabatrin even though no chronic toxicity has thus far been discovered in man. Reversible, non-inflammatory changes and vasculation in the myelin of white matter were demonstrated in some experimental animals but similar changes have not been demonstrated in man nor have any clinical syndromes emerged which might suggest the presence of such changes (Butler, 1989). Clearly, vigilance for possible long-term toxicity, especially in children, will be required for many years.

Vigabatrin is available as 500 mg tablets. The recommended starting dose in children is 1 g daily in children aged 3–9 years and 2 g daily in older children. Under

3 years of age, an initial starting dose of 50 mg/kg per day has been employed and gradually increased up to 150 mg/kg per day according to response (Luna *et al.*, 1989).

Vigabatrin is the first new antiepileptic drug to be licensed in the UK since sodium valproate became available in 1973. It may represent a milestone in the treatment of epilepsy, since it is the first new drug whose development has been based on rational principles of treatment (Reynolds, 1990). Another recently introduced drug which has also been developed by the application of neurophysiological knowledge is *lamotrigine*. This compound is believed to work by inhibiting the release of excitatory amino acids, principally glutamate, at the synapse (Porter, 1990). The drug is recommended at present for adjunctive treatment of partial seizures and generalized tonic–clonic seizures, not satisfactorily controlled by other antiepileptic drugs. Experience with the drug in childhood is limited. Liver enzyme inducers may increase its metabolism while sodium valproate reduces it. The drug is available in 50 and 100 mg tablets and the usual maintenance dose in adolescents and in adults is 200–400 mg daily but the dose should be reduced if sodium valproate is also being given. Skin rashes occur in up to 10% of patients and Stevens–Johnson syndrome has been reported. Lamotrigine may also affect folate metabolism during long-term treatment.

Other new drugs which are on trial but not available commercially include oxycarbazepine (an analogue of carbamazepine), gabapentin, zonisamide, flunarizine, felbamate, and stiripentol. The reader is referred to reviews by Porter (1990), Brodie and Porter (1990), and to a special supplement to *Epilepsia* entitled 'Research in Epileptogenesis: The Search for Tomorrow's Antiepileptic Drugs', published in 1989.

## References

BOURGEOIS, B. F. D. (1988) Problems of combination drug therapy in children. *Epilepsia*, **29**, Supplement 3, S20–S24

BRETT, E. M. (1977) Implications of measuring anticonvulsant blood levels in epilepsy. *Developmental Medicine and Child Neurology*, **19**, 245–251

BRODIE, M. J. and PORTER, R. J. (1990) New and potential anticonvulsants. *Lancet*, **336**, 425–426

BUTLER, W. H. (1989) The neuropathology of vigabatrin. *Epilsepsia*, **30** (Supplement 3), S15–17

CALLAGHAN, N., O'HARE, J., O'DRISCOLL, D. *et al.* (1982) Comparative study of ethosuximide and sodium valproate in the treatment of typical absence seizures (petit mal). *Developmental Medicine and Child Neurology*, **24**, 830–836

Collaborative Study Group (1987) Monotherapy with valproate in primary generalized epilepsies. *Epilepsia*, **28**, Suppl. 2, S8–S11

DEAN, J. C. and PENRY, J. K. (1988) Valproate monotherapy in 30 patients with partial seizures. *Epilepsia*, **29**, 140–144

DODSON, W. E. (1983) Antiepileptic drug use in newborns and infants. In: *Recent Advances in Epilepsy*. No. 1 (eds T. A. Pedley and B. S. Meldrum), Churchill Livingstone, Edinburgh, London, pp. 231–248

DODSON, W. E. (1987a) Special pharmacokinetic considerations in children. *Epilepsia*, **28**, Supplement 1, S56–S70

DODSON, W. E. (1987b) Carbamazepine efficacy and utilization in children. *Epilepsia*, **28**, Supplement 3, S17–S24

DODSON, W. E. (1988) Aspects of antiepileptic treatment in children. *Epilepsia*, **29**, Supplement 3, S10–S14

DREIFUSS, F. E. (1989) Juvenile myoclonic epilepsy: characteristics of a primary generalized epilepsy. *Epilepsia*, **30**, Supplement 4, S1–S7

DREIFUSS, F. E., PENRY, J. K., ROSE, S. W. *et al.* (1975) Serum clonazepam concentrations in children with absence seizures. *Neurology*, **25**, 225–228

EADIE, M. J. and TYRER, J. H. (1989) *Anticonvulsant Therapy: Pharmacological Basis and Practice*, 3rd Edition, Churchill Livingstone, Edinburgh

LEPPIK, I. E. (ed.) (1989) *Research in Epileptogenesis: The Search for Tomorrow's Antiepileptic Drugs*. *Epilepsia*, **30**, Supplement 1, S1–S68

FARRELL, K. (1986) Benzodiazepines in the treatment of children with epilepsy. *Epilepsia*, **27**, Supplement 1, S45–S51

GAMSTORP, I. (1976) Carbamazepine in the treatment of epileptic disorders in infancy and childhood. In: *Epileptic Seizures – Behaviour – Pain* (ed. W. Birkmayer) Hans Huber, Bern, Stuttgart, Vienna, pp. 98–103

GASTAUT, H. and LOW, M. D. (1979) Antiepileptic properties of clobazam, a 1,5 benzodiazepine, in man. *Epilepsia*, **20**, 437–446

GOLDBERG, V. D., RATNARAJ, N., ELYAS, A. and LASCELLES, P. T. (1983) Recent developments in therapeutic drug monitoring. In *Research Progress in Epilepsy* (ed. F. C. Rose), London, Pitman, pp. 462–483

HARDING, G. F. A., HERRICK, C. E. and JEAVONS, P. M. (1978) A controlled study of the effect of sodium valproate on photosensitive epilepsy and its prognosis. *Epilepsia*, **19**, 555–565

HENRIKSEN, O., JOHANNESSEN, S. I. and MUNTHE-KAAS, A. W. (1983) How to use carbamezepine. In *Antiepileptic Drug Therapy in Pediatrics* (eds P. L. Morselli, C. E. Pippenger and J. K. Penry), Raven Press, pp. 237–240

HOUTMAN, P. N., HALL, S. K., GREEN, A., and RYLANCE, G. W. (1990) Rapid anticonvulsant monitoring in an epileptic clinic. *Archives of Disease in Childhood*, **65**, 264–268.

JEAVONS, P. M. and CLARK, J. E. (1974) Sodium valproate in the treatment of epilepsy. *British Medical Journal*, **2**, 584–586

KUTT, H. (1984) Interactions between anticonvulsants and other commonly prescribed drugs. *Epilepsia*, **25**, Supplement 2, S118–S131

Leading article (1988) Sodium valproate. Lancet, **332**, 1229–1231

LEVY, R. H., DREIFUSS, F. E., MATTSON, R. H. *et al.* (eds) (1989) *Antiepileptic Drugs*, 3rd edition, Raven Press, New York

LOMBROSO, C. T. and FORSYTHE, I. (1960) A long-term follow-up of acetazolamide (Diamox) in the treatment of epilepsy. *Epilepsia*, **1**, 493–500

LUNA, D., DULAC, O., PAJOT, N. and BEAUMONT, D. (1989) Vigabatrin in the treatment of childhood epilepsies: a single-blind placebo-controlled study. *Epilepsia*, **30**, 430–437

MACDONALD, R. L. (1983) Mechanisms of anticonvulsant drug action. In: *Recent Advances in Epilepsy*, No. 1 (eds T. A. Pedley and B. S. Meldrum), Churchill Livingstone, London, pp. 1–23

MARESCAUX, C., WARTER, J. M., MICHELETTI, G. *et al.* (1982) Stuporous episodes during treatment with sodium valproate. Report of seven cases. *Epilepsia*, **23**, 297–305

MEUNIER, G., CARRAZ, G., MEUNIER, Y. *et al.* (1963) Proprietes pharmacodynamiques de l'acide n-diprophylacetique. *Thérapie*, **18**, 435–438

MORSELLI, P. L., PIPPENGER, C. E. and PENRY, J. K. (eds) (1983) *Antiepileptic Drug Therapy in Pediatrics*, Raven Press, New York

NGWANE, E. and BOWER, B. (1980) Continuous sodium valproate or phenobarbitone in the prevention of 'simple' febrile convulsions. Comparison by a double-blind trial. *Archives of Disease in Childhood*, **55**, 171–174

O'DONOHOE, N. V. (1977) Tegretol in everyday paediatric practice. In *Tegretol in Epilepsy. Proceedings of an International Meeting*, Geigy Pharmaceuticals, Macclesfield, Cheshire, England, pp. 10–12

O'DONOHOE, N. V. (1991) The epilepsies. In *Paediatric Specialty Practice for the 1990s* (eds J. Eyre and R. Boyd), Royal College of Physicians, London, pp. 51–63

O'DONOHOE, N. V. and PAES, B. A. (1977) A trial of clonazepam in the treatment of severe epilepsy in infancy and childhood. In *Epilepsy: The Eighth International Symposium* (ed. J. K. Penry) Raven Press, New York, pp. 159–162

OKUNO, T., ITO, M., NAKANO, S. *et al.* (1989) Carbamazepine therapy and long-term prognosis of epilepsy of childhood. *Epilepsia*, **30**, 57–61

OLES, K. S., PENRY, J. K., COLE, D. L. W. and HOWARD, G. (1989) Use of acetazolamide as an adjunct to carbamazepine in refractory partial seizures. *Epilepsia*, **30**, 71–78

PELLOCK, J. M. (1987) Carbamazepine side effects in children and adults. *Epilepsia*, **28**, Supplement 3, S64–S70

PORTER, R. J. (1987) How to initiate and maintain carbamazepine therapy in children and adults. *Epilepsia*, **28**, Supplement 3, S59–S63

PORTER, R. J. (1990) New antiepileptic drugs: strategies for drug development. *Lancet*, **336**, 423–424

REYNOLDS, E. H. (1990) Vigabatrin. Rational treatment for chronic epilepsy. *British Medical Journal*, **300**, 277–278

REYNOLDS, E. H. and SHORVAN, S. D. (1981) Monotherapy or polytherapy for epilepsy. *Epilepsia*, **22**, 1–10

RICHENS, A. L. (1976) *Drug Treatment of Epilepsy*, Henry Kimpton, London

RICHENS, A. L. and DUNLOP, A. (1975) Serum phenytoin levels in the management of epilepsy. *Lancet*, **2**, 247–249

RING, H. A. and REYNOLDS, E. H. (1992) Vigabatrin. In: *Recent Advances in Epilepsy*, Vol. 5 (eds T. A. Pedley and B. S. Weldrum), Churchill Livingstone, Edinburgh, London, pp. 177–195

ROBERTSON, M. M. (1986) Current status of 1,4 and 1,5 benzodiazepines in the treatment of epilepsy. *Epilepsia*, **27**, Supplement 1, S27–S41

ROWAN, A. J., MEIJER, J. W. A., DE BEER-PAWLIKOWSKI, N. *et al.* (1983). Valproate-ethosuximide combination therapy for refractory absence seizures. *Archives of Neurology*, **40**, 497–802

RYAN, S. W., FORSYTHE, I., HARTLEY, R. *et al.* (1990) Slow release carbamazepine in treatment of poorly controlled seizures. *Archives of Disease in Childhood*, **65**, 930–935

SANDER, J. W. and HART, Y. M. (1990) Vigabatrin and behaviour disturbances (letter). *Lancet*, **335**, 57

SIEMES, H., SPOHR, H. L., MICHAEL, T. and NAU, H. (1988) Therapy of infantile spasms with valproate: results of a prospective study. *Epilepsia*, **29**, 553–560

SNEAD, O. C. and HOSEY, L. C. (1985) Exacerbation of seizures in children by carbamazepine. *New England Journal of Medicine*, **313**, 916–921

VAJDA, F. J. E. and AICARDI, J. (1983) Reassessment of the concept of a therapeutic range of anticonvulsant plasma levels. *Developmental Medicine and Child Neurology*, **25**, 660–671

WALLACE, S. J. (1990) Antiepileptic drug monitoring: an overview. *Developmental Medicine and Child Neurology*, **32**, 923–926

# Chapter 26

# Adverse effects of drug therapy in epilepsy

Drug effects may be classified as desired or therapeutic and undesired or adverse. Adverse reactions may be acute or chronic or occasionally idiosyncratic. These drug-induced effects may necessitate discontinuance of treatment in up to 20% of children (Abu-Arafeh and Wallace, 1988).

## Phenytoin

The acute toxic effects of phenytoin are well known, particularly nystagmus, ataxia and tremor. These effects in association are sometimes called 'Dilantin inebriety' in the USA. Severe toxic effects, including tonic brain-stem seizures, have been described in adults taking excessive doses of the drug, and acute psychotic reactions may take place. An acute toxic encephalopathy of this nature may occasionally occur abruptly in patients on average doses of the drug who unexpectedly develop high blood levels. Apart from the tonic seizures and behavioural changes, dystonic reactions and choreoathetosis may also be seen.

Patel and Crichton (1968) pointed out that the acute toxic effects of phenytoin may easily pass unnoticed in children (particularly young children), that nystagmus may not occur and that ataxia may not be detected or may be mistaken for an epileptic manifestation in the young. Precise diagnosis may be made more difficult by the presence of drowsiness and behavioural disturbances and because excessive amounts of the drug may make the epilepsy worse. Various studies have shown that there is a correlation between the concentration of the drug in plasma and the signs of acute toxicity: the higher the concentration (100–120 $\mu$mol/l (25–30 $\mu$g/ml) the more severe the toxic signs. Acute toxicity may develop when sodium valproate is added to phenytoin. This is due to its inhibitory effect on microsomal enzyme function and also because sodium valproate displaces phenytoin from protein binding sites, leading to an increase in circulating free phenytoin. All of these acute toxic effects are readily reversible, although there are reservations about the cerebellar signs, which will be discussed later.

## Phenobarbitone

The most well-known acute toxic effect of phenobarbitone is, of course, drowsiness. However, tolerance usually develops to this effect over a period of weeks and it gradually disappears.

The stimulatory effect of phenobarbitone in young children has already been described in Chapter 6; the resulting irritability, aggressiveness and overactivity may be persistent and intolerable and necessitate withdrawal of the drug (Wolf and Forsythe, 1978). Major depressive disorder has also been reported in children taking phenobarbitone (Brent *et al.*, 1987). Phenobarbitone may have a dulling effect on attention and perception resulting in inability to maintain vigilance over long periods of time. The effects of phenobarbitone and of other drugs on the learning process and on school performance are considered in Chapter 21.

## Primidone and the benzodiazepines

These drugs have rather similar effects to phenobarbitone, although the benzodiazepines only rarely cause aggressiveness and irritability in small children. Drowsiness can be a problem, but slow introduction of the drugs and the passage of time usually lead to the development of tolerance. Primidone can sometimes produce alarming personality changes (Mysoline madness) and the EEG can be useful in distinguishing this from a consequence of a deterioration in the patient's epileptic state.

## Carbamazepine

Acute toxicity from carbamazepine is unusual and is dose related. Dizziness, drowsiness, diplopia and gastrointestinal symptoms occur with high doses. There is a curious toxic effect which has been reported in adults and which is due to the fact that carbamazepine has a potentiating effect on the action of the antidiuretic hormone 8–arginine vasopressin (AVP) on the renal tubules. In toxic doses carbamazepine may occasionally lead to water retention and even water intoxication (Ashton *et al.*, 1977). Very rarely, carbamazepine causes an acute psychosis (O'Donohoe, 1973). An important advantage of carbamazepine compared with phenobarbitone and phenytoin is that it does not seem to impair cognitive function during long-term administration.

## Sodium valproate

Side-effects from sodium valproate are relatively infrequent but troublesome when they do occur. Increased appetite and weight gain occurred in 44% of children studied by Egger and Brett (1981). Schmidt (1984) reported a maximum incidence of 9.5% in his review. Females and adolescents are the most likely victims and there is no clear relationship to dosage. A reduced caloric intake may help in preventing weight gain but, quite often, stopping the drug is the only solution. Hair loss or thinning of hair occurs in about 8% of cases. Commoner in females, the effect is temporary and may be succeeded by waviness or curling of hair. It will be appreciated that, if to the problems created by epilepsy in adolescent girls are added the problems of weight gain and hair loss, the patient may react by withdrawal and with depression, as Egger and Brett (1981) have emphasized. Furthermore, drug compliance may be compromised and alternative medication become necessary.

Drowsiness is rarely experienced with sodium valproate alone but may occur if the drug is added to phenobarbitone, due to a sudden rise in serum level of the barbiturate caused by the enzyme-inhibiting effect of valproate. An acute confusional state or even stupor can occur in consequence (Marescaux et al., 1982). It is important to remember that changes in behaviour, including hyperactivity, aggressiveness and irritability, are unusual and unexpected side-effects in some children on valproate monotherapy. Tremor may also develop in those on high dosage of the drug. Skin rashes are extremely rare. The incidence of gastrointestinal symptoms such as nausea and vomiting has been greatly reduced by the introduction of enteric-coated preparations but these may still occur with the suspension. Pancreatitis has been reported in children and adults, and should be considered if a patient develops severe abdominal pain and vomiting (Batalden, van Dyne and Cloyd, 1979).

## Idiosyncratic reactions

Before dealing with chronic toxicity a word should be said about idiosyncratic reactions. Idiosyncrasy can be defined as a peculiar or unique characteristic distinguishing an individual, and Booker (1975) wrote an excellent review of this aspect of antiepileptic therapy. Idiosyncratic reactions are very unusual and some, at least, are probably genetically determined. Booker (1972) described a group of individuals who seem unable to metabolize primidone to phenobarbitone and who develop lethargy and drowsiness on small doses of the drug. Kutt et al. (1964) described an individual with an inability to metabolize phenytoin, and there are other people who metabolize phenytoin at an increased rate. Serious individual reactions may involve the skin (e.g. rashes, exfoliative dermatitis and the Stevens–Johnson syndrome), the bone marrow (e.g. aplastic anaemia), the liver (e.g. cholestasis and hepatocellular damage) and the immunological system (e.g. a lupus erythematosus syndrome), and any one of several drugs may be responsible (*Table 26.1*). It is important to note that both the rare lymphoproliferative reaction and the lupus-like hypersensitivity syndrome induced by phenytoin regress when the drug is discontinued but are reactivated by rechallenge with the drug.

*Hepatotoxicity* is a long-recognized and rare complication of antiepileptic medication. However, no antiepileptic drug is predictably or intrinsically hepatotoxic. Hepatotoxicity with these drugs is essentially idiosyncratic and takes two forms. The first of these reactions is one of drug allergy or hypersensitivity. It occurs after a short period and the clinical features are fever, rash, lymphadenopathy and jaundice. Hepatotoxicity due to phenytoin and carbamazepine has been mainly reported in older adolescents and adults. Prompt withdrawal of the offending drug is usually followed by slow recovery although mortality rates of 10–28% for phenytoin and 25% for carbamazepine have been reported (Dreifuss and Langer, 1987; Hadzic et al., 1990).

Another type of hepatotoxicity which may happen after weeks or months of treatment is one which has been attributed to an aberration in the metabolism of the incriminated drug. Sodium valproate (and valproic acid) causes hepatotoxicity

**Table 26.1 Serious individual reactions to antiepileptic drugs (after Booker, 1975)**

| Area affected or condition produced | Drug |
| --- | --- |
| Skin (exfoliative dermatitis, Stevens–Johnson syndrome) | Potentially all drugs |
| Liver | Troxidone, phenytoin, carbamazepine, acetazolamide succinimides, sodium valproate |
| Renal | Troxidone, succinimides, acetazolamide |
| Bone marrow | Troxidone, succinimides, carbamazepine |
| Lupus erythematosus | Phenytoin, troxidone, primidone, succinimides |
| Thyroiditis | Phenytoin, troxidone |
| Initiation of a myasthenia gravis state | Phenytoin, troxidone |
| Lymphoma | Phenytoin, troxidone, primidone |
| Haemorrhage in the newborn | Phenytoin, primidone, phenobarbitone |
| Precipitation of porphyria | Phenobarbitone, phenytoin, succinimides |
| Hyperglycaemia | Phenytoin |
| Pancreatitis | Sodium valproate |

in this way. While dose-related elevations in liver enzymes may be detected in up to 44% of patients on valproate therapy (Sussmann and McLain, 1979), these elevations are not accompanied by clinical symptoms or abnormalities in the liver's synthetic functions (e.g. prothrombin time). The laboratory abnormalities resolve with dosage reduction or on stopping the drug.

Irreversible and usually fatal hepatic failure due to valproate therapy is a rare idiosyncratic reaction to the drug. Whereas the onset of hepatotoxicity with phenytoin or carbamazepine usually appears within the first 3–4 weeks of treatment, the onset of hepatic illness with valproate usually occurs within the first 90 days. The prodromal signs and symptoms are usually nausea, vomiting, anorexia and lethargy, sometimes accompanied by oedema or jaundice. A sudden loss of seizure control or even an episode of status epilepticus may be an important marker of hepatic illness (Dreifuss, 1987). In fatal cases, the histological features have been different from those reported after hepatic failure due to other antiepileptic drugs. Microvesicular steatosis, usually with necrosis, was the most prominent finding. The resemblance to the changes found in fatal cases of Reye's syndrome has been striking. Among the reported fatal cases have been cases of familial hepatic dysfunction, including ornithine carbamyl transferase deficiency, alpha-1-antitrypsin deficiency and carnitine deficiency (Scheffner et al., 1988).

The incidence of fatal hepatotoxicity is not evenly distributed among the patient population. Very young patients (0–2 years) on polytherapy with antiepileptic drugs and with other medical conditions in addition to epilepsy are disproportionately vulnerable to fatal hepatic failure. The incidence declines sharply over the age of 2 years, especially among those patients receiving the drug as monotherapy. Dreifuss et al. (1989) have reported that, despite increased use of the drug, fatal hepatotoxicity from sodium valproate in the USA is declining. In the period 1978–1984, the risk was 1/10 000; in 1985–1986 it had fallen to 0.2/10 000 and in that period, no hepatic fatalities were reported over the age of 10 years. They ascribed the fall to the fact that more patients were receiving sodium valproate as monotherapy, that more low-risk patients were being treated with the drug, and that fewer high-risk patients (0–2 years) were receiving it. Sodium valproate should not be given in a polytherapy regime under the age of 3 years, it should be avoided in patients with pre-existing liver disease or with a family history of such disease, and salicylates should not be given to a patient on sodium valproate. Fasting should be avoided in patients on sodium valproate who develop an intercurrent illness, and immediate withdrawal of the drug is mandatory if hepatotoxicity is suspected. Although it is prudent to monitor liver enzyme levels during the first 3 months of treatment when the risk is greatest, withdrawal of medication is necessary only if substantial rises occur. One-stage prothrombin time and fibrinogen levels are more sensitive than other tests of liver function in detecting hepatic compromise. Although valproate hepatotoxicity is rare, it may occur at any age and vigilance is required to detect its early onset.

## Chronic toxicity

Chronic toxicity due to anticonvulsants was brilliantly reviewed by Reynolds (1975) and his article is essential reading for anyone interested in the problem. The more recent reviews by Schmidt (1986) and by Herranz, Armijo and Arteaga (1988) are also recommended.

The fact that anticonvulsant drugs are usually administered for prolonged periods of time, often a major portion of the patient's life, allows for the appearance of chronic toxic effects which are not seen with other drugs given for limited periods of time. Furthermore, epilepsy is a symptom which begins before the age of 20 years in over three-quarters of affected individuals and it often begins in early childhood and tends to recur despite therapy. This may lead to therapy being life-long in some instances. The early onset of epilepsy may also mean that growing tissues are exposed to the effects of drugs during vulnerable stages of development. McGowan (1983), in a prospective longitudinal study of growth in children with epilepsy, was unable to show a difference in respect to height from the normal population. However, men with a long history of partial seizures in childhood and adolescence and women who had taken phenytoin before completing their growth were retrospectively found to be significantly shorter. In another longitudinal study of prepubertal children with epilepsy, many of them severely affected (Tada, Wallace and Hughes, 1986), growth was within normal limits and puberty did not occur early. It was suggested that suboptimal growth patterns previously observed in children with epilepsy attending residential schools might be due to concurrent social problems rather than to epilepsy and its treatment. Reynolds (1975) considered that there was a general lack of awareness in the profession with regard to the problems of chronic drug toxicity and that the ill-effects of overdosage and polypharmacy may be attributed to other causes, including psychological factors. Many clinicians will have seen small children on multiple drugs (for example, numbering ten in one case seen by the author) and leading a twilight zombie-like existence as a result. 'Doctors are trained to do something rather than nothing', wrote Taylor and McKinlay (1984) in a plea against the trend to prescribe drugs for every child suspected of having epilepsy. They advocated not treating epilepsy with drugs when they do not work or when they do more harm than good.

Gordon (1967, unpublished) drew attention to a fact which is familiar to most people dealing with epilepsy, namely that when treatment is stopped, for some reason or other, the fits may subsequently occur less frequently. He suggested that it was possible that anticonvulsant treatment in these patients passes over the top of the therapeutic curve and starts to have a deleterious effect on the patient. It is well known, for instance, that in temporal lobe epilepsy, the epileptic discharges are most likely to be recorded in the EEG during drowsiness and sleep. Therefore, if the patient is made excessively drowsy by treatment an increasing frequency of seizures may result. Furthermore, certain drugs, such as phenytoin, act as convulsants in toxic doses (Osorio *et al.*, 1989). At greatest risk of exacerbation of seizures are children suffering from intractable mixed seizures and showing slow spike-waves in the EEG to whose treatment regimes carbamazepine is added (Snead and Hosey, 1985). Exacerbation of seizures may also occur in children with absence seizures plus generalized tonic–clonic seizures if carbamazepine is prescribed (Lerman, 1986).

## Central nervous system effects

The chronic toxic effects on the central nervous system have received particular attention, especially the possible damage inflicted on the cerebellum by phenytoin. The acute cerebellar syndrome produced by phenytoin has already been described (see page 277). The question of whether chronic phenytoin toxicity can permanently damage the cerebellum by causing Purkinje cell loss is still *sub judice*. Reynolds (1975) thought that it did, whereas Dam (1970) thought that the Purkinje cell loss was due to frequent and severe seizures causing anoxic damage. The author sides with Reynolds in this argument and is influenced by a case seen personally. It may be that both theories are partially true and that repeated severe seizures and consequent brain damage may make the cerebellum more vulnerable to the chronic toxic effects of phenytoin (Iivanainen, Viukari and Helle, 1977). In a further review, Dam (1983) was still firmly in favour of severe epilepsy being the cause, pointing out that cerebellar lesions with degeneration of Purkinje cells were described in epileptic patients long before the introduction of phenytoin.

The production of an acute toxic encephalopathy with certain anticonvulsants such as phenytoin, phenobarbitone, primidone, sodium valproate and carbamazepine has already been mentioned. It has also been suggested that a *chronic encephalopathy*, with an insidious deterioration in intellectual functioning and in behaviour as its main characteristics, can also occur where high doses of anticonvulsants are used for prolonged periods. Such a syndrome may be mistaken for degenerative disease of the central nervous system, particularly in patients who are already mentally handicapped. The role of folate deficiency in the causation of such a deterioration will be discussed later, and it is important to remember that in this context there are many factors contributing to the development of mental illness in epilepsy including underlying brain damage, uncontrolled seizures and psychological, social and genetic influences. A chronic encephalopathic illness due to chronic drug toxicity should usually be reversible when the drugs are reduced or discontinued (Vallarta, Bell and Reichert, 1974).

Some encephalopathic drug reactions may be caused by the dopamine antagonist properties of drugs such as phenytoin (Chadwick, Reynolds and Marsden, 1976). Facial hyperkinesia, choreoathetosis, tremor, bradykinesia, and dystonic movements of various kinds may be observed. A related problem, familiar to most paediatricians, is the occurrence of *dystonic extrapyramidal movement disorders* in response to the phenothiazine drugs and to metoclopramide (Mowat, 1973). These toxic effects develop acutely at both excessive and therapeutic doses. The most common movements are sudden episodes of opisthotonus accompanied by marked deviation of the eyes and torticollis, but without loss of consciousness. Dystonic movements of the tongue, face and neck muscles, drooling, trismus, ataxia, tremor, episodic rigidity and oculogyric crises are also seen. The violent dystonic movements may mimic clonic seizures but, although the patient may be drowsy from the drug, consciousness is retained. Diagnosis rests on the history of drug ingestion. There appears to be an element of idiosyncrasy in those patients who develop the syndrome on therapeutic doses of the responsible drug. Benztropine mesylate intravenously or diphenhydramine intravenously, and later orally, act swiftly as effective antidotes. The most serious and least known reaction of this kind is the condition termed the neuroleptic malignant syndrome, characterized by opisthotonus, muscular rigidity, hyperthermia, altered consciousness, and autonomic dysfunction, sometimes lasting for weeks or months. Failure to recognize this syndrome has led to prolonged morbidity and even death. Nearly all the cases have been described in adults but Moore, O'Donohoe and Monaghan (1986) have described the condition in a child. The syndrome is thought to be due to blockade of dopamine receptor sites in the brain. The treatment of this dangerous condition has been reviewed by Turk and Lask (1991).

## Haemopoietic effects

Effects on the haemopoetic system have been recognized for many years. Aplastic anaemia and bone marrow depression have occurred rarely with the hydantoins (especially mephenytoin) and with carbamazepine and more frequently with oxazolidinediones such as troxidone and paramethadione. Megaloblastic anaemia develops in less than 1% of patients on antiepileptic drugs. Macrocytosis, without anaemia, is more frequent but of little clinical significance and can be corrected by small doses of folic acid (500 $\mu$g/day). Folate deficiency has mainly been reported in patients taking phenytoin, phenobarbitone or primidone and occurs in up to 91% of these (Reynolds, 1983a). It also appears to have little clinical significance in the absence of anaemia, and treatment with folic acid is unnecessary. It has been suggested that prolonged drug-induced folate deficiency may lead to neuropsychiatric symptoms, including depression, psychosis and dementia, and Trimble, Corbett and Donaldson (1980) found evidence of such an association in children on long-term treatment. However, Reynolds (1983b) emphasized that the statistical association between folate deficiency and psychological disorders is by no means constant and that it is probable that an interaction between the deficiency (especially if severe) and other factors leads to neuropsychiatric sequelae in some patients only.

Other haematological complications include agranulocytosis developing during the first 3 months of treatment with several drugs and lymphadenopathy occurring as a hypersensitivity reaction with phenytoin and occasionally with other drugs. This lymphadenopathy is usually benign and reversible, unlike the rare malignant lymphomas which may occur after many years of phenytoin therapy.

Thrombocytopenia with bleeding may be a complication of high dosage sodium valproate therapy (Watts et al., 1990). Coagulation defects with serious bleeding have been reported in some neonates whose mothers were taking phenytoin and/or phenobarbitone (Mountain, Hirsch and Gallus, 1970). The drugs cross the placenta and interfere with the immature liver enzyme mechanisms responsible for the production or release of vitamin-K dependent clotting factors. Prevention can be achieved by giving vitamin K to mothers at risk during the last month of pregnancy and, in addition, all babies born to mothers who are taking antiepileptic drugs should receive an intramuscular injection of vitamin $K_1$ (Meadow, 1991).

## Metabolic bone disease

Metabolic bone disease associated with anticonvulsants was first reported by Schmid (1967) in his article about rickets associated with epilepsy in children. Since then there have been many reports of osteomalacia in adults and rickets and bone fractures in children. The former may be easily overlooked and, particularly in mentally subnormal children on long-term anticonvulsant therapy, aching bone pain may also escape the notice of parents or attendants. The occurrence of metabolic bone disease is related to multiple drug therapy, to relatively high doses of drugs and to the duration of therapy. Phenobarbitone, primidone and phenytoin have been the main drugs implicated. Apart from radiological changes, investigations usually show a reduced serum calcium level, an elevated alkaline phosphatase reading and a normal serum phosphate concentration.

The bone changes are due to vitamin D deficiency brought about by drug induction of liver enzymes involved in the metabolism, especially hydroxylation, of vitamin D in the liver (Dent et al., 1970). The metabolism of the vitamin is both enhanced and diverted along pathways which result in more inactive metabolites. Treatment consists of giving vitamin D, and usually the dose required is significantly higher than that needed to correct simple dietary deficiency. It has been suggested that children with epilepsy should receive supplemental vitamin D while on anticonvulsant therapy, especially if they live in areas where exposure to sunlight is limited. A recent prospective study to determine the dose required to provide such protection showed that it ranged from 400 to 4000 IU/day but that 78% of the patients responded to a dose of 2400 IU/day (Collins et al., 1991). It is interesting that the enzyme-inducing anticonvulsants have a similar enhancing effect on the metabolism of the contraceptive pill so that increased doses may be required for the desired prophylactic effect. The same effect on steroid metabolism may occur with cortisol.

## Connective tissue disease

Long-term anticonvulsant medication, particularly with phenytoin, can affect connective tissue in various ways. This may occur as a result of an effect on collagen metabolism, or on fibroblast proliferation or may, perhaps, be related indirectly to the effects on liver metabolism as already described. The fact that phenytoin therapy is associated with a deficiency of circulating immunoglobulin A may also be important in the production of these toxic effects, but the exact mechanisms are unknown. The predisposition to development of IgA deficiency is possibly linked with an HLA-A2 antigen (Shakir et al., 1978). The best-known effect is the production of gum hypertrophy in children who are taking phenytoin (Figure 26.1).

Livingston and Livingston (1969) estimated that this occurred in 40% of patients on the drug and that it was more prevalent in children. It occurs with normal serum levels and is unrelated to dosage. It usually begins 2–3 months after commencing treatment with the drug, reaches its maximum in 9–12 months and usually regresses over 3–6 months after treatment is discontinued. Maximum hypertrophy occurs in

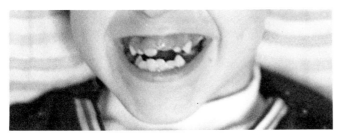

*Figure 26.1* Gum hypertrophy due to phenytoin

areas of salivary contact. Phenytoin is excreted in saliva and this may be significant in causation; the immunoglobulin A content of saliva is also reduced in such patients. Poor oral hygiene aggravates the condition so that it may also have a chronic infective basis.

Reducing the dosage of the drug is not usually successful: it must be stopped if regression is to be achieved.

Long-term anticonvulsant therapy can also cause *coarsening of the facial tissues*, including enlargement of the lips and nose. This appears to be due to a generalized thickening of the subcutaneous tissues of the face and scalp, and may be a particularly unsightly effect in adolescent girls. Those with marked changes have usually been on multiple drugs for severe seizures and this situation is especially likely to be found among the mentally handicapped. Phenytoin is the main culprit and gum hypertrophy is usually an associated finding. Falconer and Davidson (1973) reported two sets of twins in whom one of each pair developed facial coarsening while on anticonvulsant drugs whereas the non-epileptic twin was unaffected in each case.

## Hirsuties

This is another unsightly effect of phenytoin therapy, and Livingston, Peterson and Boks (1955) reported it in 5% of their patients on this drug (*Figure 26.2*) although others have reported a much higher incidence (Herranz, Armijo and Arteaga, 1988).

Hirsuties is also a particularly embarrassing side-effect in girls and alternative treatment should be considered. In the author's experience this condition usually regresses when phenytoin is stopped, although others, including Livingston (1972), disagree on this point. Some pigmentation of the skin may also be seen with phenytoin occasionally.

## Hyperglycaemia

A hyperglycaemic effect has also been reported in some patients on phenytoin or phenobarbitone, more commonly with the former drug. This appears to be due to interference by the drugs with the normal insulin response to glucose stimulation. Phenytoin should be used with caution in diabetic patients.

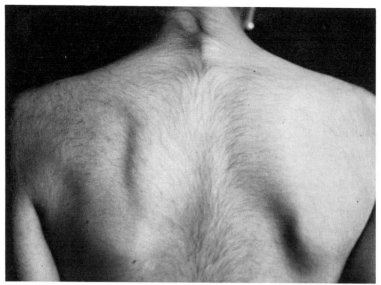

*Figure 26.2* Hirsuties due to phenytoin

## Teratogenicity

Meadow (1968) first drew attention to the association between congenital abnormalities and maternal epilepsy. He reported six infants with cleft lip and palate born to mothers who had been taken antiepileptic drugs during pregnancy. Some had other congenital abnormalities also. All had an unusual facial appearance with a prominent facial ridge, trigonocephaly, and other minor abnormalities of the face, ears and bones. Janz (1975) in a review of the subject, concluded that the risk of having a child with congenital abnormalities was two to three times higher than in the general population. If a mother has epilepsy, and is taking antiepileptic drugs, the chance of her having a child with a major congenital abnormality is just over 6%. Clefts of the lip and palate are particularly likely (10 times greater than in the general population) and congenital heart disease is four times more likely (Meadow, 1991). In addition, minor facial and skeletal abnormalities are common, and a significant degree of developmental delay occurs in a proportion of cases (Janz, 1982). The earlier reports attempted to identify specific dysmorphic syndromes associated with individual drugs, for example, the 'fetal hydantoin syndrome' (Hanson and Smith, 1975) but it is now considered that most epileptic drugs, with the exception of sodium valproate, predispose to a similar range of abnormalities in the fetus. It is also likely that similar abnormal features may be produced by a number of other toxic agents, for example, alcohol, if taken during pregnancy.

No single antiepileptic drug is completely safe during pregnancy, although some are more likely to cause problems than others. Phenytoin seems to have been incriminated most often. Carbamazepine has been regarded as relatively safe but, even with it, there have been reports of children demonstrating craniofacial defects, fingernail hypoplasia, and neurodevelopmental delay after exposure to the drug in utero (Jones *et al.*, 1989). The association between the use of sodium valproate early in pregnancy and neural tube defects, first reported by Robert and Guibaud (1982), is now firmly established. In a prospective study, Lindhout and Schmidt (1986) reported that valproate exposure during the first trimester of pregnancy is causally associated with an increased risk of neural tube defects of the order of 1.5%, a figure similar to the recurrence risk for spina bifida.

The manner in which antiepileptic drugs exert their teratogenic effect is unknown. The possible role of folate deficiency consequent on their use has been debated but there is no agreement about the value of folic acid supplements in preventing the development of malformations.

There remains the possibility that severe epilepsy in the mother may of itself be responsible for the development of congenital abnormalities in the fetus. However, comparative studies did not find an increase in the incidence of congenital malformations in mothers with epilepsy who had not taken antiepileptic drugs during pregnancy compared with the general population (Janz, 1982).

The comprehensive review of this topic by Meadow (1991) is strongly recommended to the reader.

## General remarks

It will be seen from the above that individuals with epilepsy have to contend not only with having seizures and with the psychological problems created by epilepsy, but also quite frequently with the pharmacotoxic effects of the drugs used to control their seizures. There are obviously strong arguments for keeping antiepileptic drugs to a minimum because of the risks of side-effects and toxic effects. This is not necessarily meant as an argument against the drug therapy of epilepsy, but rather as a plea that anticonvulsant medication should be carefully planned and controlled and that the dosage should not be left to chance. Accurate diagnosis of the patient's particular epileptic problem, as far as that is possible in each individual case, is a necessary prelude to wise and beneficial treatment.

Gordon (1976) has stressed that the same arguments used to limit the use of anticonvulsant drugs also apply to decisions on the *duration of therapy*. Many of the toxic effects described are more likely to occur with long-term therapy, and this is a problem of great importance in children where developing tissues may be exposed to the adverse effects of drugs. There are many factors which influence duration of therapy, including the type of epilepsy being treated, the severity of the seizures which have occurred, the evidence (or lack of it) of structural brain damage or abnormality, the association of a strong family history and the age of the patient.

Livingston (1972) recommended that effective and well-tolerated medication should be continued in all patients in full dosage for at least 4 years from the time of the last seizure and that the medication should be withdrawn gradually over a further 1 or 2 years. He recommended continuing treatment beyond the 4-year period if the end of that period coincided with the onset of puberty.

Holowach, Thurston and O'Leary (1972), and Thurston *et al.* (1982) reporting on the further follow-up of the same group of patients, favoured continuing drug treatment for 4 asymptomatic years followed by a staged withdrawal over a period of months, depending on the type of epilepsy. Shorter periods of treatment were used in uncomplicated petit mal. They found an unquestionable correlation between the epileptic syndrome present and the success or failure of withdrawal of medication. The primary generalized epilepsies (grand mal, petit mal) did best while those epilepsies with partial seizures, particularly of the temporal lobe type, and patients with multiple seizure types fared worst. More than half of their recurrences happened in the first year after drug withdrawal and, 15–23 years after stopping medication, only 28% of the cases had had a recurrence of seizures at any time. Unlike Livingston (1972), they did not find that the onset of puberty had a significant effect on the incidence of relapse after withdrawal of medication. Emerson *et al.* (1981) found that 70–75% of children who were seizure free for 4 years remained so when medication was stopped. Shinnar *et al.* (1985) noted the same outcome when treatment was stopped after only 2 years.

Summing up on this problem, the author agrees with Gordon (1976, 1987) that hard and fast rules should not apply in making decisions about withdrawing treatment. Each case should be considered on its merits and all available clinical and EEG data should be carefully considered. In view of the known risks of prolonged anticonvulsant medication, it is probably better to err on the side of withdrawing treatment sooner rather than later, provided the withdrawal is done cautiously. It is better to risk the occasional recurrence than to treat a number of children unnecessarily. It must always be remembered that the great majority of children who develop epilepsy after infancy are of normal intelligence and attend normal schools. Furthermore, no drug is free of risk although modern drugs are superior, especially where cognition and behaviour are concerned.

Schmidt (1989), who has contributed so much over many years to the study of the adverse effects of antiepileptic drugs, advised the following measures for the prevention of these effects:

1   Early adequate treatment.
2   Appropriate drug choice.
3   Single-drug therapy.
4   Drug monitoring.
5   Avoidance of acute toxicity.
6   Determination of lowest effective plasma concentration.
7   Avoidance of add-on therapy, if possible.
8   Transfer to single-drug therapy in uncontrolled epilepsy, if possible.
9   Increased awareness of toxicity.

It is to be hoped that the development of new drugs in the future, based on the application of neurophysiological knowledge, will lead to a reduction or elimination of drug toxicity.

# References

ABU-ARAFEH, I. A. and WALLACE, S. J. (1988) Unwanted effects of antiepileptic drugs. *Developmental Medicine and Child Neurology*, **30**, 117–121

ASHTON, M. G., BALL, S. G., THOMAS, J. H. and LEE, M. R. (1977) Water intoxication associated with carbamazepine treatment. *British Medical Journal*, **1**, 1134–1135

BATALDEN, E. B., VAN DYNE, B. J. and CLOYD, J. (1979) Pancreatitis associated with valproic acid therapy. *Pediatrics*, **64**, 520–522

BOOKER, H. E. (1975) Idiosyncratic reactions to the antiepileptic drugs. *Epilepsia*, **16**, 171–181

BRENT, D. A., CRUMRINE, P. K., VARMA, R. R. *et al.* (1987) Phenobarbital treatment and major depressive disorders in children with epilepsy. *Pediatrics*, **80**, 909–917

CHADWICK, D., REYNOLDS, E. H. and MARSDEN, C. D. (1976) Anticonvulsant-induced dyskinesias: a comparison with dyskinesias induced by neuroleptics. *Journal of Neurology, Neurosurgery and Psychiatry*, **39**, 1210–1218

COLLINS, N., MAHER, J., COLE, M. *et al.* (1991) A prospective study to evaluate the dose of Vitamin D required to correct low 25-hydroxy-vitamin D levels, calcium and alkaline phosphatase in patients at risk of developing antiepileptic drug-induced osteomalacia. *Quarterly Journal of Medicine*, **78**, 113–122

DAM, M. (1970) The number of Purkinje cells in patients with grand mal epilepsy treated with diphenylhydantoin. *Epilepsia*, **11**, 313–320

DAM, M. (1983) Phenytoin: an update. In *Recent Advances in Epilepsy*, No. 1 (eds T. A. Pedley and B. S. Meldrum), Churchill Livingstone, Edinburgh, London, pp. 25–34

DENT, C. E., RICHENS, A., ROWE, D. J. F. and STAMP, T. (1970) Osteomalacia with long-term anticonvulsant therapy in epilepsy. *British Medical Journal*, **4**, 69–72

DREIFUSS, F. E. (1987) Fatal liver failure in children on valproate. *Lancet*, **1**, 47–48

DREIFUSS, F. E., LANGER, D. H., MOLINE, K. A. and MAXWELL, J. F. (1989) Valproic acid hepatic fatalities. II U.S. Experience since 1984. *Neurology*, **39**, 201–207

EGGER, J. and BRETT, E. M. (1981) Effects of sodium valproate in 100 children with special reference to weight. *British Medical Journal*, **283**, 577–580

EMERSON, E., D'SOUZA, B. J., VINING, E. P. *et al.* (1981) Stopping medication in children with epilepsy. Predictors of outcome. *New England Journal of Medicine*, **304**, 1125–1129

FALCONER, M. A. and DAVIDSON, S. (1973) Coarse features in epilepsy as a consequence of anticonvulsant therapy. *Lancet*, **2**, 1112–1114

GORDON, N. S. (1976) The control of antiepileptic drug treatment. *Developmental Medicine and Child Neurology*, **18**, 535–537

GORDON, N. S. (1987) Epilepsy – to treat or not to treat. *Paediatric Reviews and Communications*, **1**, 163–180

HADZIC, N., PORTMANN, B., DAVIES, E. T. *et al.* (1990) Acute liver failure induced by carbamazepine. *Archives of Disease in Childhood*, **65**, 315–317

HANSON, J. W. and SMITH, D. W. (1975) The fetal hydantoin syndrome. *Journal of Pediatrics*, **87**, 285–290

HERRANZ, J. L., ARMIJO, J. A. and ARTEAGA, R. (1988) Clinical side effects of phenobarbital, primidone, phenytoin, carbamazepine and valproate during monotherapy in children. *Epilepsia*, **29**, 794–804

HOLOWACH, J., THURSTON, D. L. and O'LEARY, J. (1972) Prognosis in childhood epilepsy. *New England Journal of Medicine*, **286**, 169–174

IIVANAINEN, M., VIUKARI, M., and HELLE, E. P. (1977) Cerebellar atrophy in phenytoin-treated mentally retarded epileptics. *Epilepsia*, **18**, 375–386

JANZ, D. (1975) The teratogenic risk of antiepileptic drugs. *Epilepsia*, **16**, 159–169

JANZ, D. (1982) On congenital malformations and minor anomalies in the offspring of parents with epilepsy. Review of the literature. In *Pregnancy and the Child* (eds D. Janz, M. Dam, A. Richens, D. Schmidt), Raven Press, New York, pp. 211–222

JONES, K. L., LACRO, R. V., JOHNSON, K. A. and ADAMS, J. (1989) Pattern of malformation in the children of women treated with carbamazepine during pregnancy. *New England Journal of Medicine*, **320**, 1661–1666

KUTT, H., WOLK, M., SCHEMAN, R. and MCDOWELL, F. (1964) Insufficient parahydroxylation as a cause of diphenylhydantoin toxicity. *Neurology*, **1**, 542–548

LERMAN, P. (1986) Seizures induced or aggravated by anticonvulsants. *Epilepsia*, **27**, 706–710

LINDHOUT, D. and SCHMIDT, D. (1986) In-utero exposure to valproate and neural tube defects. *Lancet*, **1**, 1392–1393

LIVINGSTON, S. (1972) *Comprehensive Management of Epilepsy in Infancy, Childhood and Adolescence*, Charles C. Thomas, Springfield, Illinois, pp. 341–342

LIVINGSTON, S. and LIVINGSTON, H. C. (1969) Diphenyldantoin gingival hyperplasia. *American Journal of Diseases of Children*, **117**, 265–270

LIVINGSTON, S., PETERSON, D. and BOKS, L. L. (1955) Hypertrichosis occurring in association with Dilantin therapy. *Journal of Pediatrics*, **47**, 351–352

MCGOWAN, M. E. L. (1983) Growth in children with epilepsy. In *Research Progress in Epilepsy* (ed. F. C. Rose), Pitman, London, pp. 253–268

MARESCAUX, C., WARTER, J. M., MICHELETTI, G. *et al.* (1982) Stuporous episodes during treatment with sodium valproate. Report of 7 cases. *Epilepsia*, **23**, 297–305

MEADOW, S. R. (1968) Anticonvulsant drugs and congenital abnormalities. *Lancet*, **ii**, 1296

MEADOW, S. R. (1991) Anticonvulsants in pregnancy. *Archives of Disease in Childhood*, **66**, 62–65

MOORE, A., O'DONOHOE, N. V. and MONAGHAN, H. (1986) Neuroleptic malignant syndrome. *Archives of Disease in Childhood*, **61**, 793–795

MOUNTAIN, K. R., HIRSCH, J. and GALLUS, A. S. (1970) Neonatal coagulation defect due to anticonvulsant drug treatment in pregnancy. *Lancet*, **i**, 265–268

MOWAT, A. P. (1973) Dystonic reactions to drugs. *Developmental Medicine and Child Neurology*, **15**, 654–655

O'DONOHOE, N. V. (1973) A series of epileptic children treated with Tegretol. In *Tegretol in Epilepsy*. Report of an International Clinical Symposium (ed. C. A. S. Wink), C. Nichols and Co. Ltd, Geigy Pharmaceuticals, Manchester, Macclesfield, Cheshire, pp. 25–29

OSORIO, I., BURNSTINE, T.H., REMLER, B. *et al.* (1989) Phenytoin-induced seizures. A paradoxical effect at toxic concentrations in epileptic patients. *Epilepsia*, **30**, 230–234

PATEL, H. and CRICHTON, J. U. (1968) The neurologic hazards of diphenylhydantoin in childhood. *Journal of Pediatrics*, **73**, 676–684

REYNOLDS, E. H. (1975) Chronic antiepileptic toxicity: a review. *Epilepsia*, **16**, 319–352

REYNOLDS, E. H. (1983a) Adverse haematological effects of antiepileptic drugs. In *Chronic Toxicity of Antiepileptic Drugs* (eds J. Oxley, D. Janz and H. Meinardi), Raven Press, New York, pp. 91–99

REYNOLDS, E. H. (1983b) Mental effects of antiepileptic medication. *Epilepsia*, **Supplement 2**, S85–S95

ROBERT, E. and GUIBAUD, P. (1982) Maternal valproic acid and congenital neural tube defects. *Lancet*, **2**, 937

SCHMID, F. (1967) Osteopathien bei antiepileptischer Dauerbehandlung. *Fortschritte der Medizin*, **9**, 381–382

SCHMIDT, D. (1984) Adverse effects of valproate. *Epilepsia*, **25**, Supplement 1, S44–S49

SCHMIDT, D. (1986) Toxicity of antiepileptic drugs. In *Recent Advances in Epilepsy*, No. 3 (eds T. A. Pedley and B. S. Meldrum), Churchill Livingstone, Edinburgh, London, pp. 211–232

SCHMIDT, D. (1989) Adverse effects of antiepileptic drugs in children: the relevance of drug interaction. *Cleveland Clinic Journal of Medicine*, Supplement to Vol. 52, Part 1. S132–S139

SCHEFFNER, D., ST. KONIG, S., RANTERBERG-RULAND, W. *et al.* (1988) Fatal liver failure in 16 children with valproate therapy. *Epilepsia*, **29**, 530–542

SHAKIR, R. A., BEHAN, P. O., DICK, H. and LAMBIE, D. G. (1978) Metabolism of immunoglobulin A, lymphocytic function and histocompatability antigens in patients on anticonvulsants. *Journal of Neurology, Neurosurgery and Psychiatry*, **47**, 307–311

SHINNAR, S., VINING, E. P. G., MELLITS, E. M. *et al.* (1988) Discontinuing antiepileptic medication in children with epilepsy after two years without seizures. *New England Journal of Medicine*, **313**, 976–980

SNEAD, O. C. and HOSEY, L. C. (1985) Exacerbation of seizures in children by carbamazepine. *New England Journal of Medicine*, **313**, 916–921

SUSSMAN, N. M. and MCLAIN, L. W. (1979) A direct hepatotoxic effect of valproic acid. *Journal of the American Medical Association*, **242**, 1173–1174

TADA, H., WALLACE, S. J. and HUGHES, I. A. (1986) Height in epilepsy. *Archives of Disease in Childhood*, **61**, 1224–1226

TAYLOR, D. C. and MCKINLAY, I. (1984) When not to treat epilepsy with drugs. *Developmental Medicine and Child Neurology*, **26**, 822–833

THURSTON, J. H., THURSTON, D. L., HIXON, B. B. and VIELLER, A. J. (1982) Prognosis in childhood epilepsy: additional follow-up of 148 children 15 to 23 years after withdrawal of anticonvulsant therapy. *New England Journal of Medicine*, **306**, 831–836

TRIMBLE, M. R., CORBETT, J. and DONALDSON, D. (1980) Folic acid and mental symptoms in children with epilepsy. *Journal of Neurology, Neurosurgery and Psychiatry*, **43**, 1030–1034

TURK, J. and LASK, B. (1991) Neuroleptic malignant syndrome. *Archives of Disease in Childhood*, **66**, 91–92

VALLARTA, J. M., BELL, D. B. and REICHART, A. (1974) Progressive encephalopathy due to chronic hydantoin intoxication. *American Journal of Diseases of Children*, **128**, 27–34

WATTS, R. G., EMANUEL, P. D., ZUCKERMAN, U. S. and HOWARD, T. H. (1990) Valproic acid-induced cytopenia. Evidence for a dose-related suppression of hematopoiesis. *Journal of Pediatrics*, **117**, 495–499

WOLF, S. M. and FORSYTHE, A. (1978) Behaviour disturbance, phenobarbital and febrile seizures. *Pediatrics*, **61**, 728–731

# Chapter 27

# Surgical treatment of epilepsy

Wilder Penfield pioneered the surgical treatment of epilepsy having a focal origin during the years from the 1920s onwards. His experiences are described in a classic book (Penfield and Jasper, 1954) and the results were later reviewed by Rasmussen (1969), who reported a success rate in controlling epilepsy of between 30 and 45%. Dramatic advances have been made in the surgical treatment of epilepsy in the last decade. They have occurred through improvements in intensive monitoring techniques generally, in neuroimaging, in the use of special EEG recording techniques just prior to surgery, and in neurosurgical techniques. Physicians caring for those with medically intractable epilepsy now have available a much wider choice of diagnostic and therapeutic options than heretofore. Surgical treatment for intractable epilepsy is being used increasingly for children and adolescents as well as for adult patients. It is not proposed to deal in detail with the surgical treatment of epilepsy in childhood in this book. The reader is referred to the Proceedings of the Cleveland Clinic International Symposium on Pediatric Epileptology (1989) and to the comprehensive review edited by Lüders (1992).

The primary treatment of epilepsy in childhood should consist of the control of seizures by medical means, if possible, and of close attention to the psychological and social considerations connected with the epilepsy. It is likely that modern antiepileptic drugs will provide complete control of seizures in up to 80% of all patients suffering from different varieties of epilepsy, with varying degrees of success and failure depending on the type of epilepsy (Shorvon and Reynolds, 1982). Of the remaining 20% of patients who prove intractable to medication, only a small proportion will be suitable for or amenable to surgical treatment but, as already indicated, improved methods of investigation and more sophisticated surgical techniques are gradually expanding this number and are likely to continue to do so in the future.

## Selection of cases

The main considerations when selecting children with epilepsy for surgery are medical intractability, the degree of disability due to seizures, and lack of realistic hopes for spontaneous remission (Wyllie, 1991). Confirmation of medical intractability requires thorough trials of all major antiepileptic drugs, first singly and then in two drug combinations, to the point of clinical toxicity. The observation times necessary to demonstrate intractability vary among patients depending on their baseline seizure frequency and also on the particular epileptic syndrome which they have. It takes many months and often years to demonstrate medical intractability. The degree of disability caused by the seizures also depends on many factors, including the frequency of the attacks, their clinical type, and the presence of associated handicaps particularly mental handicap. For all children, recurrent unpredictable attacks of altered consciousness may have damaging effects on self-esteem, confidence and independence (Wyllie and Luders, 1989). Persistent psychosocial problems are commonplace in children with uncontrolled complex partial seizures, and are often complicated by parental overprotection and the decreased expectations of teachers (Vining, 1989).

Another consideration is the possibility of spontaneous remission of the patient's epilepsy. While, in general, childhood epilepsy is more likely than adult epilepsy to remit, this is not the case in those types of epilepsy for which surgery has been shown to be most effective. This is particularly true of secondary partial epilepsy resulting from temporal lobe lesions and causing complex partial seizures. Remission rates of these seizures in childhood have been reported to be as low as 10% and 18% in two series in recent years (Harbord and Manson, 1987; Kotagal et al., 1987).

The Montreal group of neurosurgeons has always emphasized that, because the seizure activity does not arise from the lesion itself but from the adjacent cortex rendered epileptogenic by the presence of the lesion, this marginal tissue must also be excised. It seems paradoxical that surgical excision, which of itself produces focal brain damage and glial scarring, should act to prevent the continuation of clinical epilepsy. However, this is the case and, although the weak epileptogenicity of surgical scars vis-a-vis other scars is not fully understood, it is probably related to the histological components of scars produced by acquired brain damage and the proportions of gliotic and cellular tissue in the immediate neighbourhood of such scars.

## Temporal lobectomy

The value of surgery for intractable temporal lobe epilepsy is firmly established and temporal lobectomy is the most common surgical procedure performed for epilepsy in childhood. Falconer pioneered resection for this type of epilepsy (Falconer, 1965) and advocated its earlier use in children who fulfilled his criteria for operation. This included failure to respond to adequate trials of drug therapy, evidence of a predominantly or wholly unilateral epileptic disorder on EEG, and a period of observation long enough to make spontaneous remission unlikely. Another criterion was that the patient should have an IQ of 60 or more but nowadays mental retardation is not regarded as an absolute contraindication to surgery (Wyllie and Lüders, 1989). Davidson and Falconer (1975), reviewing 40 children aged 15 years or younger who had been operated on and followed for between 1 and 24 years, found that 22 were seizure-free, 7 had an occasional seizures, 5 had their seizures reduced by half and only 6 subjects failed to benefit from surgery. The best results were obtained in those who were found to have mesial temporal sclerosis. Rasmussen (1983), reviewing 129 children whose epileptogenic lesion involved primarily the temporal lobe and who had undergone temporal lobectomy at 15 years or younger for refractory epilepsy, found that 60% had a complete or nearly complete remission of seizures while the great majority of the remainder were significantly improved. In a subgroup of children in which EEG and neuroimaging had been performed and in which epileptogenicity was confined to the anterior portion of one temporal lobe, Wyllie *et al.* (1987) noted a good outcome (i.e. no seizures, rare seizures, or auras only) in up to 90% of all cases and, in children and adolescents, the results appear to be at least as good as in adults (Mizrahi *et al.*, 1990).

Lindsay, Ounsted and Richards (1984), following analysis of the biographies of the children in their unique series, suggested that all children under treatment with drugs for temporal lobe epilepsy should be most scrupulously reviewed before leaving school. Some will be found to be in natural remission and should be weaned from their drugs. Others who have not remitted should be carefully investigated and considered for neurosurgery. Such assessment today requires in-patient video-EEG monitoring of their attacks and, if available, MRI scanning in addition to a CT scan. The best surgical results are obtained in patients with an identifiable lesion on CT or MRI and a corresponding seizure focus on the EEG. Since a major concern with temporal lobectomy is the possible effect on language, the side which is dominant for language and memory function needs to be determined preoperatively by intracarotid amylobarbitone tests and measures are then taken to protect areas involved in language function during resection (Wyllie, 1991).

Lindsay, Ounsted and Richards (1984) noted that a substantial number in their series deteriorated gravely in many respects between the ages of 5 and 15 years and they recommended that consideration should be given earlier in the course of the natural history of temporal lobe epilepsy to the possibility of surgical treatment. Duchowny *et al.* (1992) have reviewed their experience with temporal lobectomy for intractable complex partial seizures of temporal lobe origin in pre-adolescent children and have reported that 11 of their 16 children were seizure free, 3 were 90% better, 1 was 50% improved, and one was unchanged. All of their patients demonstrated neuropathological abnormalities on histological examination, even those five patients who had normal neuroimaging studies, including MRI, preoperatively. Prenatally acquired abnormalities of neurogenesis were the most common findings, whereas mesial temporal sclerosis was found in only two children. These authors argue that the onset of complex partial seizures in early childhood is strongly suggestive of the presence of a brain lesion, most often due to an abnormality of neurogenesis.

The case for early consideration of temporal lobectomy for intractable temporal lobe seizures is now irrefutable. Many patients who undergo temporal lobectomy are eventually able to discontinue medications. It is possible for some to achieve a totally normal lifestyle after surgery. Early surgery may avoid the development of chronic disability and enhance the chances for normal psychosocial maturation and normal integration into the social and vocational fabric of society.

## Other surgical procedures

Temporal lobectomy is the most commonly employed procedure in the surgical treatment of epilepsy. However, among the small subgroup of infants and young children who undergo epilepsy surgery, *extratemporal resections* are more common, especially frontal lobectomy. Factors resulting in earlier surgery for infants and children with frontal, parietal or occipital lobe epilepsy include earlier onset and a higher frequency of daily seizures (Wyllie, 1991). The clinical symptomatology depends on the particular cortical area affected but, quite often, the seizures appear similar to the complex partial seizures due to secondary partial epilepsy arising in the temporal lobes but with additional features suggesting an extratemporal origin. Cortical dysplasia is the commonest pathological feature in these patients and MRI scanning is usually, but not invariably, necessary for the preoperative detection of such lesions. *Hemimegalencephaly* is one such gross dysplastic lesion. Patients with this condition manifest psychomotor retardation, hemiparesis, hemianopsia, and drug-resistant seizures which often begin in the newborn period or during early infancy (King *et al.*, 1985).

Since the 1950s, *hemispherectomy* has been performed for patients with hemiplegia and frequent, intractable, focal-onset seizures. These seizures arise from multiple epileptogenic areas which are too many and too extensive for focal excision of a single lobe. Early operations included total removal of the hemisphere down to the basal ganglia. However, it gradually became clear that this procedure was followed later by the development of a delayed persistent chronic subdural haemorrhage into the operative cavity, resulting in granular ependymitis and obstructive hydrocephalus in the remaining hemisphere. Progressive neurological deterioration and often death followed. These problems have led to the development of new operative procedures. Since 1974, anatomically subtotal but functionally complete hemispherectomy has been used by the Montreal group in 20 patients, followed for an average period of 7.5 years (Tinuper *et al.*, 1988). This procedure leaves one-fourth to one-third of the hemisphere in place, usually the frontal and occipital lobes, but disconnects these areas from the rest of the brain by sectioning the white matter down to the medial pial surface and thereby separating the remaining parts of the brain from the corpus callosum and the upper brain-stem. This produced complete control of seizures in half of the Canadian cases and marked improvement occurred in a further 20%. Long-term complications were minimal. From Oxford, Beardsworth and Adams (1988) have reported similar good results in ten patients operated on since 1980. Their technique involves removal of the damaged hemisphere followed by mobilization of the dura and suturing of the dura to the falx, thereby eliminating the subdural space as far as possible. Insulation of the subdural cavity from the ventricular system is achieved by closure of the ipsilateral foramen of Munro.

Although hemispherectomy has been most frequently performed for patients with infantile hemiplegia and chronic intractable epilepsy, it has more recently been performed for patients with Rasmussen's syndrome of focal chronic encephalitis who have progressive hemiparesis, hemispheric atrophy and focal onset seizures (Hanovar, Janota and Polkey, 1992) and both it and also focal resections have been performed in a number of infants with infantile spasms who are found to have extensive lateralized or localized lesions on PET scanning (Chugani *et al.*, 1990). It has been strongly recommended for patients with hemimegalencephaly and intractable epilepsy (Vigevano *et al.*, 1989). It is argued that patients with this condition are already functionally hemispherectomized because the malformation impairs the development of higher cortical functions in the involved hemisphere. Removal of the diseased hemisphere usually leads to complete recovery from epilepsy and permits normal development of the remaining hemisphere.

Since 1940, experience with animal models has led gradually to the use of *section of the corpus callosum* in the treatment of chronic intractable epilepsy in humans. Anatomical reasoning suggested that such an interruption of the interhemispheric electrical discharges might help patients who were devastated by generalized seizures and clinical experience had shown that significant neurological deficits did not occur when neurosurgical procedures involved partial section of the corpus callosum (Wilson, Reeves and Gazzaniga, 1978). The exact procedures for corpus callosotomy have continued to evolve, and range from total commissurotomy through central commissurotomy to anterior section only. Spencer and Spencer (1989) have reviewed the use of the operation in children. They stress that it is strictly a palliative operation, unlike temporal lobectomy where the object is cure. Very rarely, all seizures may cease after callosotomy. However, the main purpose is to stop secondary generalization or reduce it by up to 90%, thereby protecting more normal cortex from involvement by repeated epileptic discharges, decreasing the number of falls and reducing the need for heavy antiepileptic medication. It is also hoped that behaviour and cognition may improve and that an increased degree of independence may be achieved. The best results are reported in focal hemispheric disease although, in that situation, subtotal hemispherectomy and disconnection is probably a better alternative. Andermann (1989) has reported favourably on the use of callosotomy in patients with the Lennox–Gastaut syndrome where the operation led to an abolition of or marked reduction in the number of disabling tonic drop attacks. The author's experience is limited to two cases of the Lennox–Gastaut syndrome, both of which have shown significant improvement over a period of 2–3 years following the operation. Taylor (1990) had cautioned against the indiscriminate use of the procedure, advising that its use should be confined to leading centres which are actively engaged in epilepsy surgery and that the operation should be carefully monitored with regard to outcome and sequelae.

## References

ANDERMANN, F. (1989) Panel discussion on epilepsy surgery in children and adolescents. *Cleveland Clinic Journal of Medicine*, **56**, Supplement, Part 1, S79–S80

BEARDSWORTH, E. D. and ADAMS, C. B. T. (1988) Modified hemispherectomy for epilepsy: early results in 10 cases. *British Journal of Neurosurgery*, **2**, 73–84

CHUGANI, H. T., SHIELDS, W. D., SHEWMON, D. A. *et al.* (1990) Infantile spasms I: PET 'identifies' focal cortical dysplasia in cryptogenic cases for surgical treatment. *Annals of Neurology*, **27**, 406–413

DAVIDSON, S. and FALCONER, M. A. (1975) Outcome of surgery in 40 children with temporal lobe epilepsy. *Lancet*, **1**, 1260–1263

DUCHOWNY, M., LEVIN, B., JAYAKAR, P. *et al.* (1992) Temporal lobectomy in early childhood. *Epilepsia*, **33**, 298–303

FALCONER, M. A. (1965) The surgical treatment of temporal lobe epilepsy. *Neurochirurgia*, **8**, 161–172

HANOVAR, M., JANOTA, I., and POLKEY, C. E. (1992) Rasmussen's encephalitis in surgery for epilepsy. *Developmental Medicine and Child Neurology*, **34**, 3–14

HARBORD, M. G. and MANSON, J. (1987) Temporal lobe epilepsy in childhood: reappraisal of etiology and outcome. *Pediatric Neurology*, **3**, 263–268

KING, M., STEPHENSON, J. B. P., ZIERVOGEL, M. *et al.* (1985) Hemimegalencephaly – a case for hemispherectomy? *Neuropediatrics*, **16**, 46–55

KOTAGAL, P., ROTHNER, A. D., ERENBERG, G. *et al.* (1987) Complex partial seizures of childhood onset: a five-year follow-up study. *Archives of Neurology*, **44**, 1177–1180

LINDSAY, J., OUNSTED, C. and RICHARDS, P. (1984) Long-term outcome in children with temporal lobe seizures. V. Indications and contraindications for neurosurgery. *Developmental Medicine and Child Neurology*, **26**, 25–32

LÜDERS, H. (ed.) (1992) *Epilepsy Surgery*. Raven Press, New York

MIZRAHI, E. M., KELLAWAY, P. M., GROSSMAN, R. G. *et al.* (1990) Anterior temporal lobectomy and medically refractory temporal lobe epilepsy of childhood. *Epilepsia*, **31**, 302–312

PENFIELD, W. and JASPER, H. (1954) Surgical therapy. In *Epilepsy and the Functional Anatomy of the Human Brain*, J. and A. Churchill, London, Little Brown and Co. Inc., Boston, pp. 739–817

PROCEEDINGS OF THE CLEVELAND CLINIC INTERNATIONAL EPILEPSY SYMPOSIUM (1989) *Pediatric epileptology: epilepsy surgery in children and adolescents.* **56**, Supplement, Part 1, S43–S91

RASMUSSEN, T. (1969) The role of surgery in the treatment of focal epilepsy. *Clinical Neurosurgery*, **16**, 288–314

RASMUSSEN, T. (1983) Cortical resection in children with focal epilepsy. In: *Advances in Epileptology: XIVth Epilepsy International Symposium* (eds. M. Parsonage, R. H. E. Grant, A. G. Craig and A. A. Ward), Raven Press, New York, pp. 249–254

SHORVON, S. D. and REYNOLDS, E. H. (1982) Early prognosis of epilepsy. *British Medical Journal*, **285**, 1699–1701

SPENCER, D. S. and SPENCER, S. S. (1989) Corpus callosotomy in the treatment of medically intractable secondarily generalized seizures of children. *Cleveland Clinical Journal of Medicine*, **56**, Supplement, Part 1, S69–S78

TAYLOR, D. C. (1990) Callosal section for epilepsy and the avoidance of doing everything possible. *Developmental Medicine and Child Neurology*, **32**, 267–270

TINUPER, P., ANDERMANN, F., VILLEMURE, J-G. *et al.* (1988) Functional hemispherectomy for treatment of epilepsy associated with hemiplegia: rationale, indications, results and comparison with callosotomy. *Annals of Neurology*, **24**, 27–34

VIGEVANO, F., BERTINI, E., BOLDRINI, R. *et al.* (1989) Hemimegalencephaly and intractable epilepsy: benefits of hemispherectomy. *Epilepsia*, **30**, 833–843

VINING, E. P. G. (1989) Psychosocial issues for children with epilepsy. *Cleveland Clinic Journal of Medicine*, **56**, Supplement, Part 1, 214–220

WILSON, D. H., REEVES, A. G. and GAZZANIGA, M. (1982) 'Central' commissurotomy for intractable generalized epilepsy: series two. *Neurology*, **32**, 687–697

WYLLIE, E. (1991) Cortical resection for children with epilepsy. *American Journal of Diseases of Children*, **145**, 314–320

WYLLIE, E. and LÜDERS, H. (1989) Complex partial seizures in children: clinical manifestations, and identification of surgical candidates. *Cleveland Clinic Journal of Medicine*, **56**, Supplement Part 1, S43–S52

WYLLIE, E., LÜDERS, H., MORRIS, H. H. *et al.* (1987) Clinical outcome after complete or partial cortical resection for intractable epilepsy. *Neurology*, **37**, 1634–1641

# Chapter 28

# Prognosis of epilepsy

## General considerations

The problems of prognosis for children with epilepsy remain controversial. This is due, to some extent, to arguments about classification and terminology, and often because of uncertainty about the long-term outcome. Essentially, the prognosis for any individual child with epilepsy depends, above all, on the type of epilepsy which the patient has. Studies of prognosis which focus only on the type or types of seizures present are flawed and not in accordance with modern views about the epilepsies and their causes. An epileptic seizure is an event, the symptom of the underlying neurological disorder, the epilepsy or epileptic syndrome. Identical seizures occur in patients destined to have very different outcomes.

The epilepsies and epileptic syndromes are subdivided on the basis of two criteria. Those with generalized seizures (generalized epilepsies) are distinguished from those with partial seizures (partial or localization-related epilepsies) and those with known aetiology (symptomatic or secondary or lesional) from those with no known aetiology (idiopathic or primary). A further category of cryptogenic refers to epilepsies where the cause is still unknown but which are presumed to be symptomatic. An epileptic syndrome has been defined as an epileptic disorder characterized by a cluster of signs and symptoms customarily occurring together (Dreifuss, 1989).

Epileptic syndromes include seizure disorders with certain clinical (ictal) and EEG characteristics regardless of a variety of causes. Epileptic syndromes tend to run a typical course with an ultimate benign, poor, or undetermined prognostic outlook. They are age-dependent and most commonly found in various epochs of childhood and adult life. Some childhood syndromes linger on into adult life and some, for example, juvenile myoclonic epilepsy of Janz, may persist throughout adult life. The West syndrome of infantile spasms is the archetypal epileptic syndrome and was the first to be described (West, 1841). However, delineation of the many other syndromes is a relatively recent phenomenon and has only been possible as a result of the advent and development of EEG technology. Age, types of seizure, and EEG constitute the essential triad of epileptic syndromes. Due to the age-determined character of epileptic syndromes, transitions from one form to another may occur. In general, severe epileptic syndromes tend to convert into another severe form with advancing age (e.g. the West syndrome may convert into the Lennox–Gastaut syndrome) while benign syndromes, based on brain dysfunction, may be followed by the development of other benign syndromes later (Nogueira de Melo and Niedermeyer, 1991a). For example, in a small number of cases, juvenile myoclonic epilepsy may be preceded by typical childhood absence epilepsy.

The delineation of epileptic syndromes has proceeded apace in recent years (O'Donohoe, 1992) and this has been of considerable practical significance, enabling the attending physician to select appropriate investigations, decide on optimal treatment and predict the outcome. Although some syndromes, notably in the case of the benign partial epilepsies, lend themselves to accurate prognostic predictions, in many others, the outlook is less predictable. Another difficulty is that the delineation of some syndromes is far from clear, leading to disagreement and confusion (Aicardi, 1988). It should be realized that the concept of syndromes is far from applicable to all types of seizure disorder in childhood. A large number of cases simply will not fit into any particular syndrome, indeed the majority in some published series (Nogueira de Melo and Niedermeyer, 1991b). A particular difficulty relates to the fact that it is often impossible to categorize a particular case in its early presenting phase and before the evolution of the disorder. So, while the delineation of syndromes has been an important advance, it is essential to continue to look at the epilepsies in a general way, that is, with primary or secondary causation and whether they are localization-based (partial) or generalized (Commission on Classification and Terminology, 1989).

## Primary and secondary causation

In general, the prognosis for childhood epilepsy tends to be better when the patient's epilepsy appears to be due to constitutional and/or hereditary factors, what Rodin (1968) called a 'specific seizure propensity', than when it is secondary to known cerebral damage or structural abnormality. This was recognized by a study group reporting to the World Health Organization on juvenile epilepsy in 1957 when it reported that: 'the prognosis of the type of epilepsy in which genetic factors predominate is better than for the other types as regards the number of fits, their responsiveness to treatment and the infrequency of undesirable psychological changes'. In this context, one may think of benign familial neonatal convulsions, febrile convulsions, childhood absence epilepsy (petit mal), photosensitive epilepsy and, above all, the benign partial epilepsies (Loiseau et al., 1983; Deonna et al., 1986). The use of the word benign to indicate eventual remission of seizures is somewhat controversial, given the social and psychological resonances produced by the diagnosis of epilepsy of whatever type. Neither can remission be guaranteed in the genetically-based epilepsies. For example, juvenile myoclonic epilepsy requires life-long treatment. Febrile convulsions, if prolonged, may result in temporal lobe damage and the development of mesial temporal sclerosis, resulting in later chronic partial epilepsy (Ounsted, Lindsay and Norman, 1966). Thurston et al. (1982), following up a large series of children 15–23 years after withdrawal of antiepileptic drug therapy, found that relapse rates were lowest in the idiopathic or primary cases and highest in the secondary or symptomatic cases, particularly those with complex partial seizures arising from the temporal lobe and in those with multiple seizure types. They found an overall relapse rate of 28% in their series, two-thirds of all relapses occurring during the first 2 years after drug withdrawal and 85% occurring within 5 years of withdrawal. Sillanpää (1983), in a study of young adults with onset of epilepsy in childhood, showed that a child with epilepsy had an 85% probability of becoming seizure-free if he or she had no organic brain lesion, presented only with grand mal seizures, and had normal psychomotor development.

## Prognosis and age of onset

Prognosis may also be looked at from the point of view of the age of the child at onset of the epilepsy. Some of the most serious seizure disorders occur in infancy and early childhood, for example, neonatal seizures, infantile spasms and the various myoclonic epilepsies. Equally true, however, is the fact that febrile convulsions, the most common seizure disorder in this early epoch of life, have a very good prognosis. This probably explains why studies showing an association between early seizure onset and poor prognosis are usually based on highly selected sources such as teaching hospitals and special clinics (Chevrie and Aicardi, 1978) while studies indicating a better prognosis for those with an early onset of seizures are more broadly based in the community (Ellenberg, Hirtz and Nelson, 1984). In those young children in whom prompt remission of epilepsy is obtained with or without treatment, the prognosis is good. Holowach, Thurston and O'Leary (1972) stressed that the possibility of stopping treatment before the age of 8 years usually implied a good long-term prognosis. Thus resistance to therapy, the chronicity of epilepsy, the occurrence of different seizure types and the association with mental defect and neurological and psychological disorders are all poor prognostic indicators in the young child. The chances for a patient to achieve complete freedom from seizures depends particularly on the intensity of the seizure disorder and its duration and both of these aspects are usually prominent when the epilepsy is symptomatic of a serious underlying brain disorder.

Rodin (1968) observed that the longer the history of epilepsy and the more seizures experienced prior to starting treatment, the less likely was complete seizure control to be achieved. Frequent recurrences of seizures, particularly during the first year of treatment, also imply a poor prognosis for seizure control (Shorvon and Reynolds, 1982). Reynolds (1981) has drawn attention to what he terms the *Gowers phenomenon*, described by Gowers in his classic book on epilepsy in 1881, as follows: 'the effect of a convulsion on the nerve centres is such as to render the occurrence of another more easy, to intensify the predisposition that already exists. Thus every fit may be said to be, in part, the result of those which have preceded it, the cause of those which follow it'. Reynolds (1990) suggests that, if this is correct, early effective treatment in the newly diagnosed patient may prevent the evolution of chronic drug-resistant epilepsy.

When considering prognosis, it is important to remember that all seizures are not epilepsy. A child may have a single seizure, unrelated to intercurrent disease or trauma, and never have another. In a common epileptic syndrome such as benign partial epilepsy with centro-temporal spike discharges, 20% or more of those affected experience a single seizure only (Loiseau and Duché, 1989). The question of single seizures has already been discussed in Chapter 8. It was pointed out there that the key risk factors for recurrence were the aetiology of the seizures (idiopathic *versus* a remote symptomatic cause) and the nature of the EEG (normal *versus* abnormal). In general, where the EEG is normal or becomes so during treatment, a favourable outlook may be expected in children.

## The secondary handicaps of epilepsy

The individual with continuing epilepsy faces many disadvantages of a social, educational, vocational, and economic nature, quite apart from the medical difficulties consequent on the seizures and the need for long-term (sometimes life-long) drug therapy. This fact is often ignored in surveys of prognosis which concern themselves with the effect of treatment on seizures alone. As Yannet, Dreamer and Barba (1949) wrote, this approach '. . . fails to take into account the many other factors that determine whether an epileptic child is living a relatively normal life in his community. It is conceivable that an emotionally well adjusted child having three to five spells a year is infinitely better off than a child having one spell a year but seriously handicapped by personality deviations resulting from untreated tensions in the home directly related to the epileptic state'. The fact that the *quality of life* for children and adolescents with epilepsy is often far from satisfactory was shown by the survey of Harrison and Taylor (1976). Their patients were originally identified between 1948 and 1953 on the basis that they had come for treatment because of having had at least one seizure in early childhood. Over 200 patients were followed up after 25 years with reference to their long-term medical, social and educational problems. Although nearly two-thirds of the sample suffered minimal ill-effects, the problems of the remainder were considerable: 10% of the patients had died, and of the survivors, 11% were confined to institutions while over 6% were invalids at home. Overall the educational achievement of the sample was good but there were also a considerable number of educational problems. Continuing epilepsy was associated with greatly reduced educational and occupational achievement in contrast to the group in remission. The authors pointed out that the consequences of epilepsy for a third of their patients were very serious indeed and that this finding correlated with the public image of epilepsy as a serious and chronic disorder, and that it revealed why the public was frightened by it and prejudiced against its sufferers.

Sillanpää (1992) points out that epilepsy has a special place among long-term illnesses because it has its highest prevalence between birth and puberty, the time of life when the onset of long-term illness invariably affects the individual's psychosocial development. An unselected population sample of children with epilepsy, aged 4–15 years, was studied and compared with normal matched controls. The prevalence of epilepsy in the study population was 0.68% and the time elapsed from the last seizure was at least a year in 62% of the cases. Another neurological deficit was present in nearly 40% of cases, the most frequent being mental handicap, speech disorders and specific learning disorders. In the remaining 60% of cases with 'epilepsy only', a handicap was experienced in over one-fifth of the children, representing a 20-fold increase in handicap compared with the controls. In this study, handicap was defined as something which limits or prevents the fulfilment of the normal role of the individual and impairment of social integration was the handicap experienced most frequently.

Henriksen (1988) has written about the prevention and treatment of such problems and about the need for the physician to be aware of their possible development. He observed that, ideally, the child and parents should be followed over the years by the same doctor and, in the case of the specialist, that he or she should be available to advise colleagues and other professionals dealing with the child on a regular basis. He stressed the importance of providing information and counselling at intervals to both parents and patient. This, he believes, will provide better understanding of the problems, relieve anxiety, and help the parents to bring up their child like any other. The parents will feel more confident and will convey this feeling to others, thus preventing negative attitudes towards the child. Vining (1989) has written eloquently about this aspect of the problem, emphasizing that lack of information plus misinformation may give rise to bizarre misconceptions about epilepsy, especially among adolescents, and that these may be a cause of poor psychosocial adaptation.

*Mortality* as a result of epilepsy is something which is of concern to everybody dealing with the child with epilepsy, and this anxiety has been well documented among parents of children with febrile convulsions (Baumer *et al.*, 1981). Kurokawa *et al.* (1982) studied the case histories of 385 patients, with epilepsy beginning under the age of 15 years, who had died. Of these, 5.7% died during the first 10 years after onset and another 2.9% between 11 and 24 years from onset. Mortality was significantly higher in the following situations: (1) epilepsy with onset before the first birthday; (2) epilepsy which was symptomatic in aetiology; (3) infantile spasms and the severe myoclonic epilepsies; (4) where there was associated developmental retardation present at the time of the first visit. *Sudden unexplained death* in people with epilepsy is a phenomenon which occurs in all ages and, in adults, accounts for up to 15% of the mortality from epilepsy (Leestma *et al.*, 1984). Marked changes in blood pressure and cardiac rhythm have been observed during both generalized and partial seizures. Interictal discharges may also produce effects on the cardiovascular system. Cardiac arrhythmias and pulmonary oedema may be associated with seizures. The phenomenon of sudden unexplained death in epilepsy is probably the result of irreversible disruption of autonomic homeostasis resulting from electrical disorganization in the central nervous system (Schraeder and Lathers, 1989). It has always been the author's practice to warn the parents of children who have frequent and severe seizures that the possibility of sudden death exists.

## Conclusion

It is appropriate to end this chapter on a hopeful and more cheerful note. Livingston (1972), in a review of approximately 20 000 patients followed up at his clinic over 35 years, found that there was complete control of seizures in 60%, that the seizures were reduced in frequency and/or severity in another 25% so that the patients were able to lead essentially normal lives, and that the seizures were refractory to all therapeutic measures then available in the remaining 15%. Annegers *et al.* (1980), in a 20-year follow-up, found that, of those with 'idiopathic' epilepsy, i.e. in patients whose epilepsy had no known predisposing cause and in whom the diagnosis was made before 10 years of age, 75% were in remission (defined as 5 seizure-free years) 10 years after diagnosis. Emerson *et al.* (1981) observed that a child with epilepsy who had been free of seizures for 4 years while taking antiepileptic drugs had about a 70% chance of remaining in permanent remission when drugs were withdrawn. Both these groups of authors found that chronic epilepsy was more likely where there was associated mental or neurological handicap from birth, where seizures had begun before 2 years of age, where initial seizure control was difficult and where complex partial seizures predominated. Similar conclusions were reached by Thurston *et al.* (1982) in their long-term follow-up study which has already been mentioned. The good prognosis for many of the idiopathic or primary epileptic syndromes, such as idiopathic grand mal, childhood absence epilepsy (petit mal), and benign partial epilepsy with centro-temporal spike discharges, has also been emphasized. As Tharp (1987) observed, it is unfortunate that this 'good news' about prognosis is not more widely appreciated by the paediatric and neurological community. He pointed out that many doctors still treat children after a single afebrile seizure, often with potentially toxic drugs, and impart pessimistic and discouraging prognostic information about epilepsy to parents. The author agrees with him that the misdiagnosis of benign partial epilepsy with centrotemporal spike discharges as 'temporal lobe epilepsy' is still all too common. The question, 'It isn't epilepsy is it, doctor?' (Brett, 1990) deserves an answer which includes as precise a diagnosis and prognosis as possible.

### References

AICARDI, J. (1988) Epileptic syndromes in childhood. *Epilepsia*, **29**, Supplement 3, S1–S5

ANNEGERS, J. F., HAUSER, W. A., ELVEBACK, L. R. and KURLAND, L. T. (1980) Remission and relapses of seizures in epilepsy. In *Advances in Epileptology: The Xth International Epilepsy Symposium* (eds J. A. Wade and J. K. Penry), Raven Press, New York, pp. 142–147

BAUMER, J. H., DAVID, T. J., VALENTINE, S. J. et al. (1981) Many parents think their child is dying when having a first febrile convulsion. *Developmental Medicine and Child Neurology*, **23**, 462–464

BRETT, E. M. (1990) 'It isn't epilepsy is it, doctor?'. *British Medical Journal*, **300**, 1604–1605

CHEVRIE, J. J. and AICARDI, J. (1978) Convulsive disorders in the first year of life: neurological and mental outcome and mortality. *Epilepsia*, **19**, 67–74

COMMISSION OR CLASSIFICATION AND TERMINOLOGY OF THE INTERNATIONAL LEAGUE AGAINST EPILEPSY (1989) Proposal for revised classification of epilepsies and epileptic syndromes. *Epilepsia*, **30**, 389–399

DEONNA., T., ZIEGLER, A-L, DESPLAND, P-A, and van MELLE, G. (1986) Partial epilepsy in neurologically normal children: clinical syndromes and prognosis. *Epilepsia*, **27**, 241–247

DREIFUSS, F. E. (1989) Classification of epileptic seizures and the epilepsies. In *Seizure Disorders* (ed. J. M. Pellock) *Pediatric Clinics of North America*, **36**, W. B. Saunders, Philadelphia, London, pp. 265–279

ELLENBERG, J. H., HIRTZ, D. G. and NELSON, K. B. (1984) Age of onset of seizures in young children. *Annals of Neurology*, **15**, 127–134

EMERSON, E., D'SOUZA, B. J., VINING, E. P. et al. (1981) Stopping medication in children with epilepsy: predictors of outcome. *New England Journal of Medicine*, **304**, 1125–1129

HARRISON, R. M. and TAYLOR, D. C. (1976) Childhood seizures: a 25 year follow-up. Social and medical prognosis. *Lancet*, **1**, 948–951

HOLOWACH, J., THURSTON, D. L. and O'LEARY, J. (1972) Prognosis in childhood epilepsy. *New England Journal of Medicine*, **286**, 169–174

HENRIKSEN, O. (1988) Specific problems of children with epilepsy. *Epilepsia*, **29**, Supplement 3, S6–S9

KUROKAWA, T., FUNS, K. C., HANAI, T. and GOYA, N. (1982) Mortality and clinical features in cases of death among epileptic children. *Brain and Development*, **4–5**, 321–325

LEESTMA, J. E., KELELKAR, M. B., TEAS, S. S. et al. (1984) Sudden unexpected death associated with seizures. Analysis of 66 cases. *Epilepsia*, **25**, 84–88

LIVINGSTON, S. (1972) *Comprehensive Management of Epilepsy in Infancy, Childhood and Adolescence*, Charles C. Thomas, Springfield, Illinois

LOISEAU, P. and DUCHÉ, B. (1989) Benign childhood epilepsy with centro-temporal spikes. *Cleveland Clinic Journal of Medicine*, **56**, Supplement Part 1, S17–S22

LOISEAU, P., PESTRE, M., DARTIGUES, J. F. (1983) Long-term prognosis in two forms of childhood epilepsy: typical absence seizures and epilepsy with rolandic (centro-temporal) EEG foci. *Annals of Neurology*, **13**, 642–648

NOGUEIRA DE MELO, A. and NIEDERMEYER, E. (1991a) Crossover phenomena in epileptic syndromes of childhood. *Clinical Electroencephalography*, **22**, 75–82

NOGUEIRA DE MELO, A. and NIEDERMEYER, E. (1991b) The limits of epileptic syndromes in childhood epilepsies. Abstracts from 19th International Epilepsy Congress, Rio de Janeiro, 1991. *Epilepsia*, **32**, Supplement 1, 86

O'DONOHOE, N. V. (1992) Delineation of epileptic syndromes. *Current Paediatrics*, **2**, 68–72

OUNSTED, C., LINDSAY, J. and NORMAN, R. (1966) Biological factors in temporal lobe epilepsy. *Clinics in Developmental Medicine*, No 22, Spastics Society/Heinemann Medical, London

REYNOLDS, E. H. (1981) Biological factors in psychological disorders associated with epilepsy. In *Epilepsy and Psychiatry* (eds E. H. Reynolds and M. R. Trimble), Churchill Livingstone, Edinburgh, London, pp. 264–290.

REYNOLDS, E. H. (1990) Changing view of prognosis of epilepsy. *British Medical Journal*, **301**, 1112–1114

RODIN, E. A. (1968) *The Prognosis of Patients with Epilepsy*. Charles C. Thomas, Springfield, Illinois

SCHRAEDER, P. L. and LATHERS, C. M. (1989) Paroxysmal autonomic dysfunction, epileptogenic activity and sudden death. *Epilepsy Research*, **3**, 55–62

SHORVON, S. D. and REYNOLDS, E. H. (1982) Early prognosis of epilepsy. *British Medical Journal*, **285**, 1699–1701

SILLANPÄÄ, M. (1983) Social functioning and seizure status of young adults with onset of epilepsy in childhood. *Acta Neurologica Scandinavica*, **68**, Supplement 96, 3–81

SILLANPÄÄ, M. (1992) Epilepsy in children: prevalence, disability and handicap. *Epilepsia*, **33**, 444–449

THARP, B. R. (1987) An overview of pediatric seizure disorders and epileptic syndromes. *Epilepsia*, **28**, Supplement 1, S36–S45

THURSTON, J. H., THURSTON, D. L., HIXON, B. B. and KELLER, A. J. (1982) Prognosis of childhood epilepsy: additional follow-up of 148 children 15 to 23 years after withdrawal of anticonvulsant therapy. *New England Journal of Medicine*, **306**, 831–836

VINING, E. P. G. (1989) Psychosocial issues for children with epilepsy. *Cleveland Clinic Journal of Medicine*, **56**, Supplement Part 2, S214–S220

WEST, W. J. (1841) On a peculiar form of infantile convulsions. *Lancet*, **1**, 724–725

WORLD HEALTH ORGANIZATION (1957) Juvenile Epilepsy. Report of a Study Group. *WHO Report Series*, No. **130**, Geneva, Switzerland, WHO

YANNET, H., DREAMER, W. C. and BARBA, P. S. (1949) Convulsive disorders in children. *Pediatrics*, **4**, 677

Chapter 29

# Prevention of epilepsy

Lennox (1960) wrote as follows:

> The preventative aspects of epilepsy have not received the attention their importance deserves. In comparison with many chronic diseases, the onset of seizures is predominantly in childhood; contributing causes are many and widely various; and the prevention of sequelae may be as important as prevention of the disease itself. Finally, and here the contrast is sharpened, the sequelae may be as much social as physical.

Thomas (1973) suggested three levels of prevention of epilepsy and its consequences as follows:

1  Prevention of the onset of epilepsy.
2  Prevention of the recurrence of manifestations.
3  Prevention of consequences of epilepsy – psychological, social and economic.

Prevention of the onset of epilepsy implies an attack on its aetiological roots, as emphasised by Aicardi (1976). He noted that seizures in children fell into two broad aetiological categories: first, those resulting from organic brain abnormalities, whether due to abnormal development or to brain insults during fetal life at birth or postnatally; and secondly, those resulting from functional disturbances in the brain and body generally, about whose nature our understanding is limited but which are, at least in part, genetically determined. These two categories partially overlap, since some genetic factors induce seizures through causing organic brain abnormalities, e.g. tuberose sclerosis.

Our attack on the aetiological roots of epilepsy should probably begin with attempts to modify the genetic origins. The genetic aspects of epilepsy have already been discussed in Chapter 2. Genetic factors can act by causing the transmission of a disease of which seizures may be a symptom but these single gene disorders, although numerous and usually associated with other gross clinical characteristics, together account for less than 2% of cases of epilepsy. Although major chromosomal disorders occur frequently and are often associated with major abnormalities of the central nervous system, they are not a frequent cause of seizures (Jennings and Bird, 1981). In Down's syndrome patients, the risk of developing epilepsy increases with advancing age, with a 1.9% prevalence rate below the age of 20 years *versus* a 12.2% prevalence rate over the age of 35 years (Veall, 1974). A variety of seizure types has been reported including a higher than expected risk of developing infantile spasms and a propensity later to manifest startle-induced seizures precipitated by sudden, unexpected stimuli, especially sudden noises (Giménez-Roldán and Martín, 1980).

In the great majority of patients with epilepsy, however, seizures are the only abnormal manifestation and, in these, when inheritance plays a part, either a gene or several genes appear to alter the convulsive susceptibility of the individual. The remarkable recent discoveries mapping the genetic linkage of certain epileptic syndromes with specific chromosomes are detailed in Chapter 2 and it seems likely that further similar discoveries will be made before long. The importance of genetic counselling in the overall management of epilepsy, with implications for prevention, is also discussed in Chapter 2.

## Brain damage

Epilepsies resulting from acquired brain damage offer greater opportunities for prevention. Prenatal infections such as rubella can now be prevented by immunization of girls before puberty, and a vaccine against cytomegalovirus infection may be generally available in the future. Congenital syphilis is rarely seen today, and toxoplasmosis can be recognized and treated in pregnancy. Perinatal brain damage, particularly that caused by anoxia, may be an important cause of later epilepsy, and improved obstetric management and better paediatric care of the neonate may contribute significantly to prevention. However, there are few studies available to prove this point. Nelson and Ellenberg (1984), in a prospective study, have evaluated the roles of late obstetric complications, especially those thought to be associated with intrapartum asphyxia, and of low 5-minute Apgar scores as possible risk factors for the later development of epilepsy in children free of motor handicap. They were unable to show that the frequency of seizure disorders was significantly higher in these children compared with those born of uncomplicated deliveries. Holden, Mellits and Freeman (1982), however, using clinical material from the same study to plot the long-term sequelae in children who had suffered neonatal seizures, found that 9% had epilepsy alone while 20% overall had epilepsy, usually in association with mental and physical handicap. The small-for-dates infant also seems at risk of developing later epilepsy, particularly when the degree of intrauterine growth retardation has been severe (Fitzhardinge and Steven, 1972). The development of neonatology has been marked, especially during the past 2 decades, by spectacular improvements in mortality and morbidity which are associated with important advances in the understanding of physiological disturbances in the newborn and with innovations in their management. It remains to be seen whether these advances will lead to a decline in morbidity from epilepsy. Perhaps useful analogies may be drawn with cerebral palsy, another condition with a multifactorial aetiology and one where perinatal factors are causative in 10% or less of cases (Nelson, 1988). There is little evidence of any recent decline in the incidence of cerebral palsy despite improved obstetric standards (Stanley, 1987). Since perinatal factors play such a small part in the aetiology of the epilepsies also, it is unlikely that improved standards of perinatal care will reduce the incidence of seizure disorders significantly. It appears, as Nelson (1988) says, that the great contribution of the improvement in both obstetric and neonatal care may lie not in the ability to reduce the incidence of handicap in the population, but rather in the ability to allow the survival of substantial numbers of infants who would have died without such care. It is important to recall that relatively simple advances and acute clinical observation, as opposed to high technology, may lead to real progress in the prevention of brain damage, as demonstrated by the early detection and treatment of hypoglycaemia in the newborn and the prevention of hypoglycaemia and hyperbilirubinaemia resulting from late feeding of low-birth-weight infants, a fashionable practice until Smallpiece and Davies (1964) pointed out its inherent dangers.

## Malnutrition in infancy

The evidence is now convincing that malnutrition in infancy permanently affects the minds of children who have been so afflicted by interfering with brain growth at a critical period (Winick, 1969). The time element is critical: both animal and human data demonstrate that the earlier the malnutrition the more severe and permanent are the effects. It appears that after infancy the brain is much more resistant to the effects of malnutrition. It also seems possible that the infant whose mother was malnourished is more at risk than the infant born to a well-nourished mother. Therefore, it would seem that the first priority should be the elimination of malnutrition in infancy and perhaps even prenatally. The problem of malnutrition is world wide, affecting perhaps half of the world's population, and is linked to the problems of intellectual impairment in general and consequently indirectly to epilepsy.

## Infectious diseases of the CNS

The young developing brain is highly susceptible to any kind of insult. Infections are very common during the first few years of life and are one of the possible causes of brain damage and seizures. Ounsted (1951) emphasized the important significance of convulsions occurring in children with purulent meningitis. He demonstrated a close association between failure of treatment and the occurrence and intensity of convulsive seizures. Age was the important determinant and purulent meningitis is commonest in infancy. He showed that status epilepticus in this age group was a relatively common complication of meningitis and was often fatal. Aicardi (1973), writing about the role of infections in the aetiology of childhood epilepsy, showed that infection was involved in causing one case of chronic epilepsy out of five. Bacterial meningitis in the neonate and subsequently is very important in this regard. Children with persistent neurological deficit after acute bacterial meningitis are at considerable risk of having epilepsy. Possibly inflammation leads to narrowing or spasm of cerebral vessels, with consequent cerebral blood-flow impairment or thrombosis (Pomeroy et al., 1990). Whether anti-inflammatory drug treatment with dexamethasone early in the course of meningitis alters this process is still uncertain (Kaplan, 1989).

Parasitic infections of the central nervous system also play a significant part in the aetiology of childhood epilepsy in large areas of the world (Bittencourt, Gracia and Lorenzana, 1988). Cysticercosis is the commonest of these and is endemic in Central and South America, South-East Asia, India, the Caribbean, and southern Africa. It is also being more frequently diagnosed in the USA, partly because of increased immigration from Mexico and also because of increased detection by CT scanning (Earnest et al., 1987). *Neurocysticercosis* causes various neurological symptoms and, in South African children, epilepsy, with or without focal signs, is the commonest presentation, followed by a syndrome of raised intracranial pressure and meningoencephalitis (Thomson *et al.*, 1984). Intraparenchymal cerebral cysticercosis is usually a self-limiting disease requiring supportive treatment with steroids for raised intracranial pressure, antiepileptic drugs for seizures, and rarely surgical intervention for relief of hydrocephalus and removal of large cysts. Treatment with the antitrematode drug praziquantel is controversial but is widely used despite some doubts about its efficacy and about side-effects (Moodley and Moosa, 1989). Clearly, the large-scale eradication of this parasitic menace would reduce the incidence of childhood epilepsy in those regions of the world where it flourishes.

## Other preventible causes

Diseases of infancy such as gastroenteritis, a world-wide problem especially in those who do not enjoy the benefits of breast-feeding, may result in brain damage through the production of hyperosmolar hypernatraemic dehydration. Mental retardation, epilepsy and cerebral palsy are sequelae in up to 11% of the survivors from this metabolic disorder (Macauley and Watson, 1967). The best means of rehydrating hypernatraemic infants remains controversial but, although there is still debate about the proper concentration of saline solution to use, all are agreed about the importance of slow reduction of hyperosmolarity if death, convulsions and irreversible brain damage are to be prevented (Chambers, 1975). Hogan (1976) pointed out that the exact nature of the rehydrating solution is not of major significance, but the volume administered and the rate of rehydration are of vital importance. If too great a volume of saline solution is given too rapidly the child becomes oedematous and develops raised intracranial pressure, and stupor and convulsions may follow. The encouragement of breast-feeding and the removal of unmodified (high sodium) milk preparations from the market has led to a marked reduction in the incidence of hypernatraemic dehydration and prevented its damaging effects (Sunderland and Emery, 1979).

There are many other situations in paediatrics where the prevention of epilepsy may be achieved by an attack on its aetiological roots. The increasing incidence of post-traumatic epilepsy in today's world has already been dealt with in Chapter 14. In early infancy and childhood vaccination and immunization may confer protection against serious diseases, thereby saving lives and preventing disability (Morley, 1989). The increasing use of *Haemophilus influenzae* type b vaccines is an important advance which should help to prevent the various sequelae of this common infection, many of which remained undetected for some years (Taylor *et al.*, 1990). Happily, so-called post-pertussis-vaccine encephalopathy is now seen to be the myth which it always was (Fulginiti, 1990). Pertussis itself remains a problem and a possible cause of permanent brain damage, especially during infancy. Febrile convulsions when prolonged are also a problem, particularly as prolonged seizures are often first seizures and affect infants especially (Lennox-Buchthal, 1973). Stopping such seizures quickly and trying to find those at risk of developing such a seizure could contribute significantly to the prevention of later chronic epilepsy.

*Health education*, in the broad sense, is also important in the prevention of epilepsy. There is increasing awareness, for example, of the special risks in adolescence in this respect when one considers the cultivation of regular and temperate habits, particularly with regard to alcohol: overhydration, especially when combined with alcoholic excess, provokes seizures. The risks of head injury and the dangers of drug abuse are also greater at this period of life. Drugs such as barbiturates, if abused, may, on withdrawal, lead to convulsions in persons who would otherwise not have suffered from them.

## Summary

In summary it can be seen that prevention of epilepsy implies attempts to avert its onset by better understanding of the genetic problems involved; by better prenatal, perinatal and neonatal care; and by more effective therapy of potentially brain-damaging illnesses in infancy and early childhood. It involves the prevention of recurrence of the manifestations of epilepsy by better case finding, by earlier and more accurate diagnosis and by better management. It implies the prevention of complications of epilepsy (the 'secondary handicaps') which may be psychological, social or economic. It requires a determined effort by all concerned with the condition to combat the public attitudes to epilepsy which are still influenced so strongly by fear and prejudice. The prevention of epilepsy and the succour of its victims should be special concerns of all physicians and others concerned with the care of children.

## References

AICARDI, J. (1973) Epileptic attacks accompanying or following acute infantile infections acquired during the first three years of life. In *Prevention of Epilepsy and its Consequences* (ed. M. J. Parsonage) International Bureau for Epilepsy, London, pp. 28–31

AICARDI, J. (1976) Prevention of epilepsy in children. *Developmental Medicine and Child Neurology*, **18**, 381–383

BITTENCOURT, P. R. M., GRACIA, C. M. and LORENZANA, P. (1988) Epilepsy and parasitosis of the central nervous system. In: *Recent Advances in Epilepsy*, Number 4 (eds T. A. Pedley and B. S. Meldrum), Churchill Livingstone, Edinburgh, London, pp. 123–159

CHAMBERS, T. (1975) Hypernatraemia: a preventable cause of acquired brain damage. *Developmental Medicine and Child Neurology*, **17**, 91–94

EARNEST, M. P., BARTH RELLER, L., FILLEY, C. M. and GREK, A. J. (1987) Neurocysticercosis in the United States: 35 cases and a review. *Reviews of Infectious Diseases* **9**, 961–979

FITZHARDINGE, P. M. and STEVEN, E. M. (1972) The small for date infant: neurological and intellectual sequelae. *Pediatrics*, **50**, 50–57

FULGINITI, V. A. (1990) A pertussis vaccine myth dies. *American Journal of Disease of Children*, **144**, 860–861

GIMÉNEZ-ROLDÁN, S. and MARTÍN, M. (1980) Startle epilepsy complicating Down Syndrome during adulthood. *Annals of Neurology*, **7**, 78–80

HOGAN, G. R. (1976) Hypernatraemia – problems in management. *Pediatric Clinics of North America*, **23**, 569–574

HOLDEN, K. R., MELLITS, E. D. and FREEMAN, J. M. (1982) Neonatal seizures: correlation of prenatal and perinatal events with outcomes. *Pediatrics* **70**, 165–176

JENNINGS, M. T. and BIRD, T. D. (1981) Genetic influences in the epilepsies. Review of the literature with practical implications. *American Journal of Diseases of Children*, **135**, 450–457

KAPLAN, S. L. (1989) Dexamethasone for children with bacterial meningitis: should it be routine therapy? *American Journal of Diseases in Children*, **143**, 290–292

LENNOX, W. G. (1960) *Epilepsy and Related Disorders*, J. and A. Churchill; London, Little, Brown, Boston, p. 1000

LENNOX-BUCHTHAL, M. A. (1973) Febrile convulsions: a reappraisal. *Electroencephalography and Clinical Neurophysiology*. Supplement **32**, 132

MACAULEY, D. and WATSON, M. (1967) Hypernatraemia in infants as a cause of brain damage. *Archives of Disease in Childhood*, **42**, 485–491

MOODLEY, M. and MOOSA, A. (1989) Treatment of neurocysticercosis: is praziquantel the new hope? *Lancet*, **333**, 262–263

MORLEY, D. (1989) Saving children's lives by vaccination. *British Medical Journal*, **229**, 1544–1545

NELSON, K. B. (1988) What proportion of cerebral palsy is related to birth asphyxia? *Journal of Pediatrics*, **112**, 572–573

NELSON, K. B. and ELLENBERG, J. H. (1984) Obstetric complications as risk factors for cerebral palsy or seizure disorders. *Journal of the American Medical Association*. **251**, 1843–1848

OUNSTED, C. (1951) Significance of convulsions in children with purulent meningitis. *Lancet*, **1**, 1245–1248

POMEROY, S. L., HOLMES, S. J., DODGE, P. R. and FEIGIN, R. D. (1990) Seizures and other neurologic sequelae of bacterial meningitis in children. *New England Journal of Medicine*, **323**, 1651–1657

SMALLPIECE, V. and DAVIES, P. A. (1964) Immediate feeding of premature infants with undiluted breast milk. *Lancet*, **2**, 1349–1352

STANLEY, F. J. (1987) The changing face of cerebral palsy? *Developmental Medicine and Child Neurology*, **29**, 263–265

SUNDERLAND, R. and EMERY, J. L. (1979) Apparent disappearance of hypernatraemic dehydration from infant deaths in Sheffield. *British Medical Journal*, **2**, 575–576

TAYLOR. H. G., MILLS, E. L., CIAMPI, A. *et al.* (1990) The sequelae of Haemophilus influenzae meningitis in school-age children. *New England Journal of Medicine*, **323**, 1657–1663

THOMAS, M. H. (1973) The ultimate challenge of epilepsy prevention. In *Prevention of Epilepsy and its Consequences* (ed. M. J. Parsonage) International Bureau for Epilepsy, London, pp. 5–9

THOMSON, A. J., de VILLERS, J. C., MOOSA, A. and VAN DELLEN, J. R. (1984) Cerebral cysticercosis in children in South Africa. *Journal of Tropical Pediatrics*, **30**, 136–139

VEALL, R. M. (1974) The prevalence of epilepsy among mongols related to age. *Journal of Mental Deficiency Research*, **18**, 99–106

WINICK, M. (1969) Malnutrition and brain development. *Journal of Pediatrics*, **74**, 667–679

Chapter 30

# Prospects for the future

Epilepsy has always been a world-wide problem for all age groups, but particularly so for children and adolescents. During the present decade, some 1500 million children will be born in the world, the great majority of them into poverty and misery. Tower (1978), speaking of epilepsy as a world problem, emphasized that increasing populations inevitably mean more epilepsy unless preventative steps are taken. At least one developing country has shown that investment in health care and education can improve health standards dramatically. Costa Rica disbanded its army and invested its resources in education and in primary health care and improved hygiene. Since 1970, the infant mortality rate there has fallen by 67% and there has also been a significant fall in the fertility rate, with stabilization of population size in prospect (Hanson, 1992).

Prevention is really of the essence if epilepsy is to be a diminishing problem in the future (see Chapter 29). In the developed countries, there is evidence that the perinatal and neonatal mortality rates can be reduced significantly by improved antenatal and perinatal care. This would seem to suggest that there should be a corresponding reduction in epilepsy resulting from brain injury at birth and this is certainly the case as far as the grosser forms of birth trauma (resulting from breech delivery, for example) and the avoidable causes of birth asphyxia are concerned. The prevalence of cerebral palsy in the population has been used as an indicator reflecting improved standards of antenatal and perinatal care and, since epilepsy occurs at least ten times as frequently among children with cerebral palsy compared with normal children, it might also serve as a guide to the prospects of reducing the prevalence of epilepsy. However, although the prevalence of cerebral palsy fell dramatically in developed countries between the 1950s and early 1970s, the result of a reduced incidence of the condition during that period (Hagberg, 1978), there has not been a further fall in prevalence since then. The prevalence among infants of normal birthweight ( > 2500 g) has remained static while, among low birthweight infants, there has been an increased prevalence. This has been particularly striking among infants of very low birthweight ( < 1500 g), where there has also been an increasing proportion of cases who are severely mentally handicapped (Pharaoh *et al.*, 1990). Parenthetically, it should be noted that up to 50% of children with associated cerebral palsy and mental handicap develop epilepsy (Hauser and Nelson, 1989). The rise in prevalence of cerebral palsy in very low birthweight infants implies either an increase in the incidence of the condition or in its duration. An increasing incidence would suggest that cerebral damage has occurred at or around the time of birth due to failure to maintain an optimal cerebral environment and this view is held by some (Hagberg *et al.*, 1989). An alternative explanation advanced by Pharaoh *et al.* (1990) is that the duration of cerebral palsy has been increased by postponing death and that infants who are abnormal as a result of prenatal factors are now surviving premature birth as a result of modern perinatal care and adding to the overall pool of cases of cerebral palsy in the community. The fact that a high proportion of infants with cerebral palsy are growth retarded at birth has been cited as indicating that there have been adverse factors affecting the development of the fetus (Pharaoh *et al.*, 1987). The various arguments about this disturbing trend have not been resolved.

Meanwhile, as far as the aetiology of childhood epilepsy is concerned, it is important to emphasize that factors related to labour and delivery appear to contribute very little to the causation of seizure disorders (Ross et al., 1980; Nelson and Ellenberg, 1987). Maldevelopment, rather than damage at birth to an initially intact nervous system, appears to be a much more important aetiological mechanism. Many epilepsies of early childhood remain unexplained by a wide variety of possible prenatal and perinatal factors. Contemporaneously, the burgeoning information coming from the application of molecular biology to genetic research is providing new facts about the primary or idiopathic epilepsies and their place in the human genome (Delgado-Escueta *et al.*, 1989).

While this type of sophisticated prevention of brain damage is engaging the attention of paediatricians and obstetricians in the developed countries, it is pertinent to remember that in countries such as India, childhood infections are still a major cause of epilepsy and that in Nigeria, cerebral malaria with associated seizures presents considerable problems. In Africa and now worldwide, the neurological complications of HIV infection, and especially the effects of opportunistic infections of the central nervous system consequent on such infection may lead to the occurrence of seizures (Belman, 1992). In many tropical and subtropical countries, the cerebral complications of parasitosis, particularly cysticercosis infestation, are a common cause of chronic seizures (Bittencourt, Gracia and Lorenzana, 1988). Malnutrition is a common problem in many developing countries and its effects mitigate against effective resistance to infection (Jackson, 1991), predispose to many epileptogenic factors, and may even interfere with the metabolic response to antiepileptic drugs. The important role played by nutrition in early life, especially successful breast feeding, in promoting optimum neurodevelopment is now well established (Lucas et al., 1992). It is certain that established public health measures providing better nutrition and hygiene play a major part globally in the prevention of epilepsy, and bodies such as the World Health Organization are of paramount importance in this area. For example, the better understanding of the use of oral glucose electrolyte solutions in the treatment of acute infantile diarrhoea in the tropics has been a major advance (Tripp and Harries, 1980) and, in developing countries also, such basic and inexpensive therapy deserves a wider application (Avery and Snyder, 1990).

*Theoretical advances* in the field of epilepsy concern concept and terminology. The concept of the epilepsies, rather than epilepsy, is gaining widespread recognition. Seizures must be seen as a behavioural manifestation of an enormously diverse group of underlying states of brain dysfunction rather than having a single cause. Such a viewpoint gives proportion to one's expectations about the epilepsies. If there is no single epilepsy then there cannot be a single cause or cure. A major advance in epileptology has been the recognition of syndromes with distinct aetiology, clinical features, treatment, and prognosis (Roger et al., 1992). There is no better example of the importance of syndrome classification than juvenile myoclonic epilepsy, which accounts for up to 10% of all cases of epilepsy at all ages yet, despite having clinical and EEG features which should lead to easy identification, the rate of misdiagnosis of this condition remains high (Editorial, 1992b).

With reference to terminology, the growing use of the International Classification of Seizures and of the Epilepsies and Epileptic Syndromes (Dreifuss, 1989) has promoted clarity of thinking and communication among those working with patients with epilepsy and in research. Increasing use of combined videotape and EEG recording of clinical seizures is affording further refinements in the categorization of seizures.

## New concepts in the pathophysiology of the epilepsies

Epileptic seizures result from the sudden, excessive electrical discharges of large aggregates of neurons, and the clinical components are determined by the site of origin of the discharges and by their pattern of spread. Epileptogenesis is a term which refers to the dynamic process underlying the development of epilepsy. It depends on the predisposition of neuronal aggregates to discharge when stimulated and on synchronization of firing within the neuronal substrate. Prevention of epilepsy requires a better understanding of the neuronal basis of epileptogenicity. Very little is known about the mechanisms that suppress ictal events during the interictal state, limit their spread once they begin, and ultimately terminate them. Identification and characterisation of these natural seizure-suppressing mechanisms should make possible the therapeutic manipulation of these endogenous neuronal processes for the benefit of the patient with epilepsy. Recent concepts concerning the action of the NMDA receptor–cation channel complex (described in Chapter 2) provide a mechanism by which recurrent epileptiform events could induce widespread enduring alterations in neuronal function. The successful cloning of a glutamate receptor in the rat brain (Hollman et al., 1989) should lead on to the identification of the structure of human glutamate receptors and to the development of therapeutic agents to block these receptors.

## New methods of investigation

When the first edition of this book was published in 1979, the section devoted to neuroimaging was small, although it was predicted that the techniques then becoming available would have a profound effect on neurological practice. Since then, the new methods of brain scanning have revolutionized neurology and have provided a handmaiden for the EEG in epileptology, by adding the delineation of brain structure to the electrical measurement of brain function. Advances in magnetic resonance imaging (MRI) techniques have led to improvements in the detection of lesions in patients with epilepsy and new insights into the aetiology of the epilepsies (Editorial, 1992a). Use of volumetric data acquisition in MRI, a technique that generates fine sections of high anatomical resolution, has revealed a high frequency of embryofetal lesions in extratemporal epilepsies (Shorvon et al., 1992). These include the neuronal migration disorders which are particularly important in childhood as causes of epilepsy and which have a characteristic distribution. The cortical dysplasias, such as macrogyria and polymicrogyria, and areas of gliosis and atrophy can be defined. A high frequency of hippocampal lesions in temporal lobe epilepsy has been revealed. These developments have given a new impetus to the surgical treatment of epilepsy (see Chapter 27).

Functional imaging, as provided by positron emission tomography (PET) and single photon emission tomography (SPECT), gives additional information about neocortical metabolism but functional MR imaging may supplant these in studying neuronal metabolism in epilepsy (Belliveau *et al.*, 1991).

It is important to remember, however, that all these techniques, like CT scanning, are extremely expensive to purchase and maintain and that they will therefore be of limited value in the service of sufferers from epilepsy worldwide. Nevertheless, they will provide new knowledge through research which will benefit all patients with the condition.

The widespread availability and use of accurate techniques for measuring the levels of *antiepileptic drugs in blood* remains one of the most significant advances in the management of epilepsy of the past 20 years. Many variables affect how these drugs are utilized by infants and children and there is also marked interindividual variation in drug-eliminating capacity (Dodson, 1987). Hence the dosing of antiepileptic drugs on the basis of the patient's weight is unreliable in paediatrics and drug levels do help to overcome this problem. The availability of rapid methods of assay using very small volumes of blood represents an important advance (Houtman *et al.*, 1990).

However, although measuring the concentrations of antiepileptic drugs can help the physician regulate therapy, these assays should not be used as a substitute for clinical judgement. The management of patients with epilepsy remains firmly rooted in clinical assessment. Certain patients will be controlled at relatively low concentrations of antiepileptic drugs while others will require concentrations well above the 'therapeutic range' to control their seizures. Paediatricians should bear these points in mind when treating the different childhood epilepsies, and should always regard the child as an individual patient and not as a laboratory index.

The 1990s have been designated 'the Decade of the Brain', and this has been endorsed by the World Federation of Neurology. The following research goals have been proposed by the National Council for Neurological Disorders and Stroke in the United States (Editorial, 1990).

1   Determine the basic cellular mechanisms of epilepsy.
2   Characterize the genetic susceptibility to epilepsy.
3   Develop new antiepileptic drugs.
4   Study further the efficacy of surgery for epilepsy.
5   Identify types of behavioural abnormalities associated with epilepsy and attempt to develop specific therapies for these.
6   Devise technical innovations including development of new lightweight ambulatory monitoring devices to warn patients of impending seizures, self regulating drug delivery systems, and more sophisticated imaging methods to measure brain structure and function.

## Holistic epileptology and the need for education

Masland (1992) has advocated what he terms 'holistic epileptology' in order to create a more general awareness that only by dealing with all aspects of the problem of epilepsy can effective remediation be provided. He points out that those providing remedial services are too often preoccupied with one or other aspect of the patient's problem and do not consider the patient's total needs. The physician, who is usually the primary source of support, tends to concentrate on the medical aspect. Working apart from the social support system, it is easy for him or her to ignore other elements of the patient's total needs. There is increasing emphasis in adult epileptology that the disabilities of persons with epilepsy stem less from the seizures than from the reaction of society to their epilepsy. For some, anxiety and depression, impairment of self-image, restriction in employment, limitation of driving and poor social relations may be more devastating than is the occurrence of even frequent seizures. To an extent, these observations are applicable to the child and they certainly apply to the adolescent patient with epilepsy. It behoves us to look at the totality of the problem rather than concentrating on seizure control only.

Ignorance, prejudice and superstition still surround epilepsy in all parts of the world, although the emphasis may differ from country to country. Even in those countries where most people smile about superstitions and old wive's tales, there remains a widespread and deep-rooted feeling about epilepsy which bars the acceptance of people with epilepsy as ordinary fellow citizens. Too often, even today, the sufferer from epilepsy may feel with John Clare (Quiller-Couch, 1939):

I am! Yet what I am who cares, or knows?
My friends forsake me like a memory lost.
I am the self-consumer of my woes;
They rise and vanish, an oblivious host,
Shadows of life, whose very soul is lost.
And yet I am – I live – though I am toss'd
Into the nothingness of scorn and noise,
Into the living sea of waking dream,
Where there is neither sense of life, nor joys,
But the huge shipwreck of my own esteem
And all that's dear. Even those I loved the best
Are strange – nay, they are stranger than the rest.

Medical care which reduces or stops the patient's seizures, and social care which helps him to adjust to society and the problems presented by his complaint, cannot have their full effect unless society changes its attitudes about epilepsy and those who suffer from it. *Education* must be the key to changing public attitudes and in this respect most has been accomplished in many countries by those people with epilepsy who have formed associations in order to take an active part in fighting their own battles. The primary aims of these associations are to combat prejudice against the disorder and to help all people with epilepsy to lead normal lives. The medical profession should be equally diligent in ensuring that medical students are adequately informed about this common and worldwide problem and that the teaching of epileptology takes its proper place in specialist training and in the continuing education of family doctors (Parsonage, 1983).

Lennox (1960) wrote: 'A convulsion is a beacon light in medical symptomatology. The path lighted by its rays reaches to the far limits of recorded medical history.' Never before has there been such intense international interest in epilepsy as there is today – in fundamental research, in the aetiology and clinical presentation of the disorder, in treatment and, above all, in the possibility of prevention.

The physician who deals with children in whatever capacity is in the forefront of the battle against epilepsy, since the majority of the potentially brain-damaging conditions occur in the paediatric age group and because the great majority of patients with epilepsy develop their initial symptoms before 20 years of age. An attempt, inevitably incomplete because of the scope and complexity of the subject, has been made in this book to provide the essential information to enable him or her to help the child with epilepsy.

## References

AVERY, M. E. and SNYDER, J. D. (1990) Oral therapy for acute diarrhoea. The underused simple solution. *New England Journal of Medicine*, **323**, 891–894

BELLIVEAU, J. W., KENNEDY, D. N., MCKINSTRY, R. C. *et al.* (1991) Functional mapping of the human visual cortex by magnetic resonance imaging. *Science*, **254**, 716–719

BELMAN, A. L. (1992) AIDS and the child's central nervous system. *Pediatric Clinics of North America*, **39**, No. 4, 691–714

BITTENCOURT, P. R. M., GRACIA, C. M. and LORENZANA, P. (1988) Epilepsy and parasitosis of the central nervous system. In *Recent Advances in Epilepsy*, No. 4. (eds T. A. Pedley and B. S. Meldrum), Churchill Livingstone, Edinburgh, London, pp. 123–159

DELGADO-ESCUETA, A. V., GREENBERG, D. A., TREIMAN, L. *et al.* (1989) Mapping the gene for juvenile myoclonic epilepsy. *Epilepsia*, **30**, Supplement 4, S.8–S.18

DODSON, E. W. (1987) Special pharmacokinetic considerations in children. *Epilepsia*, **28**, Supplement 1, S.56–S69

DREIFUSS, F. E. (1989) Classification of epileptic seizures and the epilepsies. *Pediatric Clinics of North America*, **36**, No. 2, 265–279

EDITORIAL (1990) *Epilepsy Advances in Clinical and Experimental Research.* **5**, No. 4, 1. Epilepsy Foundation of America

EDITORIAL (1992a) Magnetic resonance imaging in epilepsy. *Lancet*, **340**, 343–344

EDITORIAL (1992b) Diagnosing juvenile myoclonic epilepsy. *Lancet*, **340**, 759–760

HAGBERG, B. (1978) The epidemiologic panorama of major neuropaediatric handicaps in Sweden. In *Care of the Handicapped Child* (ed. J. Apley), Clinics in Developmental Medicine, No. 67 Spastics International/Heinemann Medical, London, pp. 111–124

HAGBERG, B., HAGBERG, G. and ZETTERSTROM, R. (1989) Decreasing perinatal mortality – increase in cerebral palsy morbidity? *Acta Paediatrica Scandinavica*, **78**, 664–670

HANSON, L. A. (1992) Weapons or welfare – the Costa Rican Experience. In: *Paediatrics into the 21st Century (Abstracts)*, Institute of Child Health/Schering-Plough International, London, p. 49

HAUSER, W. A. and NELSON, K. (1989) Epidemiology of epilepsy in children. *Cleveland Clinic Journal of Medicine*, **56**, Supplement, Part 2. S.185–S.195

HOLLMAN, M., O'SHEA-GREENFIELD, A., RODGERS, S. W. and HEINEMANN, S. (1989) Cloning by functional expression of a member of the glutamate receptor family. *Nature*, **342**, 643–648

HOUTMAN, P. N., HALL, S. K., GREEN, A. and RYLANCE, G. W. (1990) Rapid anticonvulsant monitoring in an epilepsy clinic. *Archives of Disease in Childhood*, **65**, 264–268

JACKSON, A. (1991) Nutrition in childhood. In *Paediatric Specialty Practice for the 1990s* (eds J. Eyre and R. Boyd), Royal College of Physicians of London, London, pp. 37–50

LENNOX, W. G. (1960) *Epilepsy and Related Disorders.* J. and A. Churchill, London, p. 1065

LUCAS, A., MORLEY, R., COLE, T. J. *et al.* (1992) Breast milk and subsequent intelligence quotient in children born preterm. *Lancet*, **339**, 261–264

MASLAND, R. L. (1992) Holistic epileptology. *International Epilepsy News (International Bureau for Epilepsy)*, No. **106**, 2–3

NELSON, K. B. and ELLENBERG, J. H. (1987) Predisposing and causative factors in childhood epilepsy. *Epilepsia*, 28, Supplement 1, S.16–S.24

PARSONAGE, M. (1983) Education of medical undergraduates and postgraduates about epilepsy. In *Advances in Epileptology: the XIVth International Symposium* (eds M. Parsonage, R. H. E. Grant, A. G. Craig and A. A. Ward) Raven Press, New York, pp. 1–8

PHARAOH, P. O. D., COOKE, T., ROSENBLOOM, L. and COOKE, R. W. I. (1987) Effects of birthweight, gestational age and maternal obstetric history on birth prevalence of cerebral palsy. *Archives of Disease in Childhood*, 62, 1035–1040

PHARAOH, P. O. D., COOKE, T., COOKE, R. W. I. and ROSENBLOOM, L. (1990) Birthweight specific trends in cerebral palsy. *Archives of Disease in Childhood*, 65, 602–606

QUILLER-COUCH, A. (ed.) (1939) Written in Northampton County Asylum: John Clare 1793–1864. In: *The Oxford Book of English Verse*, 1250–1978, New Edition, Clarendon Press, Oxford, p. 735

ROGER, J., BUREAU, M., DRAVET, C. *et al.* (1992) *Epileptic Syndromes in Infancy, Childhood and Adolescence*, 2nd Edition, John Libbey, London, Paris

ROSS, E. M., PECKHAM, C. S., WEST, P. B. and BUTLER, N. R. (1980) Epilepsy in childhood: findings from the National Child Development Study. *British Medical Journal*, 1, 207–210

SHORVON, S. D., COOK, M. J., MANFORD, M. *et al.* (1992) Volumetric MRI in CT negative frontal lobe epilepsy. *Neurology*, 42, Supplement 3, 206

TOWER, D. B. (1978) Epilepsy: a world problem. In *Advances in Epileptology*, 1977 (eds H. Meinardi and A. J. Rowan), Swets and B. V. Zeitlinger, Amsterdam, Lisse, pp. 2–26

TRIPP, J. H. and HARRIES, J. T. (1980) Oral rehydration of infants with gastroenteritis. *Advances in the Biosciences*, 27, 23–35

# Appendix 1

# The MCT-based ketogenic diet

The ketogenic diet is used in cases of epilepsy which have not responded to conventional medication (see Chapter 5). The effects of the diet correspond approximately to the degree of ketosis achieved. Increases in serum lipids and other metabolic changes such as disturbed water and salt balance are also thought to be significant in producing a therapeutic effect (Gordon, 1977).

The use of medium-chain triglycerides (MCT) in recent years has meant that carbohydrates need not be rigidly restricted, resulting in a more palatable and more easily prepared diet (Huttenlocher, Wilbourn and Signore, 1971). However, Livingston, Pauli and Pruce (1977) maintained that the modified diet is not as effective in controlling seizures as is the standard diet in which the amount of fat (in grams) is four times the amount (in grams) of carbohydrate and protein combined. A success rate of over 50% in controlling myoclonic epilepsies in the age range 2–5 years has been claimed but other authors (Bower, 1980) estimate improvement in a third of those treated. Readers who are interested in the details of the standard ketogenic diet should consult Livingston (1972). In the standard diet, normal dietary fats are used to supply approximately 88% of the total calorie intake in order to produce the desired effect. Because MCT oil is more ketogenic, only 50–70% of the total calories need to be supplied by this preparation. This results in greater palatability and allows a more generous allowance of protein and carbohydrate in the diet.

As has been emphasized in Chapter 5, the diet is more likely to succeed when the parents are interested, cooperative and able to gain a detailed understanding of the regimen. Initially, the children should be admitted to hospital for stabilization on the diet.

The diet is initiated by fasting the patient while allowing 50% of the normal fluid intake or a maximum of 1000 ml per 24, given as water or as low-calorie drinks (not more than 50 calories per 24). Any drugs being administered should be free of carbohydrates. Nothing else is given until the patient is strongly ketotic and this is usually achieved after approximately 36. Ketosis should be confirmed by blood and urine tests.

The next step is to introduce the MCT-based ketogenic diet while still maintaining a restriction of fluids. The basic recipe for the diet is given in *Table A1*. It has a concentration of 4% MCT and provides 65% of total calories as MCT.

The mixture is offered in small frequent drinks and the patient is advised to sip it

**Table A1 Basic recipe for MCT-based ketogenic diet**

|  | Protein (g) | Fat (g) | Carbohydrate (g) | Calories | Fluid (ml) |
|---|---|---|---|---|---|
| 8 ml 50% MCT emulsion | – | 4.0 | – | 33.2 | 8 |
| 5 g skimmed milk powder | 1.8 | 0.1 | 2.6 | 16.7 | – |
| Water to 100 ml | – | – | – | – | About 90 |
| Total | 1.8 | 4.1 | 2.6 | 49.9 | 100 |

The 50% MCT emulsion is prepared by liquidizing equal quantities of MCT oil and cold boiled water with 25 g of gum acacia per 1000 ml of fluid

slowly. Possible side-effects (vomiting, diarrhoea and abdominal pain) are usually avoided in this way, but if they should occur further water is added while still maintaining the overall restriction of fluids.

If after 24 h, the diet is being well tolerated, the concentration of MCT is increased to 5%, providing 70% of the total calories (i.e. 10 ml of 50% MCT emulsion per 100 ml of mixture instead of 8 ml). When it is clear that this concentration of MCT is being tolerated and if ketosis is being maintained, solid food may be introduced gradually.

The basic recipe with 5% MCT oil is continued as a milk substitute, flavoured if necessary with low-calorie syrups or coffee essence and the like, and the patient is encouraged to drink up to 800 ml daily, preferably before solid food is taken. The 50% MCT emulsion, flavoured if desired, is used in measured quantities before food to achieve ketosis and provide calories.

Solids are introduced slowly, and they are gradually increased in amount over approximately 5 days. Preference is given at this early stage to foods requiring small amounts of MCT emulsion in order to maintain ketosis. Fluid restriction is continued only if ketosis is not being maintained. The patient is considered to be stabilized on the diet when ketones are regularly present and when the diet is fully accepted and tolerated. MCT oil may also be used for frying and grilling and in baked foods.

A normal caloric intake and minimum recommended dietary allowance of protein are given, both based on the child's dietary history, age and weight. Approximately 60% of the total calories need to be provided by MCT oil, 1 ml of which produces 8.3 calories. Approximately 30% of the remaining calories will be provided by protein and carbohydrate, and the intake of fat other than MCT oil need not be limited unless the child is overweight. Foods are weighed and the calorie content and amounts of MCT oil required to balance their antiketogenic effects are worked out by parents from lists and specimen diets provided by the dietician. Exchange lists are used to vary the diet. Dietitians calculate the antiketogenic effects of the various foods from the knowledge that 10% of fat is antiketogenic, 58% of proteins is antiketogenic and carbohydrates are entirely antiketogenic.

The MCT-based diet is nutritionally inadequate and sugar-free Ketovite multivitamin tablets (one three times a day) and Ketovite liquid (5 ml once daily) are given, the latter providing vitamin A, choline chloride and cyanocobalamin. These supplements are essential to prevent complications such as bilateral optic neuropathy, reported in some vitamin-depleted patients on the diet (Hoyt and Billson, 1979). Calcium supplements may be unnecessary if sufficient of the basic MCT skimmed milk mixture is drunk daily. Otherwise, additional calcium is required and must always be given if the classic ketogenic diet is being used.

Sufficient iron should be provided by first-class protein foods, vegetables and cereal foods. The family doctor should be warned against prescribing additional medications with a syrup (i.e. carbohydrate) base but, if these have to be administered, then additional MCT oil to compensate for their antiketogenic effect will be required. Regular support and supervision by a dietitian are essential, particularly during the introductory stages of the diet and in the early weeks of treatment, if successful dietetic management is to be achieved.

Acceptance of the MCT is usually not a problem once the patient realizes that food will not be given until the MCT drink has been consumed. Sometimes ketosis may be difficult to maintain in the morning and this may require an increase in the daily intake of oil. As a rule side-effects are few, even when the concentration of fat is 50%; they are discussed below.

## Problems with the diet

Urine testing for ketones is performed with Ketostix. If the test is only weakly positive and especially if seizures recur coincidentally, the diet should be readjusted as follows:

1  Give 20–30 ml of MCT emulsion without any food and repeat 2 hourly if necessary until ketosis is re-established.
2  Increase the MCT allowance by 20–25% above the recommended dose for specific foods.
3  Reduce the fluid intake to 50% of the recommended fluid intake or to 1000 ml per 24 h, whichever is the lesser.
4  Reduce the food intake to three small meals a day and preferably use foods of protein origin.

If vomiting, abdominal pain or diarrhoea occur, solid food should be discontinued. The MCT basic recipe only is given to the limits of the patient's tolerance with instructions that it should be sipped slowly. The aim should be to maintain ketosis. Other fluids of minimal calorie value may be administered to sustain hydration while, if possible, avoiding a reduction in ketosis. Gradual reintroduction of solids should take place as the patient's symptoms diminish.

Some have found that gastrointestinal side-effects, especially abdominal colic and diarrhoea, preclude the long-term use of the MCT diet in many cases (Bower, 1980; De Vivo, 1983). These problems led Schwartz et al. (1983) to introduce a *modified MCT diet*. Smaller volumes of MCT than in the original MCT diet are used and some long-chain saturated fats, such as cream and butter, are incorporated in the diet. Initially, 30% of the daily calories come from MCT oil and 30% from long-chain fats and these percentages may be varied in each child depending on tolerance. Foods such as baked beans, fish fingers, beef burgers and ice cream are also given and add variety to the diet in addition to permitting a reduction in the daily amounts of expensive butter and cream. Schwartz et al. (1989a) reported that this modified MCT diet was as effective as and better tolerated than the original MCT diet.

Improvement in control of seizures has been reported in a wide variety of seizure types. Control of seizures is not always directly related to ketone levels in the blood. Schwartz et al. (1989b) reported that, although the standard ketogenic diet induced a significantly greater degree of ketosis than either the original or the modified

MCT diet, it did not necessarily produce greater seizure control. The various diets have been most effective in controlling the atonic–akinetic drop attacks of the Lennox–Gastaut syndrome which are so distressing and often traumatic and improvements in control of atypical absences and myoclonic seizures have also been reported (Sills *et al.*, 1986). Schwartz *et al.* (1983) reported that just over 40% of their patients showed a greater than 90% reduction in seizure frequency within 1 month of starting the diet. Eighty-five per cent of their children with drop attacks had a greater than 50% reduction in seizure frequency and 75% showed a greater than 90% reduction. The improvement was much less in children with infantile spasms treated with the diet, however.

Drug-resistant partial seizures, both simple and complex, and tonic–clonic seizures may also respond favourably to the diet (Sills *et al.*, 1986). In some children who show an excellent response to the diet, it may be possible to discontinue antiepileptic drugs. When the diet is well tolerated and effective, it is usual to continue with it for at least 2 years and the author has persisted with this treatment for longer periods in some very responsive cases. Schwartz *et al.* (1989b) consider that the theoretical risks of inducing early atheromatous changes with their modified diet are outweighed by the benefits of the diet, and she and her colleagues were unable to document any significant changes in blood lipid profiles in short-term studies. Neither did these authors observe any disorders of growth in children on the diet.

All who have used the various types of ketogenic diet stress that, before embarking on what is a difficult regime, assurance of parental and patient cooperation is essential, as is also continued skilled dietetic advice. The brilliant success of the diet in some cases, converting, as Sills *et al.* (1986) say, a child with numerous seizures lying in a padded bed, drooling and unable to speak or feed himself, into a seizure-free ambulant and communicating child in a short space of time, makes consideration of this form of treatment worthwhile in intractable epilepsy in childhood.

## References

BOWER, B. D. (1980) Epilepsy in childhood and adolescence. In *The Treatment of Epilepsy* (ed. J. H. Tyrer), MTP Press, pp. 251–274

DE VIVO, D. C. (1983) How to use other drugs (steroids) and the ketogenic diet. In *Antiepileptic Drug Therapy in Pediatrics* (eds P. L. Morselli, C. E. Pippenger and J. K. Penry), Raven Press, pp. 283–291

GORDON, N. S. (1977) Medium-chain triglycerides in a ketogenic diet. *Developmental Medicine and Child Neurology*, **19**, 535–538

HOYT, C. S. and BILLSON, F. A. (1979) Optic neuropathy in ketogenic diet. *British Journal of Ophthalmology*, **63**, 191–194

HUTTENLOCHER, P. R., WILBOURN, A. J. and SIGNORE, J. M. (1971) Medium-chain triglycerides as therapy for intractable childhood epilepsy. *Neurology*, **21**, 1097–1103

LIVINGSTON, S. (1972) *Comprehensive Management of Epilepsy in Infancy, Childhood and Adolescence*, Charles C. Thomas, Springfield, Illinois, pp. 380–405

LIVINGSTON, S., PAULI, L. L. and PRUCE, I. (1977) Ketogenic diet in the treatment of childhood epilepsy. *Developmental Medicine and Child Neurology*, **19**, 833–834

SCHWARTZ, R. H., EATON, J., AYNSLEY-GREEN, A. and BOWER, B. D. (1983) Ketogenic diets in the management of childhood epilepsy. In *Research Progress in Epilepsy* (ed. F. C. Rose), Pitman, London, pp. 326–332

SCHWARTZ, R. H., EATON, J., BOWER, B. D. and AYNSLEY-GREEN, A. (1989a). Ketogenic diets in the treatment of epilepsy: short-term clinical effects. *Developmental Medicine and Child Neurology*, **31**, 145–151

SCHWARTZ, R. M., BOYES, S. and AYNSLEY-GREEN, A. (1989b). Metabolic effects of three ketogenic diets in the treatment of severe epilepsy. *Developmental Medicine and Child Neurology*, **31**, 152–160

SILLS, M. A., FORSYTHE, W. I., HAIDUKEWYCH, D. *et al.* (1986). The medium chain triglyceride diet and intractable epilepsy. *Archives of Disease in Childhood*, **61**, 1168–1172

Appendix 2

# What should the child with epilepsy be allowed to do?*

Negative attitudes to epilepsy abound, both in the general community and among the medical profession (Beran, Jennings and Read, 1981). These result in the main from prejudice about, and ignorance of, epilepsy. Taylor (1973), discussing prejudice, suggested that recurring seizures reinforce the view of witnesses that the epileptic individual cannot be relied upon to participate fully in society because he is liable, unexpectedly and at any time, to go out of control. Hence the desire in the past to set sufferers from epilepsy apart. Parents, faced with a diagnosis of epilepsy, may be similarly rejecting but are more likely to overprotect the child against life's stressful and potentially dangerous situations. Recurring epilepsy and an overprotective ambiance may, however, interfere with the child's experience of normality.

The problem of how to regard the individual with epilepsy, whether child or adult, is compounded for parents and professionals by the complexity and diversity of epilepsy. The results may be a misunderstanding of the particular seizure disorder present in an individual patient, and of the risks involved to the child. Parents, friends, teachers and doctors often impose restrictions on children with epilepsy that are out of all proportion to the severity of the epilepsy, and despite the fact that the children themselves may wish to join normally in everyday childhood activities. It is reasonable, therefore, to ask ourselves what should and should not be restricted in the daily life of children with epilepsy. What may they be allowed to do or be prevented from doing?

## The risks

Generalized seizures associated with loss of consciousness are likely to be seen as presenting the greatest risks, both inherent and external, to the child. The generalized tonic–clonic seizure (grand mal) is the archetypal convulsion associated with total loss of control. Death is an ever-present fear in the minds of parents witnessing their child's first and subsequent convulsions, as studies among parents of children with febrile seizures have shown (Clare, Aldridge Smith and Wallace, 1978). Death in a febrile convulsion is now, however, a rarity, although the possibility of permanent

* Reprinted from *Archives of Disease in Childhood*, 1983, 58(11), 934–937, by kind permission of the (then) Editor, Professor Roy Meadow.

brain damage occurring in a prolonged febrile seizure is accepted (Ounsted, Lindsay and Norman, 1966). Sillanpää (1973), in a review from Finland of the medicosocial prognosis of various childhood epilepsies, found that 18 deaths occurred among 245 children studied, mainly as a result of status epilepticus and lower respiratory tract infections. The mean age of onset of epilepsy in the group was 25 months, most of the children who died were mentally subnormal, and many had neurological deficits. Molander (1982), in a recent survey of sudden unexpected death in later childhood and adolescence, reported 7 deaths over a 6-year period caused by known diseases: 2 of these were the result of an epileptic attack, 2 were due to sudden cardiac failure associated with coronary artery and myocardial disease, and 3 were caused by sudden asthmatic attacks. This study seems to establish the relative rarity of sudden death due to epilepsy in childhood. Status epilepticus, although still a serious medical emergency at whatever age it occurs and especially so in the very young, is much more amenable now to modern treatment (Delgado-Escueta et al., 1982).

# Drowning

### Swimming

The risk of drowning while swimming is something that causes particular anxiety to parents of children with epilepsy. The Brisbane drowning study (Pearn, Nixon and Wilkey, 1976; Pearn, 1977) of 149 cases of death by freshwater and saltwater drowning in children is most comprehensive, and it was concluded from it that epileptic children who swim were four times more likely to drown than were normal children but that the absolute risk of drowning was low. Furthermore, when the children with epilepsy were properly supervised while swimming, there was no evidence that they were likely to drown or suffer brain damage from anoxia after near-drowning. Some 400 epileptic children were at risk from drowning each year in Brisbane during the 7-year study but no epilepsy-induced pool or sea deaths occurred.

Livingston et al. (1980) agree that fatalities associated with swimming are relatively rare causes of death in epilepsy and that epileptic patients may swim with confidence if properly supervised. They allow patients whose epilepsy is controlled and those who have an occasional seizure to swim in a pool with an informed lifeguard present or with a competent swimming companion. They prohibit swimming under water and diving into deep water. Patients with rare seizures are discouraged from swimming in large bodies of water such as lakes or oceans, even with a lifeguard present. Children with frequent seizures are advised against any ordinary swimming but may be allowed to swim in a pool for brief periods with immediate and constant surveillance. This sensible advice is based on Livingston's experience over more than 4 decades with very large numbers of epileptic patients. He has stated that although some of the children experienced a convulsion while swimming, none drowned.

The British Epilepsy Association, in a leaflet entitled *Swimming and Epilepsy* designed for use by schools, advocates the 'pairing' system – known as the 'buddy' system in the USA – whereby all children are advised and expected to swim in pairs. This provides additional safety for weaker swimmers generally, and for children with epilepsy particularly. Children with mental or physical handicap, or both, who may also have partially controlled epilepsy are at greater risk and should be carefully supervised in the water.

## Bathing

Drowning in the domestic bathtub is a much greater hazard for the epileptic patient than is misadventure during swimming. Rose and Tizard (1968) described such a tragedy and emphasized that conversations with general practitioners, paediatricians and neurologists had indicated a lack of awareness of this particular risk. In each of the fatal cases of bathtub drowning associated with epilepsy described by Livingston *et al.* (1980) the patient had bathed alone in a bath which was completely or almost completely filled with water. They advised that older patients with epilepsy, if bathing alone, should do so in a water depth of not more than 5–7.5 cm. They also warned against the possible risks of showering alone, especially in glass- or plastic-enclosed stalls, citing accidents following seizures where unconscious patients fell through glass or plastic or against hot water taps. They recommended showering while seated as being less hazardous.

There is general agreement that young children, whether epileptic or not, should not be permitted to bathe without surveillance by a responsible person, and that older children should be encouraged to shower rather than bathe, preferably with the plughole open and the bathroom door unlocked.

## Fishing

There is yet another risk of drowning during a seizure which is associated with that most popular of water pastimes, fishing. Worster-Drought (1970) described a youth on regular treatment for epilepsy who was found drowned in a shallow river. He had been fishing from a river bank and fell forwards into the water during an attack.

### Precipitating mechanisms

The possible role of precipitating mechanisms in epilepsy-induced drownings should be remembered. Seizures triggered by a specific sensory stimulus are described as reflex epilepsy (*see* Chapter 12), the most familiar example being television-induced photosensitive epilepsy. Photosensitivity may occasionally be responsible for seizures occurring at the seaside or swimming pool and induced by the shimmer of bright light on rippling water. The part played by reflex epilepsy in epilepsy-induced drowning is uncertain. The term 'startle epilepsy' is sometimes applied to brief clonic or tonic–clonic seizures provoked by sudden and unexpected auditory or touch stimuli and might be triggered during the horseplay so often engaged in by children in swimming pools or by diving into cold water or from a height. True water immersion epilepsy (bath epilepsy) is rare at any age, although Keipert (1969) described a case induced by water immersion in an infant aged 5 months. In adults, it can be shown that, in order to provoke an attack, the bathwater must be at 37°C and that the legs and perineum must be immersed (Parsonage, Moran and Exley, 1976).

# School activities

There is general agreement that the child with epilepsy should have as normal a school life as possible but there is no ready-made answer to the question of what limitations, if any, should be imposed on his or her activities there. The advice given should be based on common sense and not determined simply by the presence or absence of seizures. Factors such as the severity and frequency of attacks, their timing in relation to waking and sleeping, and the child's judgement and perception of the risks should be taken into account. Most children with epilepsy attend normal schools, and it is important that teachers be correctly informed about epilepsy and encouraged to have an enlightened and optimistic attitude towards the condition. They should be instructed about the emergency treatment of a child having a major seizure in the classroom.

## Sports

The question of participation by the child in gymnastics and athletic activities at school needs consideration. There is general agreement that children with epilepsy should not perform activities where a fall would ensue if a seizure were experienced without warning. These include rope climbing, climbing on bars, rock climbing, the use of parallel bars and trampolining. These restraints might be waived, however, for a child who had been seizure free for a prolonged period. Factors which may operate during athletic exercise are pertinent, and hyperventilation is one such. Voluntary hyperventilation produces an alkalosis and thereby increases the susceptibility to absence seizures in true petit mal whereas, during active physical exercise, the lactate/pyruvate acidosis produced is antiepileptogenic. This may be just one of the protective factors operating during physical exercise. Berney et al. (1981) have shown that while inhibitory effects predominate in most epileptics during exercise, a minority have their epileptic discharges activated during exercise and during the postexercise recovery phase.

The question of competitive and body contact sports is also debated. Pearn (1977) believes that competitive swimming should be prohibited, since somatic stress to the point of exhaustion may trigger an attack. To some extent, however, this factor should be influenced by the physical training and conditioning of the patient. An unresolved problem is the potential exacerbation of pre-existing organic pathology by subsequent head trauma during contact sports. It has been proposed (McLaurin, 1974) that repeated head trauma may lead to further neuronal damage and loss, and thus compound the problem of epilepsy already present. This seems an unlikely event except in boxing.

As far as contact sports in general are concerned, the writer agrees with Baird (1972) when he asks 'Are they worth it?' He suggests avoiding the issue and channelling the athletic youngster with epilepsy into tennis, golf or athletics. Tennis provides adequate exercise, satisfies competitive instincts and can be continued as a lifelong pursuit. The recommendation of the Committee on Children with Handicaps of the American Academy of Pediatrics (1968) that one must strike a balance between the needs of the child to participate with his peers in their daily activities and the limitations to living a full life which any restriction may impose, is also relevant here.

Many children with epilepsy have far fewer seizures when active and engaged in normal childhood activities than when they are idle, or at rest or bored. Some may even excel in athletics and, provided their epilepsy is under satisfactory control, there seems little point in making distinctions between epileptic and non-epileptic children as far as their participation in athletics is concerned.

## Cycling

All children are subject to risks in their daily lives, especially in urban situations.

Bicycling in traffic is a hazard for the normal child, as it is also for children with epilepsy, but parents of the latter may have reasonable anxieties about the added danger of absence attacks occurring while the child is cycling on a busy road. Each case has to be judged on its merits but it is comforting to remember that it has been known for a long time that the frequency of seizures is lessened by tasks requiring some degree of concentration or arousal (Lennox, Gibbs and Gibbs, 1936). Ounsted and Hutt (1964) showed that seizure discharges occurred less frequently in circumstances which were neither boring nor excessively stressful. If the degree of attention required became too stressful, however, the seizure discharges increased and performance declined. Clinical and subclinical spike-wave paroxysms may disrupt the registration and storage of information by the brain, and focal epileptic discharges may interfere with normal functioning of the area involved. The complexity of modern traffic is such as to prohibit exposing the child with epilepsy to unnecessary risks unless his seizure control is excellent.

## Discothèques

The current popularity of discothèques has heightened parents' anxiety about the effects of loud music and flashing lights on the child with epilepsy. Berney et al. (1981) carried out a valuable study of this problem and showed that most epileptic children were not particularly vulnerable in discothèques. They suggested that photosensitive children, aware of their vulnerability and discomfort when exposed to flicker, may deliberately avoid the risk or even develop a learned aversion to discothèques. The energetic exercise of disco dancing may have a protective or normalizing effect, and the study supported this. The investigation also identified a small minority of children with epilepsy, however, whose epilepsy seemed to be activated by exercise and who were also susceptible to a wide range of other stimuli including voluntary eye closure, music, hyperventilation and intermittent photic stimulation. These children were at risk from stroboscopic illumination even at the relatively low frequency employed in discothèques.

## Conclusion

Overprotection must be avoided if possible in dealing with the school-age child who has epilepsy. As with all chronic long-term disorders, epilepsy requires adjustment on the part of the child and the family. Some aspects of the disorder cannot be altered, no matter how well they are understood or accepted. Learning from mistakes and experience and making decisions about physical and other restrictions must gradually become the responsibility of the child and not that of the parents or school personnel. The doctor who is consulted for advice should have a wide knowledge of this common disorder so that he can counsel caution when necessary or recommend when new responsibilities may safely be given to the child. A recent Japanese study among paediatricians, seeking information about allowing school children with epilepsy to join in sporting activities, showed that young, specialist and hospital doctors were more liberal in their attitudes than were older and less specialized doctors (Miyake, 1982). This suggests to the writer that the great increase in interest and knowledge of childhood epilepsies in the last decade and the availability of more effective anticonvulsants are changing the long-established and overcautious medical opinions about this common problem of childhood.

## References

AMERICAN ACADEMY OF PEDIATRICS: COMMITTEE ON CHILDREN WITH HANDICAPS (1968) The epileptic child and competitive school athletics. *Pediatrics*, **42**, 700–702

BAIRD, H. W. (1972) *The Child with Convulsions. A guide for parents, teachers, counsellors and medical personnel*, Grune & Stratton, New York, pp. 88–90.

BERAN, R. G., JENNINGS, V. R. and READ, T. (1981) Doctors' perspectives of epilepsy. *Epilepsia*, **22**, 397–406

BERNEY, T. P., OSSELTON, J. W., KOLVIN, I. and DAY. M. J. (1981) Effect of discothèque environment on epileptic children. *British Medical Journal*, **282**, 180–182

BRITISH EPILEPSY ASSOCIATION COORDINATING COMMITTEE. *Swimming and Epilepsy*. British Epilepsy Association, Leeds

CLARE, M., ALDRIDGE SMITH, J. and WALLACE, S. J. (1978) A child's first febrile convulsion. *Practitioner*, **221**, 775–776

DELGADO-ESCUETA, A. V., WASTERLAIN, C., TREIMAN, D. M. and PORTER, R. J. (1982) Management of status epilepticus. *New England Journal of Medicine*, **306**, 133–1340

KEIPERT, J. A. (1969) Epilepsy precipitated by bathing: water-immersion epilepsy. *Australian Paediatric Journal*, **5**, 244–247

LENNOX, W. G., GIBBS, F. A. and GIBBS, E. L. (1936) The effect on the electroencephalogram of drugs and conditions which influence seizure. *Archives of Neurology and Psychiatry*, **36**, 1236–1245

LIVINGSTON, S., PAULI, L. L., PRUCE, I. and KRAMER, I. I. (1980) Drowning in epilepsy. *Annals of Neurology*, **7**, 495

MCLAURIN, R. L. (1974) Epilepsy and contact sports: factors contraindicating participation. In *Epilepsy: proceedings of the Hans Berger Centenary Symposium* (eds P. Harris and C. Mawdsley), Churchill Livingstone, Edinburgh, pp. 301–305

MIYAKE, S. (1982) Opinion from paediatricians about social management of children with epilepsy. *Brain and Development*, **4**, 200

MOLANDER, N. (1982) Sudden natural death in later childhood and adolescence. *Archives of Disease in Childhood*, **57**, 572–576

OUNSTED, C. and HUTT, S. J. (1964) The effect of attentive factors upon bio-electric paroxysms in epileptic children. (abstract) *Proceedings of the Royal Society of Medicine*, **57**, 1178

OUNSTED, C., LINDSAY, J. and NORMAN, R. (1966) *Biological Factory in Temporal lobe Epilepsy*, Clinics in Developmental Medicine, No. 22, Spastics Society/Heinemann Medical, London

PARSONAGE, M. J., MORAN, J. H. and EXLEY, K. A. (1976) So-called writer immersion epilepsy. In *Epileptology*, Proceedings of the Seventh International Symposium on Epilepsy, West Berlin, 1975 (ed.) D. Janz, Publishing Sciences Group, London, pp. 50–60

PEARN, J. H. (1977) Epilepsy and drowning in childhood. *British Medical Journal*, **1**, 1510–1511

PEARN, J., NIXON, J. and WILKEY, I. (1976) Freshwater drowning and near-drowning accidents involving children. A five-year total population study. *Medical Journal of Australia*, **2**, 942–946

ROSE, J. R. and TIZARD, J. P. M. (1968) The epileptic in the bath. (letter) *Lancet*, **1**, 44

SILLANPÄÄ, M. (1973) Medico-social prognosis of children with epilepsy. *Acta Paediatrica Scandinavica*, Suppl. 237

TAYLOR, D. C. (1973) Aspects of seizure disorders. 11. On prejudice. *Developmental Medicine and Child Neurology*, **15**, 91–94

WORSTER-DROUGHT, C. (1970) Epileptic death due to suffocation during sleep. (letter) *Lancet*, **2**, 876

# Glossary

| Approved name | USA trade name | UK trade |
|---|---|---|
| Acetazolamide | Diamox | Diamox |
| Benztropine mesylate | Cogentin | Cogentin |
| Benzylpenicillin | Hyasorb, Pfizerpen G | Crystapen |
| Carbamazepine | Tegretol | Tegretol |
| Chloramphenicol | Amphicol | Chloromycetin |
| Chloremethiazole edisylate | | Heminevrin |
| Clobazam | | Frisium |
| Clonazepam | Clonopin | Rivotril |
| Dexamethasone | Decadron, Hexadrol | Decadron, Oradexon |
| Dexamphetamine sulphate, dextroamphetamine sulfate | Dexedrine | Dexedrine |
| Diazepam | Valium | Valium, Stesolid (for rectal use) |
| Diazoxide | Hyperstat | Eudemine |
| Diphenhydramine hydrochloride | Benadryl | Benadryl |
| Ethosuximide | Zarontin | Zarontin |
| Frusemide, furosemide | Lasix | Lasix |
| Imipramine | Imavate, Presamine | Tofranil |
| Isoniazid | Niconyl, Nydrazid | Rimifon |
| Lamotrigine | | Lamictal |
| Lignocaine, lidocaine | Anestacon | Xylocard |
| Lorazepam | Ativan | Ativan |
| Mannitol | Mannitol | Osmitrol |
| Methylphenidate hydrochloride | Ritalin | Ritalin |
| Metoclopramide | Reglan | Maxolon |
| Nitrazepam | not available in USA | Mogadon |
| Paraldehyde | Paral | |
| Paramethadione | Paradione | Paradione |
| Pentetrazol, leptaxol | Metrazol | Cardiazol |
| Pheneturide | not available in USA | Beneuride |
| Phenobarbitone, phenobarbital | Sedadrops, Solfoton | Luminal |
| Phenytoin | Dilantin | Epanutin |
| Primidone | Mysoline | Mysoline |
| Reserpine | Serpate | Serpasil |
| Sodium valproate | Depakene | Epilim |
| Thiopentone | Pentothal | Intraval, Pentothal |
| Troxidone, trimethidione | Tridione | Tridione |
| Vigabatrin | Sabril | Sabril |

# Index